GW00497319

THE CBT-POT

LEARNING TO PLAY YOUR MIND

Dheeresh Turnbull

Pen Press

© Dheeresh Turnbull 2013

All rights reserved

No part of this publication may be reproduced, stored in a retrieval
system, or transmitted in any form or by any means, without the prior
permission in writing of the publisher, nor be otherwise circulated in
any form of binding or cover other than that in which it is published
and without a similar condition including this condition being imposed
on the subsequent purchaser.

First published in Great Britain by Pen Press

All paper used in the printing of this book has been made from wood
grown in managed, sustainable forests.

ISBN13: 978-1-78003-636-6

Printed and bound in the UK
Pen Press is an imprint of
Indepenpress Publishing Limited
25 Eastern Place
Brighton
BN2 1GJ

A catalogue record of this book is available from
the British Library

Cover design by Claire Spinks

To my mother
Diana Turnbull
Who set me on the Way

ACKNOWLEDGEMENTS

I start with my mother (most people do!) who was completely encouraging of my intellectual and spiritual pursuits. She read first drafts of some of the early chapters, and gave helpful comments, but died before this work could be completed. She also bought me my first copy of *The Phantom Tollbooth*, an implicational CBT manual masquerading as a children's book. Colin Burgess, sometime sociology lecturer at Filton College, Bristol, was the first person to show me that what a person believes is at least partly a function of where they stand. Andrew Rawlinson started me on an intellectual understanding of Buddhism, with the clear awareness that it was always going to be more than that. Osho, formerly known as Bhagwan Shree Rajneesh, who has been pilloried for his many faults, deserves my respect and gratitude for pioneering the combination of therapy and meditation – it certainly made a difference to me. As did John Rowan, whose innovative approach to therapy served as a model for me in developing what I cheekily call fourth wave CBT, as well as helping me to make friends with my demons. Richard Gombrich, he of immense patience and kindness, helped me to be able to write naturally, while keeping a broad and grounded perspective. Thanks also to Dennis Genpo Merzel, Roshi for more than twenty years of Zen teaching, and giving the Big Mind process to the world. And to Shila and Ali at the Shuh Shuh Guh, who oversaw my most recent explorations and helped me to make my dreams – including this book – a reality.

My mental health career began in Oxford, and the support in my training from all at Oxfordshire Mind and Acorn was invaluable, as was the great teaching from all those at what is now the

Oxford Cognitive Therapy Centre, but particularly the three wise *gwydden*: Ann Hackmann, who introduced me to the idea that Cognitive Therapy might be a useful direction for me; Melanie Fennell, who directed the course with humour, inspiration and efficiency; and Gillian Butler, who continued to supervise me after the course had finished, and made supervision look effortless. Paul Salkovskis first intrigued me with the ways of OCD, and David Veale continued to stimulate my enquiries into all things obsessional. David M. Clark's name pops up throughout the book, as it should, and big thanks to Windy Dryden, whose 'Big I, little I' provides the bridge between CBT and the Big Mind process.

On the mindfulness front, Mark Williams, John Teasdale, and Jon Kabat-Zinn have all been wonderfully encouraging at different times over the last decade or so, and Jini Lavelle hooked me in to clinical mindfulness in the first place. Thanks and deep bows to all.

Many of the ideas in this book were initially developed while working with Rob Willson at The Priory Hospital North London, and the process continued with Jem Mills at Aurora. They have continued to support and encourage as this project has gone along. Many of the hand-outs were either developed jointly with Rob, or, frankly, stolen from him... Thanks, mates.

From afar, I have also been impressed by Adrian Wells' metacognitive approach. Though he, like many of the names mentioned above, may not always like what I have done with their ideas and research! I clearly take responsibility for my writings, and anything that turns out to be wrong...

For most of the time that this book was being written, Sheila Burton was my clinical supervisor, and has undoubtedly – if unwittingly – influenced the content. But please don't blame her! Her supervision groups are the stuff of legend.

It would be daft and ungrateful if I were to omit the group that has given me the most understanding of the workings of the human mind: my long- or sometimes short-suffering clients. In particular, Jane Gwynne has said that she is very happy to be known as the source of 'teapot compassion'. I should also include that group who, while not formally being clients, also taught me more than I can say: the members of Acorn day-centre, now sadly no more. Thanks to all of you for sharing your lives, problems and discoveries with me, so that what I do can benefit others.

I would also like to thank my editor at Penpress, Claire Spinks, whose enthusiasm for this project took me quite by surprise, not to mention her seemingly endless patience and consideration for my lack of technical awareness, which is much appreciated. I am greatly in her debt.

And finally, my family: Lin, Alex, Danni, Gaia and Tulip. They have had to put up with me not always being there when needed as I have pursued this particular path. Much love and thanks.

Dheeresh Turnbull, Hove, April 2013

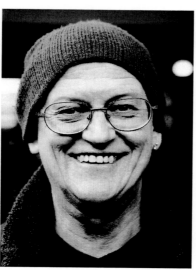

author photo © Martijn Mulder

CONTENTS

PART 1: HOW IT ALL WORKS

INTRODUCTION[1]

The CBT-Pot: Learning To Play Your Mind, as well as being a bit of a mixed metaphor (we don't usually play teapots!) is a new departure in self-help psychotherapy. Following in the footsteps of its ancestors (CBT, mindfulness, Zen), it is an attempt to help you learn how to work with your mind rather than fighting it, to control better that which can be controlled, and to stop trying to control that which can't. The teapot idea gives a sense of resource, and also the idea of 'teapot compassion' (see chapter 11). And just like a musical instrument, as we get more familiar with its workings, we can become more skilled in releasing the tunes – including your 'life-tune', if you like – that are locked inside. As you learn to listen, using a variety of methods, then you can discover what you're really about, with profound effects on your life: your work, your relationships and perhaps your spiritual development, if that's something that interests you.

Aaron T. Beck, the founder of cognitive therapy, is reputed to have said (Christine Padesky in Grant et al., 2004) that he hoped that cognitive therapy as a separate discipline would disappear in time, as the insights which he did so much to bring to the world of psychotherapy became common knowledge. This may be the last turning of the wheel of CBT, wherein that discipline is recognisably separate, and probably only just. So let us see where it has come from...

THE BRIEFEST OF BRIEF HISTORIES OF COGNITIVE AND BEHAVIOURAL PSYCHOTHERAPY

The first 'wave' was the arrival of behaviour therapy, as a reaction against psychoanalysis, which at that time – the early 20th century – was the dominant force in psychotherapy. The second wave was the

---

1 If you're not interested in the theory you can skip this bit. Or you might want to come back to it later, when you've tried some of the techniques.

cognitive revolution, spearheaded by Albert Ellis and Aaron T. Beck in the 1950s and 1960s, which, incorporating the best of behaviour therapy, gave us Cognitive Behaviour Therapy (CBT), now recognised as the treatment of choice for a whole range of emotional problems in much of the western world.

A few brief paragraphs will serve to introduce CBT:

Beck sees the Stoics, and particularly Epictetus, as the philosophical forerunners of cognitive therapy, as evidenced by this statement:

"Men are disturbed not by things but by the views which they take of them." (from the Enchiridion). So CBT is about challenging our *interpretation* of events.

A key phrase in CBT is *collaborative empiricism*. This puts the therapist less in the role of guru, and more as the more experienced partner in an experimental investigation of the problems the person is facing. One metaphor that is used is that of the driving instructor. So together we come up with alternative explanations to those you have been using, and then find ways of testing them out. In the end, you become your own therapist.

At a master class in Oxford (1997), Beck described cognitive therapy as being like a stool with three legs: one leg is the *cognitive and behavioural techniques* (this is often mistaken for the whole of CBT), and another is the *art of therapy*, which is common across different kinds of therapy. So CBT is a therapy in its own right. The third is the *psycho-educational* element: there is quite simply a lot of information about how human minds work, the ignorance of which leads people to make mistakes in how they live their lives. Naturally this book aims to be helpful in this department. So this is (second-wave) CBT in a nutshell.

The third wave, still just emerging into the mainstream, shifted the focus away from changing the *content* of what we think towards *metacognitive* processes: thinking about thinking; looking more at the focus of attention. It is very influenced by Buddhist meditation, in particular *mindfulness*.

This follows naturally from the second wave: once you see that what you are thinking is an interpretation and can be challenged, then sooner or later it dawns on you that much of what goes through your mind is not the *truth* but a *particular version* that need not be unquestioningly accepted.

In one of its most organised forms, Acceptance and Commitment Therapy or ACT, the focus is on noticing how, because of language, we have lost touch with the difference between a thing and its label. In another discipline, Neuro-Linguistic Programming, this is expressed as "The map is not the territory." So our ability to abstract the label from the thing itself, while being incredibly useful on the one hand, often leads to a confusion on the other, as, for example, we become frightened of scary words or pictures because they carry the association with the event that scared us.

Another prominent third-wave member, Mindfulness-Based Cognitive Therapy (MBCT), focuses primarily on teaching the practice of meditation to promote living in the here and now, accepting and appreciating the moment (even if you don't like it!) as an alternative to the processes of worrying and rumination. Interestingly, this also usually involves some practice of body-type disciplines such as yoga or chi gong as well as sitting meditation. In fact, one definition of mindfulness (given by the CBT therapist and tai chi practitioner Nigel Mills[2]) is "Putting the mind where the body is". Thus body disciplines become very helpful for people to have and maintain this awareness: as the body is always in the present, if you can keep your attention *in* the body, then your awareness is in the present.

These two schools (ACT and MBCT) have taken slightly different views on how to deal with the content of our thoughts. In summary, ACT says that all thoughts and feelings are just private events of which we need not take much, if any, notice; the point being to *act in line with what you want to achieve*, i.e. valued goals. MBCT focuses mainly on watching thoughts go by, but also uses some cognitive therapy techniques to help us recognise that the thinking may be faulty.

THE FOURTH WAVE?

This work could be described as the beginnings of a fourth wave of CBT. So what, you ask, could possibly be added to the third wave which would in any way improve the quality of therapy? The rest of this book is, in a way, an attempt to answer that question. But in summary the principles are these:

1. We (i.e. this new kind or fourth wave of CBT therapists) retain an empirical and pragmatic approach. That is, we do not automatically accept *or reject* any psychological dogma,

---

2   At a British Association of Behavioural and Cognitive Psychotherapies (BABCP) spring conference

whether it derives from CBT, traditional meditation practices or other sources. This experimental attitude will hopefully not fall into the traps that some of our predecessors fell into, who sometimes unthinkingly rejected approaches from non-western cultures for no scientific reason.

2. For this reason, we *include* tried and tested orthodox CBT techniques. Unlike (for example) ACT, we see fourth wave techniques as complementing and expanding traditional cognitive behavioural therapy.

3. Building on the insights of third wave therapists such as John Teasdale, Mark Williams and others, and the dictum of Marshall McLuhan ("The medium is the message"), we seek, if necessary, to take therapy beyond the verbal, and even beyond the imaginal. Those familiar with CBT will recognise the oft-repeated refrain, "I know what I'm meant to feel, but I just don't feel it." We could say that in such cases, *emotional mind* has not been engaged. We wish to engage whichever mind is needed, and use whatever we need to use in order to make that happen. So we encourage you to try a range of creative techniques in order to keep the therapy personal to you, rather than just doing some dry intellectual exercise.

4. It's time to stop running away from the word 'spiritual', while definitely not implying that anyone has to adhere to any particular *religious* viewpoint. But the main barrier that the fourth wave is encouraging you to cross is the illusion that *all we are* is contained in this 'skin bag', as Zen masters are wont to describe the body – revealing the fallacy that the boundaries of the physical body are the boundaries of the self. An appreciation of the *unbounded* is needed. A contemporary and very helpful trend in current applied psychology is the awareness of *emotional* intelligence as distinct from *intellectual* intelligence. Yet much that is highlighted under the heading of emotional intelligence is that which we would actually describe as *spiritual* intelligence. All three are distinct and useful.

5. While it is likely that most people reading this book are doing so to 'get better', I would rather you view this process as the beginning of a journey, in the course of which your life can become immeasurably richer and more fulfilling, and during which, as one of my many teachers said, "Your personal difficulties become less significant." (Mao Shih An, 1996)

So, a story:

Imagine you have been driving a train around a circular track for some time – perhaps most of your life. You see the same sights come and go, but also, outside the circle, you glimpse a far more interesting land. But you are driving this train, and are therefore condemned to go around in circles. Suddenly – and this is very strange, because it has never happened before – the train stutters and comes to a stop. You get out (also something you can't remember having done before), and to your astonishment, you discover that the machine you are driving is actually a car, and that the 'tracks' are merely drawn on the ground as guidelines. Because of this, there are actually a great variety of choices as to where you could go, including some roads that lead off to the more interesting lands that you had glimpsed, but thought unavailable. You look down and see that a stick has become caught in the wheels, but now (with your new-found manoeuvrability) it is an easy task to dislodge the stick, and off you go.

The circular journey is the unnecessarily restricted life that we often live. The stop is what we in CBT call a *critical incident*, which brings us to question our lives, and perhaps come to therapy, during which we learn how to get out of the vehicle (our pre-existing mindset) and discover how it works and its real potential. Discovering and activating the true potential of the organism – that's you – is a task that is central to fourth wave CBT. Perhaps dislodging the stick could be interpreted as short-term therapy, while the freer journey that follows may be fuelled by the practice of meditation, longer-term therapy, or both. Sometimes people remove the stick and go back to driving only on the tracks. This is unfortunate. As the Chinese saying has it (vegetarians look away now) "The fat of the pheasant is not eaten" – that means you missed the best bit.

In essence, the problem we all face is that we don't see things as they are. We mostly see the representations of things in our heads. In our computer-dominated age, we might call them 'programs' . On a good day we may check out the evidence in the real world, whether or not whatever it is we perceive out there actually conforms to our picture of it. ("It has four legs and a tail and is barking at me, so it must be the creature called 'dog'.")

We come to therapy or meditation, usually because either the world isn't conforming to our picture of it in one way or another, or because it is, but the picture is horrible! This is significant, because as psychologists of attachment theory (like John Bowlby and Donald Winnicott) have shown, it is having a representation – an inner working model – of mother that enables her to go away (initially for short periods) without the baby thinking it is going to die. Because I can hold this image, I know I'll be all right! From this most important start, we therefore learn to invest a great deal of emotion in our representations or images, to the point that sometimes we are relating to the representation instead of the real person, even though the real other is in the room. Of course, we are not aware that the other that we are seeing is not the real other, except when the person seems to act 'out of character' i.e. not according to our preconceptions of how they should act. Hence the well-known unpredictability of spiritual teachers, as they attempt to wake us up to just how programmed we are by surprising us into a deeper appreciation of what is actually happening.

There are obviously many kinds of psychological treatment methods available, not all of which appear to operate from an understanding that programming is at least one of the core problems. Those that do can help us in (usually) one of three ways:

1. To see that, because of particular circumstances, our inner working model of the world (or some aspect of it) is inaccurate and/or unhelpful. Perhaps we can then come to understand the origin of the inaccuracy, and then put together a model that works better, so that there are fewer glitches in our interaction with the world.

2. To see that our inner working model is not only inaccurate, but that *it is only a model*, and to learn to distinguish between the model and reality by *dis-identifying* – standing back – from the model.

3. To see that some aspects of one's inner working model have taken on a life of their own, and to work to reintegrate them in light of the bigger picture by first identifying with each aspect and finding out what it wants or needs, and what it is trying to tell us. From there we can 're-own' it, so that it ceases to work undercover, which has been the cause of the trouble.

Without attempting to be all-inclusive, most short-term cognitive therapy falls into the first category; mindfulness (and mindfulness-based approaches like acceptance and commitment therapy) falls largely into the second; and more psychodynamically-oriented psychotherapies, particularly (for example) those of a Jungian persuasion, have elements from both first and third.[3] What I am suggesting is that in taking CBT to a place where it can use all three methods, a new, or fourth, wave is born.

Clearly, all of these methods can be useful in different circumstances and according to the needs and wishes of the person pursuing them. However, many therapists are only aware of one or two of these ways – or, at best, know of the others but cannot practise them. This is an unsatisfactory state of affairs which cannot be remedied all at once, but this book is an attempt at a user-friendly manual that provides at least a skeleton upon which the client or practitioner can put his or her own flesh.

CONCLUSION

Fourth wave CBT is a development of Cognitive Behavioural Therapy which incorporates elements of non-CBT systems and practices into CBT to enhance the methods and understanding of that discipline, and to enable it to help you play your mind more effectively and beautifully. You will learn 'standbackability' (the ability to stand back from your mind's contents), while also being able to connect with that from which you have become disconnected, some of which you would probably think of as 'negative' (e.g. difficult past events), and some 'positive' (e.g. a sense of connection with the boundless). As we shall see, the values we put on these experiences often determine how we feel about them.

---

3 On a more transcendent level, some more visualisation-oriented meditation practices (for example, those described in the *Tibetan Book of the Dead*) are also working in the third way.

CHAPTER 1: FORMULATING YOUR PROBLEM

Hot cross bun – Safety behaviours – Vicious daisy – Problems and goals

Although CBT works alongside (and usually in co-operation with) the medical model of psychiatry – you may have been given a medical diagnosis, for example – we set great store by looking at the person's individual *formulation* or *conceptualisation*. What this means is that we look at your individual situation, both in the present as well as the recent and more distant past, to see how you've got to the state you're in at the moment. So, as a therapist I'm looking to get to the place where I can say something like, "No wonder! If I'd been through what you've just been through, given what already happened to you before, I'd probably be feeling just like you're feeling right now." There are various tools we can use to do this, and I'm going to show two here: the 'hot cross bun' and the 'vicious daisy'. Later on we will look at the historical formulation. In addition, each 'disorder' has its own particular model, which you can find in *Part 2: Some applications*.

THE HOT CROSS BUN

This has been popularised in Greenberger and Padesky's very well-known self-help book *Mind Over Mood*. CBT based on this technique is sometimes known as 'five areas CBT' because its main function is to break down the person's problem into five areas:

1. Trigger (can be external or internal, i.e. in our heads)
2. Cognitions (thoughts or images)
3. Bodily sensations
4. Mood or emotion
5. Behaviour

In early CBT, e.g. Burns (1980), it was alleged that you had to understand something in order to feel it, implying that *thoughts cause feelings.* We know now that this is not always so, and that sometimes it can be the other way round, or that the different components influence each other. This is represented in the diagram below. It corresponds to the idea of 'conditioned co-production' in Buddhism, which holds that different aspects of the mind influence each other. So when we think something, that will inevitably bring with it certain emotions and body sensations, which, if we follow through and don't question them, will lead to us acting in certain ways (behaviour). But sometimes our primitive emotional equipment – the *limbic system* – will pick up a threat long before thinking mind gets hold of it, so the emotion and body sensation will come first, sometimes even generating the behaviour before thought has woken up to what has been going on. Daniel Goleman talks about this as 'emotional hijacking' in his 1995 book *Emotional Intelligence.*

Sometimes the first thing we become aware of is the *body sensation,* and it is our *interpretation* of that which influences our mood. In setting out what is happening in a 'hot cross bun' we can see how the parts interact, and that helps us to see what is going on.

Trigger Situation (mental/physical):

Hot cross bun diagram

Here is a filled-in example of someone's situation who is depressed.

Trigger Situation (mental/physical): *Thinking about going back to work*

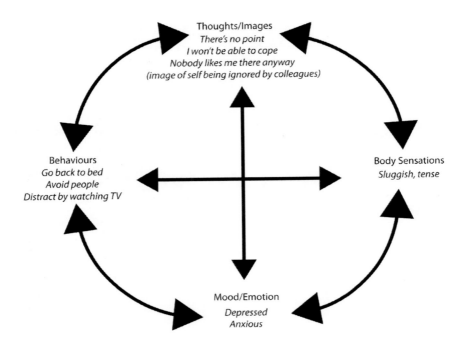

Thoughts/Images
*There's no point
I won't be able to cope
Nobody likes me there anyway
(image of self being ignored by colleagues)*

Behaviours
*Go back to bed
Avoid people
Distract by watching TV*

Body Sensations
Sluggish, tense

Mood/Emotion
*Depressed
Anxious*

Filled-in hot cross bun

Notice that all this is set in the present; unlike some other therapies, CBT doesn't go delving into the past for the sake of it. If the problem can be sorted in terms of what's happening right now, we will try to do that. On the other hand, we do usually need to find out a bit about your personal historical context (how it was when you were brought up, what mattered in your family and so on) to get a sense of how your current problems are going to feel for you. But we will look at that later.

For now let's find out a little more about the different categories, starting at the top of the diagram and working clockwise:

1. Trigger situation: whatever it is that sets off the train of thought or body sensation or mood shift. It could be an actual external situation – in some thought records, this is described as 'environment' – but it may not be. Here the person's drop in mood is set off by them *thinking about going back to work*. So it can be an unwanted thought just

popping up in your head, but it might be an unexpected body sensation, or even a shift in mood for no apparent reason.

2. Thought/Image: this is whatever it is that's going through your mind when your mood starts to shift, or perhaps just a short time before. In a book like this we tend to show thoughts as written content, but we're very visual animals, so it's probably more likely – for some of you, anyway – to come as a picture. You may also notice a sort of negative running commentary on the initial thought or image, like "That shows you're screwed, then" or "See? You always knew she didn't love you."

3. Body sensation: this is sometimes very obvious, like the sensations experienced during panic or anxiety about health, but often you may not be able to find anything to put in this box, or it may seem unrelated to what's going on in the situation. Never mind – put it in anyway, and it may turn out to be relevant.

4. Mood or emotion: more on this in the next chapter, but for now think of it as the kind of feeling that happens when you think in the way you're thinking in 2.. It's usually expressed in one word, and comes with an associated body state: happy, sad, depressed, anxious, angry, guilty, joyous, ashamed etc.

5. Behaviour: this is what you *do* in the situation, either as a result of how you're feeling, or sometimes as the trigger which sets off the feelings/thoughts, or both. This can be a physical action or an avoidance – deliberately *not* doing something – or it could be a mental action, like *worrying*.

So now is (as always) a great time to start. Either drawing a hot cross bun of your own, or using a photocopy from the back of the book, see if you can separate out the different elements of a situation that is causing you problems at the moment or was an issue recently. In CBT we try to be very specific, so if you can, keep it to one particular thing, like "what happens to (or in) me when I think about going to that party?", "What will happen when my boss sees me tomorrow morning?" or "What do I think and feel about how my children have turned out?" Don't worry about getting it right! After all, we haven't even really explored what thoughts or feelings are yet. This is just to get you used to the idea that problems have different elements, and that if you can separate them out, it becomes a little easier to see where you can change something if you need to.

As we have seen, one of the five categories is behaviour. CBT lays great emphasis on the things we are unwittingly doing that *keep the problem going*. Again, we have noticed that these doings can be of different kinds: they can be physical actions, like checking the door repeatedly as you leave the house; they can be mental actions, like worrying for hours about a meeting before or after the event; or they can be avoidances, like not revisiting the scene of an accident. All of these things may seem sensible or prudent at the time, but can serve to make the problem worse. This is especially true if the thing you're doing is an attempt to head off the situation you're afraid of, or is something that *prevents* you from finding out if the thing you're afraid of is really a threat or not – we call that a *safety-seeking behaviour* or 'safety behaviour' for short.

The idea of a safety behaviour is illustrated by one of my favourite stories, featuring Mulla Nasrudin, that well-known holy fool from the Middle East.

Sprinkling Breadcrumbs

One day a neighbour came across the Mulla sprinkling breadcrumbs outside the front of his house.

"Mulla, what are you doing?" the neighbour asked.

"Can't you see, I'm sprinkling breadcrumbs," the Mulla replied.

"Yes, I know," replied the frustrated neighbour, "but why?"

"Ah," said the Mulla, "to keep the tigers away."

"But we don't have tigers round here," replied the neighbour.

"Yes," said the Mulla, "effective, isn't it?"

So what does the Mulla need to do in order to find out if there are in fact tigers in the area? Of course, he has to stop sprinkling breadcrumbs. But is he going to do that if he genuinely believes there would be tigers in the area if he didn't? Of course he won't![4]

This brings us to our next formulation tool, which is especially useful in understanding how anxiety disorders work. This is called the vicious daisy.

---

4 Some very interesting recent research (by Jack Rachman and others) has pointed out how judicious use of safety behaviours can help the person get close to whatever it is they're afraid of, but these behaviours do not usually *prevent* you from discovering what's going on. In our example, it would be like the Mulla going outside wearing some protective gear in case the tigers did approach – but still *not* sprinkling breadcrumbs. So, he would still discover that tigers didn't come.

THE VICIOUS DAISY

Some of you may have grown up with the *Asterix* comics. These tell the story of a village in Gaul at the time of the Romans; the heroes, Asterix and Obelix, are resistance fighters against the Roman occupation. A continuing subplot concerns the villagers' worry that the sky was going to fall on their heads. Interestingly, this was apparently a real fear of the ancient Celts. It is also a great example of the sort of belief that, if you really thought it was true, would make you feel anxious! So think for a minute – if you really thought there was a likelihood of this happening, what sort of precautions might you take?

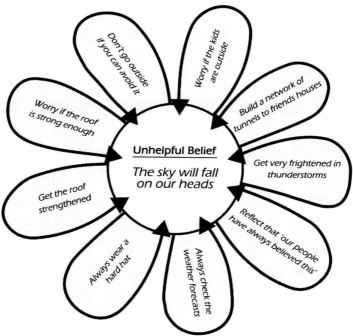

Filled-in vicious daisy

Probably you have come up with a few suggestions, like: don't go outside unless you have to (avoidance); get the roof strengthened and always wear your helmet (physical action); worry if your kids are outside for more than a few minutes (mental action). However, each time you take the (apparently sensible) course of action to take care of this problem, you also set off *unintended consequences* or by-products, the most obvious of which is to *confirm the 'truth' of the central belief,* i.e. the sky being likely to fall on our heads. But there are other things which will keep this belief going, too. How do you think you would feel during a thunderstorm? "It's happening, by Tutatis!" – panic! And taking into account the set of sensations that come with the panic, surely that must mean the threat is real... And of course there are cultural inputs: haven't our people always believed that the sky might fall on our heads? And now it's coming to pass!

So you can see that each of these actions (which seem like obvious steps to take if you believe that the sky will fall on our heads) has the effect of confirming the 'truth' of that idea. So we can represent this on the vicious daisy [see filled-in diagram on the previous page].

The point is this: **that we can maintain and strengthen a belief that has not a shred of real evidence in its favour by what we do and how we think about it.**

Of course, unintended consequences can be positive as well as negative. I call them *metamessages*: the (usually unintended) message that an action or series of actions sends *to* the person *about* him- or herself. A positive example might be in the well-known cosmetic ad: "Because you're worth it."

Again, have a go. Using a blank from the back of the book, or drawing one yourself, see if you can do your own vicious daisy. Start with the fear that you suspect may be irrational or at least overstated (e.g. *one only* taken from the following list: everybody hates me; I'm ugly/worthless/ unlovable/bad; I can never succeed at anything; there's no point; if they knew what I was really like they'd leave me) and place that at the centre of the daisy. Now draw or fill in the petals, which represent anything you do *because of* this belief, either to confirm it (like sprinkling breadcrumbs) or somehow to compensate for it. Also put in anything else that makes you think the belief is true, like getting anxious whenever you think of it, or because in your family you were always treated this way and/or "We always worry about stuff like that"; or "If I do think about that I get these weird feelings so it must be true", etc. Sometimes there are so many petals it's more like a vicious chrysanthemum. That's OK!

Good. Well done. Now let's go back to the *Asterix* diagram. I suppose with your superior knowledge of science compared to those poor Gauls, you probably think that the sky is space and cannot fall. So let's try it. If we replace the 'sky will fall on my head' belief (at the centre) with 'the sky is space and cannot fall' what happens to the petals? Do we need to strengthen the roof? No. Is it the end of the world if there's a thunderstorm? Probably not. Does it matter if our people have always believed this? No. And so on. And what are the 'positive' petals we can put around the new belief to make a 'kindly' daisy? We *can* go out if we want to. The kids *can* play out (as long as there aren't other real dangers!). I *can* take my helmet off outside. And maybe I need to buy granddad a book on astronomy, so he doesn't get so anxious during thunderstorms. And when you do a *kindly* daisy, what are the positive metamessages 'hidden' in each petal?

Now we're doing CBT. So what is the belief that is akin to 'the sky is space and cannot fall' for *your* situation? Try doing your own vicious and kindly daisies. Don't worry if it doesn't solve the problem straight away – we're only formulating at the moment. But at least in theory, you may be able to see what you are doing that is unwittingly helping to keep your problems going.

Warning! Stop! Don't blame yourself! You didn't know this till now!

Let us gently unpick this situation. We'll come to the historical formulation in a bit, but let us first think about why we're reading this book, and what we might want from therapy.

PROBLEMS AND GOALS

Aaron T. Beck, whom we've already mentioned, said that cognitive therapy is whatever the therapist does to help the client get from where they are to where they want to be. But in order for that very broad description to work, we need to know where the 'want to be' is, and sometimes that's not as easy as it sounds. Most people say what they don't want: "I don't want to be depressed anymore", or "I don't want to feel anxious." Of course you don't. But CBT of whatever kind isn't about 'thinking positive'.

Take a moment to think about this. Suppose a friend is absolutely devoted to his dog. Time passes and the dog dies. Would it really be a sign of mental health if, when you asked him how he was feeling, he said "Fabulous, never better!"? I think that you'd be more worried about him than if he said he was feeling very sad. But if he's still spending a huge amount of time grieving over Fido ten years hence, then there would also be something wrong. So it's about having the emotion that is *appropriate* for the situation.

MICRO AND MACRO

To start with, though, let's accept that you come to therapy feeling 'crap' and you want to feel 'great'. Of course. We all want to feel great. And by now, hopefully you've at least had a go at doing a hot cross bun or a vicious daisy (or both) around at least one of your problem situations. This means you've been able to break down the problem into its component parts, which will help you to see where you can reasonably do something different or see things in a different way. That is working at the *micro* level. For each individual problem you need to do this.

But we also need to work at the *macro* level – that is, to look at your life as a whole. So the next thing is to try and get all your major problems down on paper. That may seem a little disheartening, but it can be helpful just to write them down – however long the list, it is finite! So to start with, just do a spidergram: write headings for the problem areas randomly over a sheet of paper (e.g. work, relationship, social situations etc.), and then join them up if they're connected, or don't if they're not. So you might have a diagram that looks something like this:

Problem Spidergram

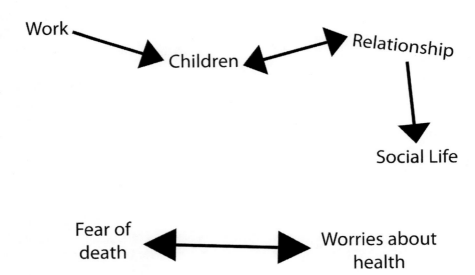

Where the different topics are joined up, try to see if it's actually the same problem popping up in different situations (e.g. getting anxious with other people), or if it's really a problem in one area that's having some kind of fallout in another, like feeling stressed at work because of a difficult relationship with your boss, leading you to work too hard and that having a damaging effect on your marriage (even though the problem is not primarily with the marriage). Some problems may just be separate, like having a fear of heights, for example. So now, use the skills you learned at the micro level – hot cross bun or vicious daisy – and apply them to each one of the separate problems. What are the different components of *each* different problem (thoughts, feelings, body sensations, behaviours)?

If you like, you can do a problem and goal hot cross bun, as below:

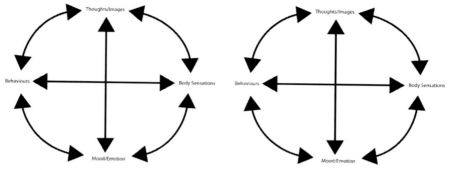

Problem hot cross bun   Goal hot cross bun

Now you should be in a position to have a stab at doing a problem list. So on the *left-hand side* of a piece of paper – or in the 'problem situation' column in the table provided on page 21– write a list of the problems that are troubling you. Be as specific as you can, and try to include thoughts, feelings and what you are doing, and body sensations, too, if relevant (like in panic, or feeling sluggish in depression). Some examples might be:

- *Thinking there's no point in doing anything, feeling depressed and/or lethargic and mostly staying in.*

- *Being frightened to go out in case I have a panic attack, getting really horrible sensations as if I'm going to have a heart attack.*

- *Thinking I look weird and that no one will like me, and staying in and feeling depressed because of that.*

- *Worrying that if I've touched something that feels dirty I will somehow contaminate others, or that something bad will happen to those I love if I don't wash my hands a lot.*

Now, what are the solutions? On the middle 'goals' column, think about what the more rational or appropriate thoughts, feelings and behaviours might be in your situation. Don't worry if they don't seem obvious to start with. What might you say to a friend who was in your shoes? What have other people said; the ones you know really care about you? We are only at the beginning of this process, so you're not expected to be able to come up with all the answers, but you may be able to see, at least in theory, what a better way of looking at this problem might be. If you can't think how you 'ought' to think or feel, just put down what you would like to be able to do, that you can't do at the moment. In the end, that will probably turn out to be the most important thing anyway, and definitely the best yardstick of your progress as you go through therapy, whether that's self-help or being guided by a therapist.

There are different aids to setting good goals (usually expressed as acronyms like SMART or PACER! as shown below), which can help you formulate your goals in a way that is more likely to work, but don't be put off if your own idea doesn't totally conform to their rules. Nonetheless, it's worth briefly reviewing them:

SMART

S: Specific – making what you want to achieve narrow enough in focus to allow you to know when you've achieved it. For example, 'being happier' wouldn't qualify, but 'being able to talk to other parents at the school gates' would. This links to the next one:

M: Measurable – you know when you've got there. This doesn't necessarily mean you can quantify it physically, but someone else should be able to tell that you've got there.

A: Achievable – you know that whatever it is, is in your gift. If I am a politician and I want to be elected, I can try to put forward my best possible case for my policies (achievable), but I can't technically have 'getting elected' as a goal, because that's not down to me.

R: Realistic – if I struggled with basic biology at school, maybe that career as a neurosurgeon will have to wait...

T: Time-limited – not always possible, but it's good to have benchmarks so that the process is grounded in reality, otherwise you don't know when you're 'supposed' to get there.

This is all good sensible stuff. The other acronym, PACER! (from Neuro-Linguistic Programming), operates similarly:

PACER!

P: Positive
A: Achievable
C: In my Control
E: Ecology
R: Resources
! Review, evaluation points

What PACER! adds to SMART, in my view, is really the E word – *ecology* – which is nothing to do with green politics or biology, but refers to your integrity: does this goal correspond with who you are and/or who you want to be? In one hospital where I worked, a great proportion of the patients were suffering burnout from working in the banking or IT industries. Most had going back to work as their stated goal; for some this was just right, but for others I knew that if they did go back, in a few months we'd see them again. That work situation just wasn't suitable for who they were as people.

As the ACT (Acceptance and Commitment Therapy) people have it, what do you want written on your tombstone? If the way you're currently living isn't going to attain that, then now is probably as good a time as any to change direction! Therapy is a chance to review how we're living our lives. That said, it is important not to make rash decisions if you're in the middle of a profound depression – you almost certainly won't be seeing things quite straight! But you want to end up with the right tombstone, or it might be very confusing for the gravediggers...

Of course, the hypothetical problems listed above, being hypothetical, aren't specific in the way that real problems are, so I can't keep to SMART or PACER! in formulating possible solutions. With some problems you can't always put a timeframe around them, anyway. But partly for the sake of symmetry, let's look at some possible goals to go with our examples:

Problem	Goal
Thinking there's no point in doing anything, feeling depressed and/or lethargic and mostly staying in;	Not questioning the point of things unless I'm in a philosophy class (after all, you didn't before you got depressed, right?), but getting out and doing stuff. Having more energy.
Being frightened to go out in case I have a panic attack; getting really horrible sensations as if I'm going to have a heart attack.	Being able to go wherever I want to go without being afraid of panicking; knowing that I'm not going to have a heart attack.
Thinking that I look weird and no one will like me, and staying in and feeling depressed because of that.	Going out socially without worrying what I look like any more than the next person does.
Worrying that if I've touched something that feels dirty I will somehow contaminate others, or that something bad will happen to those I love if I don't wash my hands a lot.	Just paying as much attention to hygiene as people normally do; not restricting my life because of contamination issues.

The next bit, as you can see from the box overleaf, is to work out some steps leading to the goal. Put these on the right hand side of your paper. This is always work in progress, and it is good to come back to your problems and goals every so often, as what you want and what you consider realistic may change as you go through the therapeutic process.

Problem and Goal Table

Problem Situation	Goal	Steps to get there
Example: being afraid to go out in case I have a panic attack.	Being able to go wherever I want without being afraid of panicking.	Expand the range of places I can go (use a hierarchy); challenge my fear of panic using an ABC or panic diary; experience panic and see what happens.

So now you've got the beginnings of a formulation:

- Some idea of the thoughts, feelings and behaviours in at least some of the problems you're struggling with;

- Some idea of how it might look at the other end of the therapy process;

- And some idea of the steps you might need to get there.

Well done! If you're just reading and haven't done it yet, *please go back and do the exercise*. Research shows that just reading self-help books has very limited help value. But if you actually *do* the stuff, you may be surprised at how much can change...

CONCLUSION

In CBT (fourth wave or otherwise) we need to formulate our situation. This means breaking it down into its component parts. That way, we can see more clearly where the problems are and what we might be able to do about them. We also need to develop a clear and realistic vision of what we want instead, and be prepared to have that change as we go deeper into investigating how our lives work. It is also interesting to see what we are doing that may be unwittingly taking us in directions we don't want to go. It will also be useful to identify actions that carry positive metamessages.

CHAPTER 2: EMOTIONS

Different families of emotions and what they are there for – Body sensation in emotion – When is a feeling not a feeling? – Accepting emotions – Allowing processing – Rating moods

Most people come to therapy to feel better: to feel happier, more in control, less anxious or depressed. And although CBT tends to work *indirectly* with the emotions (by focusing on other parts of the hot cross bun and changing those), it is important to get to know the emotions and what their job is when they're working properly. Also, we should remind ourselves that these emotions were 'laid down' in the brain at a very early stage in the evolution of our species. In fact, some of them have not changed that much since we were lizards! So it is not surprising if we sometimes act a bit 'primitive' if we get swept away by them.

We can categorise emotions as falling into eight or nine 'families': happy, love, sad, anxious, angry, disgust, guilt/shame, and envy/jealousy. The last two pairs are close to each other, but not identical. These groupings are not definite and absolute, but seeing them as families helps us to find our way around them. Notice they nearly all have associated body sensations (which helps us to tell them from thoughts, which don't). Let us take each family in turn and look at some of its members:

Happy:
Joyful, content, at ease, relaxed, ecstatic etc.
All of these emotions are self-reinforcing, that is, if we do something that makes us feel one of these emotions, we are likely to want to do more of it. If we are feeling like this, we are more likely to shift into the next family:

Love:
Kind, generous, compassionate etc.
This not only makes *us* feel good, it also cements the group, family, tribe

Table of Emotions

Emotion	Function	Typical body sensations
Happy	Reward helpful behaviour	Warmth, lightness
Loving/compassion	Increase solidarity in the group	Warmth, softness
Sad	Helps to process hurt/loss	Heavy feeling, often in stomach or chest; tears
Anxiety	Protection (in panic – fight/flight/freeze; in worry, heading off problems in advance)	Sweaty, nauseous, heart racing, 'butterflies' etc. Body aches in generalised anxiety
Anger	Protection (of self/ others you care for/ property etc.)	Extreme tension, readiness for attack, heightened arousal
Disgust	Protection (preventing poisoning, literally or metaphorically)	Nausea, retching
Guilt/ Shame	To punish 'bad' or inappropriate actions	Reddening (shame), feeling in pit of stomach (guilt)
Envy/Jealousy	To get what you want and to keep what you have	The 'green-eyed monster', takes you out of the here-and-now

etc. so that we are not just concerned about our personal survival and well-being, but also that of the group to which we belong.

Sad:
Downcast, disappointed, dejected, hurt, despondent, low, grief-stricken etc.
These emotions, of course, have the opposite effect to the first two families – that is, we don't deliberately do things that make us feel like this – but allowing ourselves to feel these emotions can help us to let go of events which have hurt us in some way. If we *don't* feel sadness it can lead to depression. Rational Emotive Behaviour Therapy (REBT) portrays sadness as a healthy negative emotion. On the other hand, *ruminating* leads to unhealthy emotional states (dejected, despondent, depressed etc.).

Anxious:
Scared, frightened, panicky, nervous etc.
This is our alarm system. In its most extreme and physical version, panic, our fight/flight/freeze reaction is triggered, causing a wide range of uncomfortable sensations. In a more low-level but continuous version caused by constant worrying, it causes a different set of physical reactions (body aches, digestive upsets or raised blood pressure, for example) and also lowers the threshold at which panic attacks can occur.

Anger:
Raging, irritated, cross, grumpy etc.
These emotions protect us, but in a different way from anxiety. However, they're closely related to anxiety, in that both trigger raised arousal levels. Anger is showing our teeth and claws when we feel under threat, but at some level we're prepared at least to stand our ground - we back ourselves to keep what we've got, if you like. Imagine fighting over a kill on a hunting trip. Often anxiety kicks in first →fight or flight →anger →fight.

Disgust:
Repulsed, yucky etc.
This probably comes from the reaction we get if we eat something we need to get rid of, but it can also be felt in a range of other situations. Again, it has very strong physical attributes, making you want to spit or retch. Combined with anger and directed against the self, it causes self-loathing. We could see it as the ultimate aversive emotion.

Guilt/Shame:
Ashamed, embarrassed, guilty etc.
In a way, mixing guilt and shame is not helpful, because they are different. Yet they are both emotions which make us turn away, either from others (shame), or from something we've done (guilt). While guilt says, "What you've *done* is unforgivable", shame says, "*You're* bad, go away and hide", although shame can be external (how it feels when you are excluded from a group) or internal (feeling embarrassed about how you've behaved in a given situation, for example). One can of course feel both! Ultimately, they both act to stop us behaving in certain ways, whether in relation to our own laws and rules, or those of the group (clan, tribe, society etc.).

Envy/Jealousy
Greedy, possessive etc.
These are another pair that are close but not identical to each other. Technically envy is about things and jealousy about people, but the central quality for both is wanting something you haven't got, or think/ fear you haven't got (as in possessiveness). In reasonable measure envy can be a motivator; jealousy is harder to find a 'positive' function for, except in evolutionary 'selfish gene' terms.

EMOTIONS AND BODY SENSATIONS — WHEN IS A FEELING NOT A FEELING?

Cognitive Behavioural Therapy works well when it is specific about how the different elements of a problem interact, as we have seen in the hot cross bun, for example. Yet our everyday language is not so precise! So people talk about feelings in a number of different ways, and it is helpful to be clear about what we mean. At the very least there are two uses of the term. We use the word 'feeling' to describe anything that is related to sensation or touch: if we are aware of physical pressure, or internal body sensations like hunger or thirst, we say 'I feel...'. So feeling is obviously appropriate for the body sensation 'arm' of the hot cross bun. Unfortunately for those of us who like things clearly defined, we also use the term 'feel' for anything that touches us emotionally – like sadness, anger, happiness etc. In my view this is no accident, since as we have seen, *every emotion comes with its own signature set of bodily sensations.* So we can obviously use the term 'feel' for the mood or emotion arm of the hot cross bun too. For the sake of clarity, I will therefore try to use the ambiguous term 'feeling' as little as possible in this book, but rather use sensation (for the body stuff) and mood or emotion for that area.

However, some people, especially therapists (!), often use 'feel' when they mean 'think' (e.g. "I *feel* you're putting me down", when they mean "I *think* you're putting me down, and that's making me *feel* angry/ hurt/ sad"). This leads to confusion about thoughts and emotions/ feelings. It has to be said that some are a bit ambiguous: what about 'vulnerable', for example – is this an emotion; a sort of cousin of anxiety, or an expression of the self-judgement 'weak' and therefore a thought or belief?

So perhaps this exercise cannot be perfect, but if we are as clear as we can be about whether something is an appraisal/ thought/ judgement on the one hand, or an emotion with a felt sense on the other, this will help us to break down problem situations into their different parts and therefore understand them better.

Two little tricks that can sometimes help us tell the difference between thoughts and emotions are these:

1.   Remember that an emotion is a quality, usually described in a single word, which carries accompanying physical sensation(s)

2.   If you can follow "I feel" with the word "that", it's probably not a feeling but a thought, e.g. "I feel (that) you're putting me down", or "I feel (that) I'm going to have a panic attack."

In the second example the person is undoubtedly feeling something – some body sensations – which are making them *think* they are going to have a panic attack (and therefore making them *feel* anxious).

ACCEPTING EMOTIONS AND ALLOWING PROCESSING

The emotional brain – the limbic system and its components – is something we have inherited from our mammalian ancestors, or sometimes from our reptilian ones. Our distinctly human characteristic, the huge forebrain, is an evolutionary afterthought. It is as though the basic model brain is a Sinclair ZX computer (which some readers may remember), and on top of that was grafted an old 1990s IBM using Microsoft DOS, and on top of that each subsequent program until we get to - where are we presently, Windows 8? OK, I know they're operating systems rather than programs, but you get my drift. So this incredible human brain is actually built on very primitive basic hardware, and yet is a miracle of cognitive sophistication. Unfortunately the emotions often seem to belong to the Sinclair ZX bit, so it helps to think of our emotions as definitely animal. *This doesn't mean they're bad.* They are absolutely vital, in that they prime our bodies for particular kinds of action, and are thus known as 'action tendencies'. But we as humans have possibilities which are unique in the animal kingdom. If an animal feels an emotion, it *has to follow through* with the action if it can (unless there's a stronger inhibiting emotion, or with the possible exception of reconditioned domestic animals). As humans, we sometimes – and only sometimes – have the ability to override what the emotion is telling us to do.

And here is a principle of mental health, which in my view should be taught in schools, put out in public health announcements and so on. It is this: *it is not usually, in the long run, helpful to suppress unwanted emotions. Nor is it always good to act on them.*

Emotions are there to tell us something. On the other hand, it may well be that it is not a good idea to follow through with the action that the emotion is priming you for – that can land you in prison! But if we can:

1. acknowledge the feeling,
2. find out what it wants,
3. and feel the accompanying bodily sensations (whether or not we want to act on them), then
4. the emotions can be processed, and
5. will not turn into the secondary bodily reaction known as *stress* – leading to the variety of complaints that are so common and well-publicised in modern western society.

In fact a great proportion of the work that therapists of all persuasions are engaged in is unpicking the consequences of unprocessed emotion from earlier experiences.

Emotions, then, are the action tendencies that prime us for various kinds of (usually protective) actions. Uniquely in the animal kingdom, we humans have the possibility of not doing what they say, at least sometimes. But that energy has to go somewhere, and if we choose not to do what the emotion is saying, then we have at least to *feel* it, which means listening to what it has to say. Otherwise there may be consequences for us in terms of increased stress caused by our not being able to process the emotion.

Sometimes – as psychotherapists from Freud onwards have noted – the suppression of emotions is outside of our consciousness, and is then known as *repression.* Another term that is used – e.g.in Voice Dialogue and D. Genpo Merzel's Big Mind process (see below) – is *disowning.* So we can say that particular emotions that we don't like or which seem too dangerous to us become *disowned*, either consciously (suppression) or unconsciously (repression), because they don't fit the picture of who we think we should be or how the world is supposed to work.

But emotions don't happen in a vacuum. As we saw in the hot cross bun exercise, they are one element in a situation, along with thoughts, behaviours, body sensations and whatever the trigger is that is coming from the environment (outside or in our heads). Usually in CBT we don't try to change emotions directly; rather we examine them to see whether they seem appropriate in kind and intensity for the situation we find ourselves in. One of the things that we therefore need to be able to do is measure or rate the emotion or mood: how strong is it? We can do this on a scale of 1–10 or 1–100 – it doesn't really matter, as long as you know what the scale is. Sometimes people don't like putting numbers on things; if you feel like that you can try a scale with words, like 'very much', 'quite a lot', 'somewhat', 'not much' and 'very little'. In general it's easier with numbers! But let's try rating our moods, and linking the emotion with a situation:

Rating Moods

Situation	*Mood/Emotion (0-100)*
Boss being critical in performance review	*Ashamed 60, Angry 75*

Try putting in two or three of your own – use things that have happened recently so you have a clear memory of how strong the emotions were or are. In fact, I suggest keeping a mood-rating log like this over the next week, so you get used to noticing which emotions are present and how strong they are. Then you'll be ready to make the most of the next chapter!

SUMMARY

On one level, emotions are our instinctual programs which prepare our bodies to behave in particular ways in certain kinds of situation;

each one has a function, and is there to give us a message of one sort or another. However, emotions can be and are influenced by thought or interpretation, which is how Cognitive Therapy works: change the interpretation and the intensity and/or type of emotion may change. As we will see, it's not always as simple as that. But what is not helpful is to try to prevent ourselves from feeling those feelings. Instead, we can learn to accept the emotions as messengers whose messages we need to hear, although we may choose not to act on them.

CHAPTER 3: COGNITIONS: WHAT ARE THEY?

Appraisals – Interpretation – Automatic, intrusive and deliberate – Depression FM and other inputs – Am I my thoughts? – Image work

Remembering Aaron Beck's nod to the Greek Stoic philosopher Epictetus ("Men are disturbed not by things but by the views which they take of them") it is not surprising that the main drift of traditional cognitive therapy is all about seeing that it is what we *make* of what is happening; our *appraisal* of the situation (and then the behaviour that our appraisal leads to) that may be giving us problems.

> Paul Salkovskis tells the story of the dog poo on the path leading from this particular house to the street: Coincidentally, living in this house are four people: one suffering from anxiety, another from depression, a third from anger problems, and a cognitive therapist. So one morning the first of these walks out of the house to go to work, and treads in the dog poo. "Oh my God," he says, "if that's how my day's starting, who knows what the rest of it's going to be like. If I go in, I'll probably say the wrong thing to the boss, get fired and heaven knows what else." So he goes back in and goes back to bed. The second one comes out and does the same thing, "I knew there was no point in getting up today. That just shows the futility of me trying to do anything." And he too goes back to bed. The third one comes out – by now the mess is across the path – and also treads in it. "I'm going to kill those damn neighbours who let their **** dog into our **** garden!" and he goes off to accost the neighbours. The cognitive therapist comes out, also treads in it, and thinks to herself, "Just as well I had my shoes on." We could add that if any of them had been practising mindfulness, they might have seen it on the path and cleaned it up... or at least not trodden in it!

Sometimes clients say that they often don't know what the thought was that made them feel a certain way. Often it may be an image, or just an interpretation of whatever else is going on: the body sensation, the unexplained drop in mood, the seeming lack of energy for 'no good reason'. But what are we making of *that*? What does it mean? The answer to that and similar questions will give us the way to explain what is going on.

In CBT we can distinguish various kinds of thoughts: deliberate, automatic, intrusive and metacognitive. In addition to these there are underlying beliefs of different kinds.

Deliberate thinking is the useful kind, when in the right place and proportion. It's what we do to figure stuff out, to do the calculations, to answer 'how' questions. When we try to use it to answer 'why' questions (at least in the world of psychotherapy), we're on shakier ground.

Automatic thoughts are those that just pop into our heads without us doing anything. Sometimes they seem like a never-ending running commentary on what is happening ("Oh you stupid idiot, why did you do that?"), and are often negative, as in that example. They are the target for the techniques we will see more of later, because once we see what these thoughts are doing, we can see whether or not they are helpful. They are sometimes abbreviated to NATs (Negative Automatic Thoughts), which I suppose makes CBT a sort of insecticide, although we don't actually need to get rid of them, which leads me to the next category:

Intrusive thoughts. These come into our mind against our will; they are the ones we desperately *don't* want to think. They may start out as NATs, but our very attempt to keep them out, paradoxically keeps them there. There is a story about this:

> The earliest version of this story goes back to ancient India, and the Buddhist philosopher-mystic Nagarjuna. One day, a disciple came to him with a problem. "I have been working very hard at this enlightenment stuff," said the student, "but I just can't empty my mind."
>
> "Oh that's easy," said Nagarjuna. "Just don't think about monkeys."
>
> Of course the poor man went away, and whatever he tried to think about, monkeys were there. And if, out of sheer exhaustion, he managed to forget them for an instant, India being India, there was always a real one trying to get in the window to remind him.

Recent CBT versions of this involve the exercise of trying not to think of white bears or pink elephants. Funny how it's always animals. Although a friend of mine once had a set of tattoos which completely covered both arms, and when asked why he had had them done, he said, "To forget" which inevitably prompted the response, "Forget what?" To which he just as inevitably replied, "I don't know, I've forgotten." This silly story hopefully shows us that one can only *deliberately* remember, for the very act of *trying* to forget involves putting the very subject that you're trying to forget in the forefront of your mind – so you can forget about it!

The upshot of all this is really that suppressing thoughts doesn't work. Now that is an example of a kind of *metacognitive* idea. I'm sorry about the jargon, but it is a useful label for *thinking about thinking*. Many of our problems come, as Epictetus said, from what we make of stuff. Even more come from what we make of what we make of stuff:

- "If I'm thinking like that, things must have got really bad."
- "If I don't worry about her, who's going to?"
- "If I'm worrying a lot, I'll make myself ill."
- "Thinking something is as bad as doing it."

...and so on. Of course we can have helpful metacognitive beliefs too, like, "It's just a thought, don't sweat it."

Underlying beliefs are fundamentally of two kinds: unconditional or *core* beliefs ("I'm worthless"; "Life's a struggle": "Other people are dangerous") and conditional beliefs, including rules for living ("If I can please everybody, then I won't be in danger"). We will come back to underlying beliefs in Chapter 7 under *Schemas and rules*.

DEPRESSION FM AND OTHER INPUTS

We saw in Chapter 1 how CBT gains much from separating out the different parts of a problem situation, and in particular trying to distinguish thoughts from emotions or moods. Aaron Beck noticed that particular conditions tend to produce particular kinds of thought. Depression, for example, gives rise to ideas like "There's no point" and "It's too much effort", while anxiety, not surprisingly, produces thoughts of a catastrophic nature. So the condition produces the thought, and then we fall down the ready-prepared hole by *believing it* – which then makes the condition (depression, anxiety etc.) stronger.

One way of developing the necessary detachment to begin to get some freedom from this conundrum is to recognise and name the origin of the thought. In fourth wave CBT we use the metaphor of a radio or some other identifying marker to help us see that this is not our *rational* appraisal of the situation, but an *automatic* input coming from a condition: "This is not me, this is Depression FM broadcasting in my brain" or "Hello, panic lizard" or "Is this Radio OCD?"

AM I MY THOUGHTS?

In psychosis, people sometimes hear their thoughts as though they were voices coming from outside. In fact we know they are really thoughts because it is the part of the brain which produces thoughts that is activated when these 'voices' are heard. Most people with depression or anxiety, on the other hand, are well aware that the negative thoughts they are hearing are coming from inside their own minds. However, this often leads them to the conclusion that they *are* their own thoughts and thus should be in control of everything that happens in their own brains, and if they're not, well then frankly that must mean they're barking. Woof!

This in my view is a mistake, because although thoughts may happen inside one's own mind (where else could they really happen?), it turns out that one's mind is much greater than we know, and that it is not remotely helpful to identify with its contents as 'me', never mind try to be in control of all of it. Let's try some exercises:

Look at the Furniture

Sometimes it is important to see what is around us. Now, how do you know you are not that chair (or table, or other piece of furniture in the room where you are reading this)? No, don't go all philosophical on me, I mean how do you stop yourself bumping into it? Ah, now you've got it. You see it, right? You are the one over here, and the chair (table etc.) is the one over there. So you are the one looking at the chair, and the chair is the one being looked at. Of course all our senses give us information like this. We could sum up this information with the concept of awareness. So I am aware of the chair – it's not me – and the chair is the thing that I am aware of. So I don't trip over it.

So far so good.

It follows from this that if I can be aware of something (like the chair), I am not it. OK?

Now, can you be aware of your thoughts? (I don't mean perfectly or all the time) Yes? Well, if I know I'm not the chair, because I can be aware of it, and I can be aware of my thoughts, what does that say about me and my thoughts?

You mean I'm not my thoughts?

The American philosopher Ken Wilber puts it succinctly: "Suffering is the misidentification of 'I am-ness' with an object" (see his video on YouTube: "I am Big Mind"). Thoughts are one kind of object, in this sense.

The Fridge

We can come to the same idea with another domestic metaphor. I want you to imagine that you're a fridge (as if you didn't have enough problems). There you are, and somebody comes along and puts some milk in you. What do you do? Keep it cold, right? Somebody else comes along and puts some butter in you. What do you do? The same? OK. Now, another person comes along and puts a dirty old boot in you. Of course you don't like it! But what can you do? You're a fridge. That's right, you've just got to keep that dirty old boot nice and cold.

So why is there no point in you getting upset about the presence of that dirty old boot in you? Who is in charge of what comes in to you and what goes out? It's not you, is it? Your door gets opened and stuff comes in and goes out, not in your control...

But do you think you are the milk, or the butter, or the old boot? No of course not, you're the fridge. And in this way, fridges may be more intelligent than human beings!

So we are the fridges, and the milk and the butter are thoughts and feelings we like, and the dirty old boot is one that we don't like. We can think of ourselves as containers for these thoughts and feelings.

In this area there is only one major difference, actually, between us and fridges, and that is that while fridges really don't have any control at all over what goes into them or comes out, we have one peculiar mechanism. And this is that if we really want something to go away, then it stays there. So if you really don't want to think about monkeys, pink elephants, or sex with camels (!) then guess what's coming into your mind...

But if we're containers, then I guess the main thing is to make sure there's enough space for all the thoughts and feelings, whether we like them or not. Why don't you have a look and see how big your mind is? Can you find the edges?

And here's the third:

Sky and Clouds

Buddhists have a metaphor for the relationship between our minds and thoughts and feelings. They say the mind is like a clear blue sky, while thoughts and feelings are like clouds. Of course some days the sky is completely overcast. Does that mean the sky isn't there? Of course not, as any of you who've ever flown will know: above the clouds, just infinite sky. Is there any point in trying to make the clouds disappear, by force of will? Of course not, it's just the weather. Are clouds always changing? Naturally. Do I have to like them? No. Do I have to accept that they are there? It makes sense to, if they're there.

So what do you want to identify with, as being you? The ever changing and tempestuous clouds of thought and emotion, or the clear blue sky of awareness (which contains the thought and emotion anyway)?

So while our thoughts definitely occur within our minds, our minds are bigger than we know. And to help us look at our thoughts and emotions, it is helpful to take a perspective that is 'outside' of them, and not confuse the *one who is looking* with the *object that is looked at.*

IMAGES

When we talk about thoughts, we often think of them as though they were sentences; trails of words informing us. Of course those exist, especially in those of us who work a lot with words. But for many – and probably most people – the more powerful and evocative thoughts are actually experienced as images. The word-thoughts may come second, as a commentary on the image, and our earliest memories may even be encoded in a bodily felt-sense. So whenever we talk about thoughts in this book, we don't just mean strings of words in our heads. As we will see, it is often in image and felt-sense that the real 'juice' is found.

SUMMARY

There are four different kinds of thought: deliberate, automatic, intrusive and underlying belief. We may experience thoughts in different ways: as words, images or even felt-senses. Fundamentally, a thought is not a thing, but a representation. However, we become identified with our thoughts, and that causes us trouble. To learn to identify with the 'one who knows' rather than what is known helps us to avoid getting caught up in our own nonsense. "Don't let the sound of your own wheels drive you crazy..." (The Eagles).

CHAPTER 4: DIFFERENT WAYS OF DEALING WITH UNHELPFUL THOUGHTS

Challenge or accept – Thinking errors – Faulty feelometer – Thought records – Letting thoughts go by – Thoughts and feelings as my children – Two kinds of distraction

In essence, learning how to deal with unhelpful thoughts can be seen as the most basic and necessary skill of CBT. Sometimes cognitive therapy is reduced in popular imagination to 'changing the way you think'. As we shall see, fourth wave CBT is a great deal more than that, but it is still important to consider our thinking, and to adopt the traditional CBT approach where appropriate. In the previous chapter we distinguished two kinds of unhelpful thought: *negative automatic (NATs)* and *intrusive*. Whichever kind it is, the first thing is to question what is happening: "What kind of a thought is this?"

Just by doing that we have created the space between ourselves and the content of our minds. We then have a choice between *believing* what our mind may be saying, or *mistrusting* it. If the thought is after all useful, then great, go with it. ("Yes, I really do need to fill out my tax return, thank you, mind.") But if it isn't, then we need to find out what it is: "Ah, here we have a NAT/ intrusive thought...now what do we do?"

The choice now is between simply accepting that this is an unhelpful thought and letting it go (which, as we shall see, often really means letting it be there), or questioning it in some way. If we're not sure whether it's true or not, we may need to go through the process of challenging to find out. Sometimes the thought or image may seem relatively innocuous on the surface, but it provokes strong and unpleasant emotion. In that case we may need to dig a little deeper through Socratic questioning, to which we will return in a bit.

One of the key tools we have in CBT to help us distinguish between accurate and inaccurate thoughts is the list of thinking errors or thinking distortions.

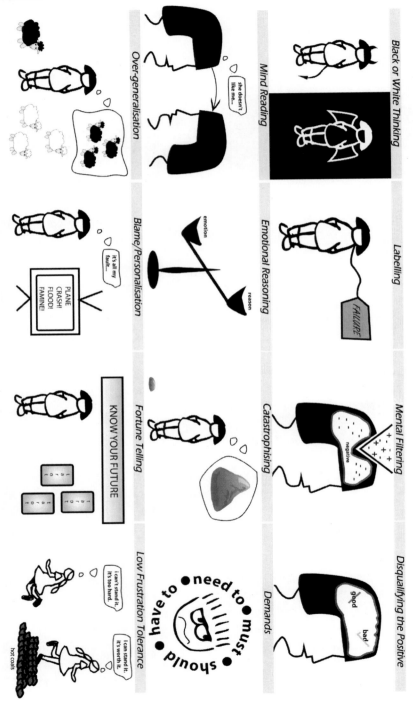

THINKING ERRORS/DISTORTIONS

All-or-nothing family

The most basic of all distortions is the tendency toward *All-or-Nothing* (also known as Black-and-White) thinking. It's common in children – things are either wonderful or terrible; all good or all bad. When we extend this through time and/or space we get *Overgeneralisation* – one policeman gives us a parking ticket and we think all policemen are horrible and that definitely we need to treat them as the enemy.

Taking Black-and-White thinking to the next level we get *Labelling*, in which we reduce the person – self or other – to the quality we abhor: "I'm an idiot"; "He's a prat"; "She's lazy." What we are doing when we say this is making an equivalence between that person – often oneself – and the label:

- He = Prat
- I = Idiot
- She = Lazy

Of course the person is much more than that...and we're all lazy, idiotic prats sometimes!

Another member of this group is *Disqualifying the Positive*. This is very common in people with depression, who have a tendency to discount what they have managed to do, and only focus on what *didn't* work. In fact this is a particular kind of *Mental Filtering*, in which negative inputs get through, but positive feedback can't (unless it is somehow changed to negative). So when you get a great mark in an evaluation, you beat yourself up for not doing even better, and only concentrate on those aspects you need to improve on, thus turning a success into a failure (subjectively speaking).

Jumping-to-conclusions family

There are enough problems in the world without us manufacturing any extra ones, but we do. Sometimes we imagine what others think of us – usually with a negative slant, right? – when of course we can't *know* what is going through someone else's mind, or even if they're thinking about us at all! This is called *Mind-Reading* and is one of the *Jumping-to-Conclusions* family. When our imaginations are less about what others are thinking and more about the future in general, we call it *Fortune-Telling*. If the imagined consequences are dire, it may even count as *Catastrophising*– 'molehills into mountains', the favoured error of choice in anxiety.

Demands

This one stands by itself as the tyrant it is. This is the 'hardening of the oughteries'; an excess of living rigidly by the rules. Sometimes we live by them without even knowing that we're doing so. As we'll see in the chapter on schemas, these unwritten rules may be causing us difficulties precisely because we didn't know that we were their prisoner! In general, the more we can learn to live in the moment and respond to circumstances as they arise, the less rule-bound we need to be. Listen for 'shoulds', 'have-tos', 'musts' and 'oughts'. If you can turn it into 'want to', i.e. "I don't feel like doing this, but I know that to do it is in my own best interests", then that particular demand is probably not a problem. Actually there are very few *real* demands: if you're not being threatened with a machine-gun or similar, there are only choices. The Rational-Emotive Behaviour Therapy (REBT) people suggest trading in your demand for what they call a *full preference*: "I would much prefer it if (whatever it is) didn't happen, but I can tolerate it if it does."

In this way, demands overlap into the next group: *Low Frustration Tolerance*, where we shoot ourselves in the foot by telling ourselves we 'can't stand' something, or that it is 'intolerable'. Mostly these are overstatements; the REBT line, again, is that sometimes events are very unpleasant, upsetting etc., but we *can* stand them. Learning to tolerate the unpleasant physical sensations of anxiety, for example, is one of the key skills in learning to overcome it.

Personalisation and blame

This is where we attribute responsibility unwisely – blaming ourselves for something that at best was only partly our fault, or blaming others when we don't really know how much of the action we dislike was really up to them. Personalisation leads to excessive guilt, while blame leads to anger. A helpful technique to deal with taking excessive responsibility is the 'responsibility pie', where you divide up all the possible causes (personal and impersonal) in a pie chart; attribute all other factors with a percentage, and only then add what you think is the right proportion for yourself. Ninety-nine times out of a hundred, you will find that you blame yourself less when you do this exercise. A close cousin to this one is *Arbitrary Inference*. Despite its rather highbrow-sounding name, this simply means joining two ideas together which actually have no necessary connection with each other: "Just because I don't have a driving licence" (idea one) "it doesn't mean I'm a complete failure as a human being" (idea two).

Emotional reasoning

This is when we mistake the strength of our feeling for the truth of what we think: "I'm feeling very anxious so it must be dangerous to go outdoors." That we feel something strongly is not necessarily a sign that what we feel is the case. In fact, if you have been given a diagnosis of anxiety or depression, remember that these are known as 'emotional disorders'. What that means to me is that you have a 'faulty feelometer'(see overleaf), and therefore what you feel may well be unreliable, so don't accept it as the truth straight off – give yourself some time to look more carefully from a more objective point of view.

You may like to peruse this list; we all use most of them sometimes, but there are usually some that are our particular 'favourites'.. It is important also to recognise that originally these are *processing shortcuts* which are really useful when everything else is working OK. When hungry and confronted by a pile of manure and a pile of chocolate, all-or-nothing thinking is great! Likewise, unless employed on road maintenance, one absolutely shouldn't (*Demand*)go walking on the motorway. However, we know that emotional disorders like anxiety and depression pollute our thinking, which means that it can be worth checking our thoughts against the list of thinking errors quite frequently. What some people have found helpful is simply sticking the list up somewhere prominent – on the kitchen notice board, for example, or attached to the fridge with a magnet – and whenever you feel that your mood has dipped a bit or that you've got overly anxious, going and having a look to see if what you're thinking has any thinking errors in it. Charlotte Joko Beck talks about 'emotion thoughts', which is a way of emphasising that we all suffer from emotional disorders in our thinking. It's a bit like having a faulty feelometer (see box overleaf).

Once we have established that our faulty feelometer has been giving us inaccurate messages, then we need a way of finding out what is actually going on – how fast are the trees going by? Most commonly, the kind of inaccurate thinking that will be going on is *automatic thinking*. The technique for dealing with NATs is different than for intrusive thoughts, which we will examine below. For now let us go back to an examination of automatic thinking in more detail.

The Faulty Feelometer

Imagine you're driving along and you look down at your speedometer and see that it's reading 0 mph. Then you pull up at some traffic lights and again look down at it. It's reading 70, and you're completely stopped. How much longer are you going to believe what your speedo is telling you? Not long, I guess!

If you've been given a diagnosis of (or are otherwise convinced that you have) depression or anxiety, these are emotional disorders. We can liken those to having a faulty feelometer.

If your speedo isn't working, how are you going to judge your speed – at least until you can get to the garage to get it fixed? Maybe by how fast the trees are going by? Or by how fast other drivers appear to be going? In any case, you need to use more objective criteria.

So it is with the faulty feelometer. If you have anxiety or depression, your 'instincts', or what you 'feel' like doing, or what you 'feel' is going to happen – these are all likely to be unreliable for the time being. The list of thinking errors can act as a double-check to see whether what you feel is going on is actually the case, or is a biased view coming from Depression FM or the well-known Panic Station.

We are not trained to identify Negative Automatic Thoughts, yet they can fill our heads like some kind of unwanted running commentary to our lives, affecting our moods, often without us realising. If you are depressed, the thoughts will tend to be unduly negative about **yourself** ("I'm not good enough"); the **world** ("There's no point"); and the **future** ("I will never get better"). If you are anxious, on the other hand, the thoughts will tend towards the catastrophic ("I'm going mad"; "The world is dangerous"; "I will never cope").

NATs have several characteristics:

- They are **automatic** – they just pop into your head without any effort on your part.

- They are **distorted** – they do not fit the facts.

- They are **unhelpful** – they keep you feeling the extreme feelings you are experiencing.

- They are **plausible** – you accept them as facts, and it does not occur to you to question them.

- They are **involuntary** – you do not choose to have them and you can't switch them off.

Using the *ABC* form

The main method of challenging your negative automatic thoughts is to use a thought record. The one I favour[5] is called an ABC form, but the principles are similar whichever type you use.

The ABC Form

Activating event or trigger situation	Beliefs/negative automatic thoughts (NATs)	Co-productions	Dispute your beliefs & NATS and devise better alternatives	Effects of alternative thought...
Anything can be an 'A' – external or internal events	What went through your mind? What did 'A' mean to you?	What came with the thought?	Remember compassionate mind	...on your body, emotions and actions.
		Emotions: list and rate 0-100 intensity		Re-rate emotions 0-100 – any new emotions?
		Body sensations: list intensity 0-100		Body sensations: list intensity 0-100
		Behaviour: what did you do? Did it confirm beliefs in B?	What might I tell someone else in this situation?	New behaviour? Plan behavioural experiment(s)
	Remember: thinking errors?			

---

5 The ABC reproduced here has the advantage over other thought records in that it contains a space for both the unhealthy maintaining behaviour and the new alternative behaviour, as well as both automatic thought and the alternative (dispute). It also includes body sensations. It differs from the REBT original in that body sensations, emotions and behaviours are seen as Co-productions rather than Consequences (of thought).

These are the instructions:

A:
The first step is to identify – if you can – what was going on when you started to feel bad. That could be a situation in the world, or what was going through your mind at the time. It doesn't matter which: *anything can be an A (Activating event.*). So write in what was going on in the A column.

C:
Next we go to the C column to see what, apart from the thought, was generated in you by the event – how it 'made you' feel, both bodily and emotionally, and what that led to you doing. This particular form calls the C column 'Co-production'; although we are looking at the effect of thought on the other components, we do not say that thoughts 'cause' them, rather we can say that body sensations, emotions and behaviours *come with* particular thoughts as a package. By making the package accessible to consciousness, we can take it apart and see where we can make changes. As you can see, the C column is actually divided into three: body sensations, emotion and behaviour. So we need to know what the **body sensations** were, as well as the **emotion** that was triggered by the event in the A column, and what you did as a result – the **behaviour**. We also need to rate how strong or intense the body sensations and emotions were; you can do it on a 1–10 scale or 1–100. It doesn't matter as long as you are consistent on each form.

B:
Then we can come back to the B Beliefs column to find out *what was going through your mind that 'made you' feel that way.* Sometimes it just seems like a thought; other times an image. Sometimes it may be what you *made of* the physical sensations, like in panic. It may be that you find it difficult to 'catch the thoughts'. In that case it may be more helpful to look at the *co-productions* of the mood or emotion; for example, try putting an unexplained mood-drop in column A and see what you make of that in column B.

It may not be immediately obvious why the thought made you feel so bad (anxious, low, angry), in which case it will be helpful to do some questioning of the beliefs, images or thoughts. There are various questions you can use, but three that usually work well are:

1. What does (this thought) mean to me?
2. What is particularly bad about it for me?
3. What would it say about me (or others or the world) if it were true?

So with each negative automatic thought (NAT) that you come up with, you ask one or more of these questions about it. For example, if I have been having an argument with my partner, I might think, when I ask what that means to me, that perhaps "She doesn't love me any more." If I then ask what is so bad about that, I might guess that "She's going to leave me." And possibly, if I ask what would that say about me if it were true, I might also conclude that "I am unlovable." This would probably be the bottom line here, which would be what is driving all the other NATs.

Having got to the bottom line of each thought or image (you know you're there when it makes sense to you why this particular thought made you feel so bad), then it's worth checking the thoughts all the way down against the list of thinking errors or distortions. These are not 'bad' – remember they are actually processing shortcuts, which usually save us time and energy! But if we're suffering from depression or anxiety, then our feelometer is probably not working very well, and we need to switch back from automatic to manual and re-examine whether our thinking has been distorted by the mood disorder.

D:
Now that we have identified the distortions in our thinking which made us feel so bad, we are now in a position to Dispute these thoughts in the D column. To put it another way, we can now try to talk about the A in a way that is not distorted.

We could summarise disputes as being of four (overlapping) kinds:

1. The pantomime dispute: seeing the thinking error, and otherwise examining the evidence, we can see that the original statement in B is simply not true; hence 'pantomime' ("Oh no it isn't!").

2. The metacognitive dispute: thinking about our thinking, we can see that the thinking is just a mental event – possibly a product of the condition or illness – and not 'the truth'. Are you tuning into Depression FM? This resembles what people who are not depressed/ anxious tend to do when they have barmy thoughts. ("It's just another barmy thought, take no notice.") Another angle on this is to see that you are the person who is aware of the thought, and not the thought itself, so you don't have to identify with your mind-contents.

3. The compassionate dispute: people who are depressed or anxious are often very hard on themselves, that is, their inner

self-critics tend to get overly activated. So it is useful to ask yourself: if your best friend came to you with this problem, how would you respond to him/her? Even more powerful, especially for parents, is to imagine that ten, twenty or thirty years down the line, one of your children comes to you with this problem. What do you say to them? Most people recognise that they as parents will try to act in their children's best interests, so what they would say to their kids will tend to be what is actually in their own best interests. Or try it the other way round: what would your best friend/coach/mentor/guardian angel/in fact anyone else who has your best interests at heart say to you in this situation?

4. The schema dispute. Schemas are longstanding patterns of belief and emotion usually deriving from childhood. They get activated when we enter a situation that in some way resembles difficult situations we encountered in our youth. Our buttons get pressed, and we go into schema mode. Working on this level is usually long-term, but at this stage it is helpful to recognise that our buttons have been pushed ("Oh, that's triggered my worthlessness/abandonment stuff") so we can learn to step back from acting as though these childhood-derived thoughts were true.

In fact, all of these disputes are ultimately about 'standbackability': bringing the NATs and other submerged material to the surface, we can examine it all carefully and decide whether we want to believe any of it. Is it helpful? Does it enhance my understanding of the situation? Does it work? Sometimes the alternative that you come up with will simply be one version or another of "I don't know." Great! At least that way you don't have to believe that the worst will happen (or has already happened), The truth is that often we *don't* know, and it may be that the most helpful thing you can do is learn how to live with the uncertainty.

E:
Finally we need to evaluate what Effect disputing has had. Have we hit the spot? So we look at the emotions to see if they are still the same, both in intensity and in type. Maybe doing the dispute has triggered some different emotions – these could be 'positive' emotions like hope, but might also be healthy 'negative' emotions like sadness – emotions which need to be felt in order for emotional processing to take place.

Also, have our new perspectives in D enabled us to *do* anything different? Sometimes the new behaviour has to happen before there is any change in the intensity or type of emotion. So the last stage in the process is to plan a behavioural experiment. We may have a new take on the situation or the activating event, but until we test it out it's still just theory. So once you've come up with a new interpretation, then you can do a behavioural experiment and then feed back the results into your worldview (use the behavioural experiment sheet – see next chapter). In many situations you may find that the emotion scores on the ABC don't reduce much if at all until you have done the behavioural experiment(s).

Examples

Two examples follow. The first one is a fictional example of a social anxiety situation. In the Disputes section, the various kinds of disputes are indicated by numbers. You will notice (in Effect) that the anxiety doesn't go down very much. This is OK – it's still movement, and the anxiety is only likely to go down once the person has gone to a party and successfully tried out their new strategies. Also, in a situation like this, the self-conscious image revealed at the bottom of the B column will need to be addressed, possibly through imagery rescripting, in a separate session. Once this has been worked through, the person may find it easier to enter the feared situation.

The second example is about depression. Again, the numbers in the D column refer to the type of dispute. 'Depression FM' is a metaphor for the mechanism in depression which generates typical depressed thoughts like "There's no point" etc. Depressed people often are put off social interaction by the thought that they will bring others down. The 'worthless' belief referred to in D may be a core belief derived from childhood experiences. An additional behavioural experiment might be to exercise first to lift the mood, and then meet some friends.

The cognitive therapist Christine Padesky has suggested that you need to do 25 or 30 thought records before you can do them in your head. After a while, you will come to recognise that a particular thought is the same or similar to one you have already challenged, so of course you don't need to do it again! In fact, once you start to see patterns in your ABCs, you are close to uncovering the underlying beliefs and rules which may be driving your problems at a deeper level. For more on this, go to Chapter 7: *Schemas and rules*.

The ABC Form

Activating event or trigger situation	Beliefs/negative automatic thoughts (NATs)	Co-productions	Dispute your beliefs & NATS and devise better alternatives	Effects of alternative thought...
Anything can be an 'A' - external or internal events	What went through your mind? What did 'A' mean to you?	What came with the thought?	Remember compassionate mind [Numbers refer to type of dispute: 1 pantomime, 2 metacognitive, 3 compassionate, 4 schema]	...on your body, emotions and actions.
Lying in bed, finding it hard to get up and get going.	There's no point getting up, I haven't got anything to get up for- [mental filtering; disqualifying the positive]	Emotions: list and rate 0-100 intensity Depressed 85 Anxious 60 Shame 70	I've got lots of friends who've been encouraging me to get in touch. When I'm better I've got a good job to go back to. (1) This sounds like Depression FM. How do you know you won't enjoy it, at least a bit? (2)	Re-rate emotions 0-100 – any new emotions? Depressed 40 Anxious 50 Shame 20
	Even if I go to the park or meet some friends I won't enjoy it- [fortune-telling/all-or-nothing thinking]	Body sensations: list intensity 0-100 Sluggish 90 No energy	Their emotional well-being is their responsibility. They can leave if they don't like it- (1)	Body sensations: list intensity 0-100 Sluggish 40 Energy 40
	I don't want to see my friends because I'll bring them down and that's not fair- [Personalising/demand]	Behaviour: what did you do? Did it confirm beliefs in B? Stayed in bed till it was too late to do anything; ruminated about how bad it was and why depressed? (3)	They know you're depressed, you don't have to be the life and soul! (3) Would someone who was really rooting for you call you lazy? Or just think might help rather than how I feel. Encourage	New behaviour? Plan behavioural experiment(s) Even when I'm depressed, act according to what I think might help rather than how I feel. Encourage
	All this shows I'm not really ill, just lazy. [mental filtering/labelling]	Watched TV.	Maybe 'lazy' is just another version of your 'worthless' belief. (4)	rather than berate myself and see what happens to my mood. Go to the park!
	Remember: thinking errors?		What might I tell someone else in this situation?	

48

The ABC Form

Activating event or trigger situation	Beliefs/negative automatic thoughts (NATs)	Co-productions	Dispute your beliefs & NATS and devise better alternatives	Effects of alternative thought...
Anything can be an 'A' – external or internal events	What went through your mind? What did 'A' mean to you?	What came with the thought?	Remember compassionate mind [Numbers refer to type of dispute: 1 pantomime, 2 metacognitive, 3 compassionate, 4 schema]	...on your body, emotions and actions.
Thinking about going to a party where I don't know many people.	I'll come across as awkward and shy. [mind-reading] I won't be able to think of anything interesting or funny to say. [fortune-telling/demand] I'll make a fool of myself and won't be able to face any of them again. [catastrophising] I'm totally inadequate (image of self aged about 7, crying at a children's party and being scolded by parents). [labelling] Remember: thinking errors?	Emotions: list and rate 0-100 intensity Anxious 70 Shame 80 Body sensations: list intensity 0-100 Butterflies in stomach 45 Heart racing 30 Behaviour: what did you do? Did it confirm beliefs in B? Phoned up and made excuses not to go. Spent the afternoon worrying about what they would think.	I don't know how I'll come across. (1) Maybe the idea I have to say something is a product of my social anxiety. (2) If you feel a bit awkward at a party where you don't know anyone, that's normal; it doesn't mean you're a fool, give yourself a break! (3) The situation has triggered a core belief "I'm inadequate"; this is about the past not the present. (4) What might I tell someone else in this situation?	Re-rate emotions 0-100 – any new emotions? Anxious 40 Shame 20 Hope 40 Body sensations: list intensity 0-100 Butterflies in stomach 20 Heart calm New behaviour? Plan behavioural experiment(s) Go to party with friend as first step. Try to engage with people there rather than thinking of how I'm coming across.

INTRUSIVE THOUGHTS

Intrusive thoughts sometimes start out as automatic thoughts. What sets them apart is that we really hate them being there in our minds – their very presence has some particular meaning for us that we cannot tolerate. They are actually there for most if not all of us, although most people can bear them, or at least dismiss them as just some barmy thought. But for those of us who genuinely find them intolerable, they cause a lot of problems, particularly in disorders of an obsessional nature.

These thoughts carry a different set of thinking errors. They are usually to do with mistaking a thought for a thing:

- Thought-event fusion: thinking something means it will happen (or is more likely to);
- Thought-action fusion: thinking something is the same as/as bad as doing it;
- Thought-object fusion: e.g. thinking that something is contaminated means it *is* contaminated in reality.

The key here is that a thought or image is *only a representation* of something. If you draw a picture of a cup, you can't drink out of it, no matter how hard you try...

Intrusive Thoughts

The main thing about intrusive thoughts is that they are only intrusive if you don't let them in. And as they are already in anyway, you may as well offer them a cup of tea by the fireplace...

So we have to accept that an intrusive thought (image/urge/tune – "I just can't get you out of my head") is there. Does that mean I have to do what it says? No. Does that mean I have to like it? No. Does that mean it will be there forever? *Only if you try to stop it being there.* Once it feels welcome, it will be free to go whenever it likes.

> ### The Tortoise
>
> When I was a boy I used to have a tortoise that kept escaping from her pen, a rough enclosure made of coated wire. It would take her on average about two hours to clamber over it – she was very determined. It used to worry me if I was going out for any length of time. Eventually I worked out what to do. Before going out I would place her just on the outside of the pen. By the time I got back she would just have managed to clamber back in – thinking she was getting out! Dealing with intrusive thoughts is a bit like this, we have to use the same sort of reverse psychology – once we really let them in, they are happy to go. But if we try to keep them out they will always find a way of getting in. Fortunately, once we discover that thoughts only have the power we give them, and that by themselves they are harmless, then we can open the doors wide.

LETTING THOUGHTS GO BY

We have now seen that there is little point in trying to control our thoughts directly. On the other hand, if we get 'hooked' by an idea or a belief that we suspect may be unhealthy, it can be helpful to apply the fine perspective afforded us by the thinking error list, with or without an ABC, to help us unhook or detach. We want to get to a stage where non-deliberate (automatic or intrusive) thoughts are just viewed as mental events: transitory blips on the mind-screen with no essential reality, or passing clouds in the clear blue sky of your infinite mind. So let them float, for what else is there to do with them?

THOUGHTS AND FEELINGS AS MY CHILDREN

Yet some people somehow manage to turn the attitude in the previous paragraph into "I must try to push the thoughts away by thinking of them as clouds." No. They are, as we have seen, *already* detached from you (otherwise you couldn't be aware of them), but any effort to push them away will rebound on you – we're back to pink elephants again! So to counter this pushing away or *disowning* tendency, think of *all* thoughts and feelings as your children – I'm thinking perhaps of a primary school classroom as much as a family – and they all have to have a say.

If you try to send one child out of the class, it may be necessary for a short time, but ultimately the racket they make hammering on the door from the outside trying to get back in, will be more trouble than it's worth, and you'll have to let them back in to sit on the carpet with the others. However, human nature being what it is, we're going to like some 'children' (thoughts and feelings) better than others. Does that mean we should allow some to speak and not others? No. Does that mean we should try to make one into another (fear and anger into love and kindness, for example)? No! Each has its song to sing, and all are necessary and should be allowed.

However you feel about them, it is your job to give them *all* compassion, whether you like them or not! Must you do what they say? No, of course not, although if it seems like a good idea, then it's probably a good idea. But – and this is very difficult – try not to favour one automatic or intrusive thought over another. They're all thoughts.

TWO KINDS OF DISTRACTION

There is a long history of controversy around distraction in CBT. John Teasdale and Melanie Fennell, two CBT researchers in Oxford, discovered that distraction could lift the mood in depressed people for as long as they remained distracted, so it can have its uses in depression. On the other hand, after quite a long period of using distraction to control anxiety, it was discovered that distraction in anxiety was often a safety-seeking behaviour – that is, it prevents you from finding out whether the thing you fear is going to happen or not. So in this case, it is 'bad'.

Fortunately there are two things we can draw on to help us here. One is the fact that there are two kinds of distraction: one is the purely abstract trick to take your mind off things, like counting backwards in threes from one hundred. In this case it is clear that we are not connected with the here-and-now, but are away 'in our heads', doing an imaginary problem. But the other kind is the distraction *into* reality: we reconnect with the here-and-now, and thus are operating in *a more real world* than whatever may be going on in our heads. The other principle is that of 'function over form'. Is the distraction (or anything else you may be doing) serving to prevent you from discovering what is really going on ('bad'), or is it helping you to *stay with* whatever it is, precisely so you can discover how this situation turns out if you don't interfere with it ('good')?

In the case of distraction, these two things often come together – if, while walking round the supermarket, I am having frightening images of passing out and everyone looking at me, it may be helpful to distract myself from those images by focusing on the here-and-now (distracting into reality) so that I can discover that I *can* actually manage to get round the supermarket and do my shopping. On the other hand, it may well be a good idea at some time to fake passing out in a supermarket as a behavioural experiment to see what happens! You might want to have a friend on hand to support you afterwards...

In CBT it is often not just what we do that counts, but *why* we are doing it. More on this in the next chapter.

Distraction itself is really a way of manipulating our attention, and we will come back to that topic again in Chapter 6.

SUMMARY: WHAT TO DO WITH THOUGHTS

- Stage 1: Noticing that we are having thoughts! Sometimes they work on us so subtly, we don't notice them having an effect. Even if you don't spy the trigger, what does the situation *mean* to you?

- Stage 2: Challenging; reframing; re-attributing; disputing. When we are first troubled by thoughts, we need to discover that the content of thoughts may not be the literal truth. We can get a more objective understanding by using the thinking error list and thought records like ABCs which will help us to come up with alternative understandings. Sometimes we will need to go into different layers of belief, like *rules* or *core beliefs* (see Chapter 7: *Schemas*).

- Stage 3: Discovering detachment. Realising that there is more than one way of viewing what is going on takes us into a different space. We can use exercises like "I am not that chair" or "the fridge" exercise to change our identification. Combined with the practice of mindfulness meditation, we can learn to view our thoughts as passing clouds which need not trouble us. This is particularly useful for intrusive thoughts, the challenging of which only tends to make them louder. This is the stage of "This am I not, this is not mine, this is not myself."

- Stage 4: Re-owning thinking mind (with compassion). In detaching ourselves from thoughts, we may unwittingly disown the thinking mind itself. If we do this, we make ourselves stupid – not all thoughts are unhelpful! Our thoughts are part of us in the *wider* sense (thoughts and feelings as my children). Once we have gone beyond identifying with them, we can listen fully to what they have to say.

CHAPTER 5: BEHAVIOURS: THE BIT YOU CAN CERTAINLY CHANGE!

Mental and physical behaviours – Behavioural experiments – Exposure and response prevention – Hierarchy – Activity scheduling – Doing and being – Training the mind and body – The metamessage

MENTAL AND PHYSICAL BEHAVIOURS

When we think of behaviour we tend to think in terms of what we do physically – that is, visible actions 'out there'. But a behaviour is anything we *do* (or deliberately don't do) physically or mentally. This can include worrying about something, deciding not to call someone or making a mental note to do something later, as well as digging the garden or putting the cat out. And while we all have worries, we can engage in the behaviour of worrying more or less, but all of our behaviour is open to change, with more or less effort and difficulty according to how attached we are to the behaviour, and in the case of addictions, how attached the behaviour is to us.

BEHAVIOURAL EXPERIMENTS

'Behavioural experiment' is the CBT term for what we do when we try something out in the 'real world', although that may include something we do or don't do in our heads. It is the means by which we get to know what is really the case, rather than just a competing theory. Actually, in reading this book you are already carrying out some kind of behavioural experiment – probably you think that if you read it then you might learn something of use. I hope you're right! But the thing about calling these deliberate shifts in behaviour 'experiments' is that, as in a scientific laboratory, there are *no wrong outcomes*. Rather, there is just what happens. Of course we have to do the experiment as best we can, but as long as we have done that, the outcome is what it is – this time.

The other thing that we should know about behavioural experimentation is that it is where change happens. If we just do cognitive work without actually doing anything different 'out there', the chances are that nothing will change. It seems as though the thinking mind can provide a complete loop so that we can carry any kind of theory in our head without it actually touching us emotionally at all! And then of course the problem (whatever it is) just carries on as before. On the other hand, if we really do something different, it involves more systems, so we are more likely to be genuinely touched by the experience, and then change can happen.

That is not to say we should be trying to ignore our thoughts (although sometimes that might be a good idea). One of the things to consider when planning a behavioural experiment is what *level* of cognition is being tested. Are we working at the level of automatic thoughts, or somewhat deeper; perhaps at the level of rules or core beliefs (see Chapter 7)?

Basically, there are two kinds of experiment. One is where we don't have the faintest idea what is going to happen. Perhaps we've never ridden a horse/travelled to a foreign country/said something good about ourselves in public/kissed a member of the opposite or same sex. We don't have any specific fears, but we've never done it before, so it's new. These are called *discovery* experiments.

The other kind are called *hypothesis-testing* experiments: that is, we have an idea of what might happen, but we don't know for sure if it's true. We might be finding out whether the thing we scared of actually happens (Theory A); or we might be seeing if the alternative (Theory B) that we've worked out – perhaps on an ABC – is actually closer to the truth. Or sometimes we can set it up so that we can see which of two (or more) possible outcomes actually turns out to be the way things are. So, for example, if I am having a lot of panic attacks and I have a thought that if I let a panic attack just take its course I will go mad (Theory A), but then after doing an ABC I decide that that thought of going mad is catastrophising, and in fact another version might be that I will feel very uncomfortable, and perhaps afraid of going mad, but in all probability will be just as lucid as normal afterwards (Theory B). Now I have two competing hypotheses to be tested next time I have a panic attack.

Sometimes, as I said, we do a behavioural experiment after doing a thought record. But sometimes you may already know what it is you want to test out. It is necessary to be as clear as possible about what that is, and also when you are going to do it, for how long and so on.

Of course the real world cannot be as controlled as a science lab, but we can do our best to be sure that the outcome is giving us accurate information.

SAFETY BEHAVIOURS

As well as being too vague, the other thing that can get in the way is any *safety behaviour* that we've overlooked. (You may remember that we introduced the idea of safety behaviours above in Chapter 1 with the story about Asterix and Obelix.)

For example, Bert suffers from panic attacks in supermarkets following one incident years ago when he was in a tearing hurry to get the shopping done first thing before work, having drunk about a pint of strong coffee, and had a panic attack. After a number of sessions with his therapist, he is persuaded to go back into a supermarket with the objective of buying a couple of items and proceeding through the checkout as normal. He takes a trolley and holds tightly to it all the way round. He manages to get round, but has a strong feeling that he is just on the edge of a panic attack. When he discusses how it went with his therapist, she questions him about the trolley. After all, he was only going to buy a couple of things. It was only at that point that Bert realised that holding the trolley was a safety behaviour, and that by the very act of holding on tightly to it, he was telling himself that he was in a dangerous situation, and thus felt anxious. So it is worth thinking about possible safety behaviours when you are at the planning stage.

However, the key aspect of a safety behaviour is whether it prevents you from discovering whether what you are afraid of is actually true. Sometimes if the thing you're afraid of is so scary that you couldn't do it at all unless you hold on to a trolley (or whatever the equivalent is for you), then you need to consider whether it's better to do the experiment with a safety behaviour *as a halfway stage* towards doing it without. So in the example above, it may be better for Bert to discover (while holding the trolley) that nothing terrible happens to him in the supermarket than for him not to go round at all. That way he gets some new and useful information, which can then help him go round without a trolley next time.

STAGES OF BEHAVIOURAL EXPERIMENTS

There are four stages to carrying out a behavioural experiment:

1. Deciding what it is you want to test. At what level (automatic

thoughts, rules or core beliefs) do you want to work? Is it a discovery or a hypothesis experiment? If the latter, are you testing the negative or feared outcome, the positive or alternative outcome, or comparing the two?

2. Planning the actual experiment – time, date, how long, with whom etc.

3. Carrying it out and noting what actually happens.

4. Feeding back the results into your theory and drawing conclusions. That may lead you back to step 1 for more experimentation.

We will look at particular behavioural experiments under the specific applications in Part 2. But why not try filling in the blank form provided on the next page?

EXPOSURE AND RESPONSE PREVENTION

Exposure and Response Prevention (ERP) is the treatment inherited by cognitive therapy from behaviour therapy. It is based on conditioning theory; essentially the early 20th century work of the Russian psychologist Pavlov. His landmark experiment involved ringing a bell whenever he fed his dogs. He discovered that, after a while, if he rang a bell and didn't give them any food, they still salivated. Putting ourselves in the dogs' minds (something no self-respecting traditional behaviour therapist would ever do), we could say they were conditioned to expect food at the sound of the bell. Pavlov also found that if he continued to ring the bell and repeatedly and consistently *didn't* give them food, they no longer salivated – that is, the response was *extinguished*.

Now we can draw some conclusions from this experiment for our purposes.

1. Two things that have no intrinsic relation can become associated through conditioning.
2. In order for this to happen, there has to be some kind of 'glue' – in this case, hunger.
3. The link can be broken through de-conditioning.
4. This process doesn't have to be rational (or conscious?) – it happens outside thinking.

Behavioural Experiment Record Sheet

Theory you want to test	Planned experiment	Safety Behaviours you might use	What happens when you carry it out	Results	What can I do now?

This kind of treatment is particularly useful when you know that your anxiety is not rational; that the fear you may have can't be true logically, but still the symptoms arise and either prevent you from entering the feared situation or make it a very unpleasant experience. In fact, the behavioural side becomes two-phase, in combination with behavioural experiments: first, you do the experiment (e.g. going into the supermarket where you have had panic attacks) to discover that it's possible, and that even if you feel panicky, it's not life-threatening (or whatever the 'threat' belief was). When you've achieved that, you then devise a plan of going in every day (exposure), ideally without doing any of your safety behaviours (response prevention), and gradually watch the anxiety diminish.

Another way of looking at what you're doing in exposure, as compared to behavioural experiments, is that you're training *the body*. Behavioural experiments can convince rational mind and sometimes intuitive, poetic mind as well, but often the body remains untouched, so you still get the body sensations of anxiety, which then start the cycle all over again! One of my clients helpfully used to distinguish between her 'mind-mind' and her 'body-mind'. ERP touches the 'body-mind'. Or, even more accurately, we could just admit that we're not that different from Pavlov's dogs after all, and accept that what we're doing is retraining the animal.

One of the key points in using ERP is that it should happen repeatedly, consistently and without exception. If you occasionally reinforce the thing you're afraid of, that is like the occasional reward you get on a slot-machine game – it keeps you playing! And in this case we want to stop the game. So ideally, we need to face whatever it is daily, allow the anxiety (or whatever other feeling is there) to come up, and stay in the situation long enough for the feeling to come down by itself, and repeat until the situation provokes no further anxiety.

Traditionally in CBT it would have been said that you need to do the exposures without recourse to any safety behaviours. But recent research by Jack Rachman and others has shown that *judicious* use of safety behaviours can be helpful, in that it enables people who could not otherwise do the exposures (and so would otherwise drop out of treatment) to engage and get better. I would suggest that for people using this book on a self-help basis, the best strategy is to try without safety behaviours if you can manage it. However, if whatever you are attempting is too difficult, build in doing it with the safety behaviour as an intermediate stage on the hierarchy.

For example, a client had been on the receiving end of an unfortunate golf ball accident (it had hit her on the head and injured her quite badly). To take her dogs for their normal walk (important to her recovery for all kinds of good reasons) meant walking by the golf course. She only felt able to do this initially while wearing her cycle helmet, but through walking repeatedly with the helmet on, she discovered that no flying golf balls came anywhere near her head. She was then able to discard the helmet – it hadn't prevented her from discovering that golf-balls were most unlikely to hit her on the head after all.

Although we have seen that this conditioning and de-conditioning is not a thinking process – that is, it seems to happen in an old part of the brain – nonetheless we can still interfere with it by thinking and/ or mental behaviours. Sometimes therapists have said, in an attempt to reassure patients who are worried about doing an exposure, "Don't worry, the anxiety will come down after 20 minutes or so; half an hour at worst." So then the poor client, already distinctly uncomfortable sitting in a tank of spiders or whatever, keeps checking his watch, and thinking, "But the anxiety should have gone down by now!" But it is the safety behaviour of watch-checking, and the demand that the anxiety *should* have gone down, that has kept it up!

Another particular pitfall is to say, "This isn't conscious, so I don't need to engage my conscious mind; I'll do the exposure, but distract myself while I'm doing it, so that I don't feel (so much) anxiety." No, that won't work, because although this is about training the 'body-mind', the 'mind-mind' needs to be there too. And if you're saying to yourself "I need to be distracted" then at the metamessage level you're telling yourself that the situation must be really scary – or why would you need to be distracting yourself? It is also important to emphasise that, for exposure to be effective, the anxiety *needs* to come up! The body/animal can't discover that anxiety isn't needed unless it's there.

Finally, and again commonly in this kind of therapy, the person says to themselves, "I shouldn't feel anxious." This, unfortunately, is the red rag to the proverbial bull. It is as though you are saying to your (vital, necessary, helpful) alarm system, "You shouldn't be there; I'm going to ignore you if I can." Now how does the alarm system, the protector, feel about that? It just wants to do its job of keeping you safe, and you're saying you're going to ignore it? No wonder it presses all the alarm bells it can, so, as is so often the case in fourth wave CBT, the first step is to *accept the feelings.* They are there because some part of you is trying to have its say.

Sometimes in doing ERP we uncover a deeper layer of meaning in the feared situation. A much earlier association, perhaps, between some traumatic event in the past and something about your present situation that's giving you trouble – the 'glue' in that case being the emotional charge attached to the original event.

Let us summarise the method of ERP:

1. Identify the situations you tend to avoid, or wish to reduce the anxiety in. Rate in order of scariness on a hierarchy – that is, a list of situations graded in order of how anxious they make you feel. You could use a scale from 0–100, where 0 means no anxiety, 70 means marked anxiety, and 100 is blind panic. The guideline principle should be that you tackle situations that are *challenging but not overwhelming*. Doing each lesser task gives you more confidence to attempt the next one. Think of it like training a frightened animal – go too fast and it will be harder even to get them into the training enclosure next time.

2. Enter the feared situation frequently, repeatedly and consistently. If possible, just focus on the one you're working on. Drop all safety behaviours if you can (or at least the ones that get in the way of you discovering what happens) and allow the anxiety (or whatever other emotion emerges) to come up. Stay with the sensations of anxiety; if anything move *towards* them – breathe into them if you like, not to try and make them go away, but to see if they have anything to tell you! Or just connect with them, as they are what's happening for you right now. You may have thoughts about going mad, losing control etc. These are thoughts, not the truth.

3. When you can enter the situation without undue anxiety, move on to the next one. Give yourself a reward for doing it – use *compassionate mind* (see Chapters 7 and 11).

Here is a form you can use for a hierarchy. We will come back to it in the section on anxiety in Part 2, where there are some filled-in examples. There is a blank one for photocopying in the appendix at the back of the book. If you have some different areas you are working on, you may wish to have a different hierarchy for each one:

Note: sometimes people get caught up in working at a level below what they could be doing. A client of mine was coming to the end of her allotted sessions, and we still had some way to go – we were

Hierarchy			
Situation	How scary? 0-100	Working on it? (Tick)	No longer gives anxiety (Tick)

about halfway up her hierarchy – with only a couple of sessions left. She decided, in a bold strategic move, that she would go to the top of her hierarchy and work on that, on the grounds that if she could cope with that, she could do all the lesser stuff by herself after we had finished. She did fine. You just have to know what your animal can put up with....

ACTIVITY SCHEDULING

One of the things that nearly always happens when we get depressed, and sometimes even when we get stressed is that we stop doing stuff. Mostly that's about 'saving energy' because if we're depressed it *feels like* we don't have any energy. But before we know it, we can end up not doing anything at all, or having any of the experiences that make our life what it normally is, and that makes us even more depressed. And when we get more depressed, even ordinary tasks like brushing your teeth or making a snack can feel like huge mountains to climb.

So activity scheduling is the first-line treatment against depression; indeed, its related cousin, behavioural activation, offers itself as a complete treatment for depression. However, in fourth wave CBT we see activity scheduling of one sort or another as a helpful area of work for everybody. When we come to therapy, whether that is as a result of a 'breakdown' or at an earlier stage of feeling stressed, depressed or anxious, this is a chance to review how we are living our lives. The way we live our lives is expressed in what we do and how we do it, as well as how we feel and what we think. As we have seen, we are not fully in control of what we think, and nor should we try to be. Even this far into CBT it must be clear by now that what we feel is heavily influenced by what we think, which in turn is influenced by all kinds of programming. So in a way, what we *do* is the only area in which we have real choice. Also, what we do confirms belief at a much deeper level than merely thinking about it, as we saw in behavioural experiments and exposure.

So the route back, rather than continually questioning *why* we got depressed or beating ourselves up for being depressed (both of which will make us worse), is to restart our activities, even if we don't feel like it.

We will look at activity scheduling in more detail in Part 2 under depression (Chapter 13), but we can introduce it briefly now so that you can have a shot at it.

The first step is to monitor our activity levels. The criteria we use in CBT are *Mastery* and *Pleasure*. We rate all our activities on a scale from 1–10.

Mastery means, roughly, achievement: the amount of effort it takes you to do anything. This, it is important to state, doesn't mean how much effort you think it *ought to* take when you're well; if you're feeling really low, for example, it might be a serious effort to get up before 9am. So if you manage it, then you give yourself a high mastery score, say 8.

Pleasure, of course, means what it says: the amount of enjoyment you get from doing something. Often people who get depressed stop doing things for pleasure, because they think they won't get any pleasure out of it. While it may be true that you don't get *as much* pleasure from whatever it is as you used to, it may be that you can get *some* pleasure from it. On the other hand, you certainly won't get any if you don't do it at all!

On this form, we also include an overall mood rating (0–10), where 0 is the worst you've ever felt and 10 is the best.

ACTIVITY SCHEDULE

Week beginning: /   /

Rate each activity (0-10) for M (mastery = effort) and P (pleasure), according to how *challenging* or *pleasurable* the activity was for you.

Days→ Time	Monday	Tuesday	Wednesday	Thursday	Friday	Saturday	Sunday
6am – 8							
8 – 10							
10 – 12							
12 – 2pm							
2 – 4							
4 – 6							
6 – 8							
8 – 10							
10 – 12							
12 – 2am							
Overall mood rating (0-10)							

So for the first week, or whatever your therapist suggests, don't try to change anything – just rate your mastery and pleasure levels for each activity on this timetable-like form we call an activity schedule. You don't have to write in a lot of detail, just a couple of words: "Watched TV" or "Went for a walk", and an M (mastery) score and a P (pleasure) score for each activity. If you want to look at it in more detail, see the chapter on depression below (Part 2, Chapter 13).

Now that you've filled in the Activity Schedule for a week or two, what do you notice? Is there a balance of mastery and pleasure? Was your overall mood rating the same every day? Was that affected by what you did? What sort of things seemed to make the most difference? Write them here:

....
....
....
....

Mastery and pleasure remind us – as does the attempt to balance them in the activity schedule – of the old saying "All work and no play makes Jack a dull boy." And where this duality of work and play holds sway, it is vital to make sure that play has enough space. But when the poet composes her sonnet, or the musician just reaches that peak of performance, is that work? Certainly it may have taken much work to get there, but at that point? We say that we 'play' music. One of the old dicta of the hippies was that work + love = play.

DOING AND BEING

One of the contributions that the fourth wave of CBT is seeking to make is to reintegrate parts of ourselves that have become alienated from each other. Now it is a truism to say that we cannot all be musicians or have vocations, but how then can we make our ordinary tasks such that they no longer feel so much like chores?

One solution is structural. I have heard that in Bali, traditionally everyone had two jobs: one 'ordinary' job and one creative – everyone, according to temperament, was either a visual artist, a dancer or a musician in addition to being a dustman, a doctor or an office clerk. This is like mastery and pleasure on an institutional scale.

There is a parallel here to the concepts of *doing* versus *being*. When we work behaviourally, we sometimes think it is all about doing; but non-doing, or being, has a place too. But that doesn't necessarily mean sitting still, although as we shall see in the chapter on mindfulness, doing that sometimes is definitely a good idea!

There are two points here: one, we know from basic CBT (and Epictetus) that it is the attitude that we bring to something that largely affects how we feel about it. And in essence the attitude of 'work' is that it is done for an ulterior motive: the pay packet in the first instance (how many people would go on doing what they do if they weren't paid for it?). But money aside, we do a (work) project to *get it done.* That is, there is a definite point or outcome to our actions. Even if we are not at work, we tend to approach household chores in the same fashion, so we can get them done in order to a) have them done, and b) do something else that we consider pleasurable. Now while that duality exists, as I have said, it *is* important to have these things in balance. But what if there really were a way of approaching ordinary tasks that made them feel less like chores and more like play?

This is the second point: this attitude is that of mindfulness, a way of living in which only the present is real; thus there is no 'point' in anything beyond its own sake. The Vietnamese Zen master Thích Nhat Hanh recounts how when a friend was round for dinner he asked if he might do the dishes afterward. Nhat Hanh said there were two ways of doing the dishes: one, doing them to get the dishes done, or two, to do the dishes for the sake of doing the dishes. He only wanted his friend to do them in the second way!

On Zen retreats, there is a period every day called *samu* or the work period, when all the participants roll up their sleeves and help clean up the place. This is considered as much a part of the meditation as the sitting or the talks, and the idea is to bring that moment-to-moment mindful awareness to the everyday tasks. There are numerous stories in Zen of enlightenment experiences happening whilst engaged in doing ordinary stuff. Concentrated, but off-guard![6]

We can summarise all this as the contrast between the attitude of doing, and the attitude of being. Doing or achievement is fine! And there is of course a time to sit down and plan strategy, to think about goals, and both what we want to get out of doing something and also, hopefully, what we want to contribute, or put in.

Being, on the other hand, is not seeking anything else other than how it is right now. That doesn't necessarily mean inactive. The Chinese Taoists have a concept known as *wu-wei* which means 'empty action' or 'acting without acting' – that is, doing the doing, but with an *attitude* of

---

6   As well as Thích Nhat Hạnh's many books, Gary Thorp has provided a helpful reminder of how to apply this attitude to everyday life in his *Sweeping Changes – Zen and the Art of Household Maintenance*.

being; of total absorption in whatever it is. It is paralleled in the Olympics of Ancient Greece, wherein a runner who showed more grace might receive the laurels over the one who came first. He was more at one with the activity. In everyday language we talk about 'losing oneself' in something – that is *wu-wei*; there is no longer any self, or any effort. Young children are often like that when they play. The challenge then becomes whether we can train ourselves to bring this attitude even to things we don't like.

TRAINING THE MIND AND BODY

Robert Winston, in his TV programme on the mind a few years ago, illustrated how habits work in neural terms. He took some children to a cornfield. At first they had to work really hard to even get through the corn and establish a pathway. That is like a new behaviour, very effortful. After a while the children had trampled down wide paths through the corn, and could run up and down with ease. That is like habits or addictions; it is the easy and automatic route to take. In fact, we don't even think about it under certain circumstances – it just happens, and has become the default option.

So the more we repeat something, the stronger and easier to access are the neural pathways connected with that course of action or pattern of thought.

This has several implications for our lives. The one that I noticed first was the impact of our daily work on our non-work lives. Whatever it is that you do – your work mode – will probably become the default setting for your mind at other times, at least until you become aware of and act on that fact. So a security guard gets panic attacks because he is always checking for threat; a top-level IT executive develops generalised anxiety disorder because her focus is always to look for a problem coming and head it off before it actually arrives – worrying, by any other name.

What this means is that *we are training our minds and bodies all the time, whether we intend to or not.* If we react habitually, we are reinforcing our habits. So when we think about doing therapy or doing the homework associated with therapy, or doing mindfulness practice, then it is worth remembering that how we are *now* is in no small part a result of acting on the patterns of thought and behaviour that we have been encouraging (probably unwittingly) in the time before now. So if we want to carry on as we have been, then we should carry on training our minds in the way we have been. If, on the other hand, we want something different, then we need to start choosing different options of action and of deliberate thought. For while (as we saw) we are not in control of automatic thought, it is up to us how we think deliberately, and which thoughts we choose to 'buy'. Similarly, we need to think about what tendencies are being reinforced by the actions we take: this is the *metamessage*. This should be, I suggest, *the main therapeutic criterion for action.* That is, deciding what it means to *us* (not anybody else) to take a particular course of action.

CONCLUSIONS

We have seen that there are a number of different ways of working with our behaviour:

1. We can test out different ideas by running behavioural experiments, which work best if we drop all our safety behaviours (eventually) and are prepared to accept whatever the outcome is.
2. 'Retraining the animal', or exposure and response prevention: this is working at the level of conditioning, and is helping the old brain catch up with the new.
3. Activity scheduling: this is about acting in our own best interests (AIYOBI! See Chapter 13) if not (sometimes) doing what we feel like! There are different qualities we can learn to keep in balance: mastery and pleasure; doing and being; or using the 'activity window' (see Chapter 13) the four categories of: physical; creative; social and nature.
4. Trying to act, at least sometimes, in *being* mode – that is, doing stuff for its own sake, and not just to get a certain outcome. It's called playing, and life is more fun that way!
5. At all times we need to recognise that *we are acting* – that is, we are reinforcing certain patterns by repeating them. This is what the Buddhists and Hindus call *Karma*, which happens on a mental as well as a physical level, in terms of the patterns of thought we encourage.

Whatever you find yourself doing, it is worth asking yourself, "What is the metamessage of this activity? What does it say to me *about me* that I am doing this? Does it mean I am taking care of myself? Operating at the optimum level of risk? In line with my valued directions in life?" Take some time to consider...

CHAPTER 6: ATTENTION

Can I control this? – The attention dial – Dimensions of attention –
Techniques to operate your own dial – Samadhi

ATTENTION

Many of us remember being at school, our minds wandering, and suddenly the voice of the teacher: "Pay attention!" And you reluctantly returned to the exposition of long division or whatever it was. But apart from that, most of us have had precious little training in the deliberate manipulation of attention. If we think about it at all, we may have noticed that it's easier to concentrate when we're enjoying something; equally, we also have 100% concentration if our lives are in danger.

The Attention Dial

When I was little, I used to go pond-dipping, looking for little creatures that I would take home and look at under a not-very-powerful microscope.

Subsequently, with the more high-powered equipment at school, I made a discovery that was almost more fascinating than the various wiggly organs of the water-fleas I spent so much time observing: what you see under a microscope depends on the degree of magnification you are using. It could be at the level of organs, or it could be cells. You just had to twist the dial, and you got two different pictures even though you could be looking at the same thing.

What has only come to light in the West relatively recently, is that we have an attention dial that is just like this – what we see is a function, at least in part, of how we are looking at stuff. Indeed, as the cognitive therapist Adrian Wells has shown, the content of our thoughts may be largely determined by the way our attention is directed. So how can we learn to use the dial?

So what are the ways in which we can be in control of our attention? As we have seen, there is little point in trying to control thoughts and feelings once they're actually 'up'. But what we can do is look at how we direct our attention. There are various techniques which have been developed by psychologists in the west, and there are techniques of meditation which have been around for rather longer, and usually come from either the Indian sub-continent or the Far East.

We can think of our attention as having three different but related dimensions, which we can learn to influence if not completely control. These are:

1. Narrow-to-wide (like changing the lens to wide-angle on a camera) or near-to-far.
2. Outside-looking-in to inside-looking-out.
3. Standing-back-from to becoming-absorbed-in.

All of these can potentially work both ways. If we take the first example (narrow/wide or near/far), we can notice various possibilities. Traditional concentration-based meditation, and in fact any kind of deliberate focusing, involves a narrowing-down of attention. You shut out any distractions by restricting your attention to a particular point or task. In Indian meditation of a *concentrative* nature (whether Hindu or Buddhist), this is called developing *dhyana* or one-pointedness. In problems like anxiety about health, or panic, becoming too focused on body sensations, (for example), can sometimes work against us, so we need to find a way of broadening our attention. For this reason Adrian Wells (psychologist and cognitive therapist) has developed the Attention Training Technique (ATT). This involves learning to shift attention away from inside the body, which is equated with being inside the self, to an externally focused direction. He uses a scale from −3 (entirely externally focused) to +3 (entirely self-focused) to measure this. The method involves concentrating on different sounds, e.g. the therapist's voice, other close-by sounds, and more distant sounds.

The therapist gets the client to focus initially on the first sound – the voice – exclusively ("No other sound matters"), and then the second – the therapist tapping on a book or the desk and so on – for the first six minutes. For the second six minutes, the therapist jumps from sound to sound (rapid attention switching), and finally divided attention, wherein the client has to try to hear as many of the sounds as possible at once. The instructions for this part of the exercise are particularly interesting:

Finally expand your attention, make it as broad and deep as possible and try to absorb all the sounds simultaneously. Try to focus on and be aware of all the sounds both within and outside of the room at the same time. [Pause] Covertly count the number

of sounds that you can hear at the same time. [Pause] Try to hear all the sounds simultaneously. Count the number of sounds you can hear at the same time.
(Wells 2000 p146)

Normally we just shift our attention without thinking – if we need to concentrate on something, our focus just narrows automatically. When the task is finished, we relax and our attention naturally broadens out – we hear the birds singing again. They may have been singing all along, but our attention was restricted so we couldn't hear them. Sometimes we narrow our attention out of threat – something seems 'not right' so we focus on it. We can look at different forms of anxiety as being stuck in a pattern like this panic, health anxiety (obsessive compulsive disorder, body dysmorphic disorder etc.). But when we're in this state of anxiety, we don't deliberately narrow our attention – it 'just happens'. However, we can learn to broaden it deliberately, as Adrian Wells has shown.

The second 'dial' is similar to the first, but not identical. Outside-looking-in (or observer perspective, to give it its formal name) is a particular problem in social anxiety. We talk about becoming self-conscious, and in order to become conscious of ourself as a whole, we have to imagine what we seem like from the outside – that is, how we think others see us. It is as though we put ourselves in the other's shoes and look back at ourselves. That's usually an uncomfortable experience, rather like the first time you play back your own recorded voice. But by focusing on ourselves we are preventing ourselves from discovering what others' reactions are – are they really acting like I'm a blithering idiot, or is it just my anxiety telling me that? Because in order to see what their reactions are, I have to pay attention to them, not to how *I* look.

So here we are not just expanding and contracting our attention, like in the narrow-to-wide dimension, but crossing the self/not-self boundary. In outside-looking-in, we're in *not-self* (what we imagine others are thinking) looking in on *self,* while in its opposite, inside-looking-out, we're in the self, looking out at *not-self.* There are two techniques to help us get from outside-looking-in to inside-looking-out, namely Situational Attention Refocusing (SAR, also from Adrian Wells) and Task Concentration Training (TCT, from Sandra Mulkens et al.). Here is Wells' basic instruction for SAR:

When you enter a feared social situation, you tend to focus your attention on yourself. For example, your anxiety symptoms become the centre of your attention, and because they feel bad you think you must look bad. Focusing on yourself prevents you from getting a realistic sense of the social situation. In order to overcome your anxiety, you have to go into the situation and allow yourself to discover that your fears are not true. To do this, you should observe other people closely in order to gain clues about their reaction to you. For example, when you are self-conscious and it feels as if everyone is looking at you, you should look around and check this out. By focusing attention on what is happening around you, you will become more confident and discover that your fears are not true. (Wells and Papageorgiou 1998, in Wells 2000 p152)

Task Concentration Training, on the other hand, helps you to focus attention on *anything* other than yourself: the other person or people in the situation, for example, but also the task in hand and the environment. You will find a blank form for this in the forms section of the appendix.

So to start with you note what proportion of your attention is directed towards the self (outside-looking-in), and what proportion is directed towards others, the task and the environment. You note how you're feeling – how anxious, for example (0–100). You then start practising ways of redirecting your attention outwards – that is, away from the self, and towards other people, whatever you're trying to do (the task) and your external environment.

Naturally it is more difficult to do this in some situations than others. Most people feel self-conscious if they suddenly discover that their trousers are undone! But as we're trying to learn the skill of becoming other-directed, it works better if you start by choosing situations in which it is easy to be unselfconscious.

This is where the second dimension of attention training overlaps with the third, because it is easiest to be unselfconscious when you are totally absorbed in something. Indeed, in ordinary language we talk about 'losing yourself' in things, whether that is entertainment, or playing a musical instrument, or performing some manual task that you enjoy, or a sport and so on. So we can modify that scale to being from self-conscious to absorbed. What we are intending to develop here is the ability to take the state of being absorbed in something and transfer something of that state to situations where you are (unnecessarily) self-conscious. We will come back to this in more detail in Part 2 when we look at social anxiety, and if you like you can go straight to Chapter 21 to read more about this. Otherwise, you may wish to try out a Task

Concentration Training form relating to a situation in which you feel mildly self-conscious.

I am aware of two ways in which you can shift your attention from outside-looking-in to inside-looking-out:

1. Deliberately focusing on some aspect of the other person (their dress, what they're saying etc.) or on some detail of the environment (the texture of the bark on the trees, for example).

2. Refocusing, initially, inside your own body: using the sensations of your feet on the ground, or your bottom on the chair, or your breathing, to relocate yourself *inside yourself.* Then you are inside and can 'look out'. If you use this technique it is important that you are *really* in your body, non-judgementally, as opposed to being in your head, looking down at your body and scanning for signs of anxiety!

Finally, there is the third dimension of attention which we can describe as going from detachment to absorption. Whether one wishes to be detached from or absorbed in something depends (unsurprisingly) on what it is. In general, mindfulness techniques help us to be detached from our mental contents while becoming more absorbed in the sensory world and beyond. This is usually done via an initial narrowing of attention onto the breath to provide a sort of stable platform from which simply to watch one's mental contents, ideally without engaging with them. This is known as access concentration. One's sensory experience then seems richer without so much yammering from the thinking mind.

What happens then is that in becoming detached from one's thoughts and feelings, one can become more absorbed in that which is not self, but 'inside' as well as 'outside'.

> In Buddhist (and Hindu) meditation, the term *'samadhi'* is used to denote states of absorption. These can be in something 'with support' *(vikalpa)*, or objectless *(nirvikalpa)*. Fundamentally, we can describe *samadhi* as states in which the self disappears and one is 'lost' in whatever the object of awareness is. For the moment, we can think of it as a sort of concentration, although in the Indian terminology concentration is better reflected by the term *'dhyana'* – of which the Japanese word *zen* is a direct translation.

Now that we have had a glimpse of how we might use each of these dimensions in therapy, let us look at them more generally to gain an overview of their wider use. It is important to state that none of these attentional states are good or bad in themselves; it is more about being able to move freely along whichever scale according to what is helpful.

The first dimension, which Wells uses in ATT, is that from near-to-far or narrow-to-broad. In therapy we tend to use it to help people to broaden their focus to combat obsession, rumination or worrying: all states where the attention has become 'stuck'. However, sometimes it is necessary to work at the other end: in concentrating on something specific, we are productively narrowing our attention. In meditation, this leads us to the state which in Sanskrit is known as *dhyana*, or one-pointedness of mind.

In the second dimension, we mostly think of being self-conscious as 'bad'. But if we had no ability to imagine how we might seem to others (and didn't care at all), we would be approaching states known as schizoid or psychopathic! Unfortunately our culture has become obsessed with appearance and making a good impression – celebrities are perhaps best at that – so we are encouraged to be self-conscious. So again it is about having the appropriate level of self-consciousness – there is nothing unhealthy in looking in the mirror to (briefly) check one's appearance before going out. It is when that becomes the most important thing, or one gets stuck in having to do it repeatedly, that it becomes a problem. That said, unselfconscious is a much healthier state to rest in; to have as the default option.

In the third dimension, as we said before, it is a question of what you are trying to detach from and what you are trying to become absorbed in. This is, of course, a matter of choice, although most of us don't have complete control over this. In meditation, one usually seeks to detach from the content of thoughts and become absorbed in the object of meditation. You start with a narrow focus of awareness (developing *dhyana*), and depending on the kind of meditation, either stay with that narrow focus (thereby intensifying it), or, as in mindfulness, broaden out to include more and more.

> What did the Zen student say to the hot-dog man?
> *"Make me one with everything"*

When we do that, we are in a way combining all three. As we expand our consciousness outward, concentrically if you like, we are moving along the near-to-far scale. At some point we go beyond what Zen teachers have called 'this skin bag' – the boundaries of the physical self. So we are no longer really looking in as there is no longer any 'in' or 'out' (the second scale). As we continue, we include more and more until there is nothing we exclude, and so we are absorbed with everything! This is *nirvikalpa samadhi* (absorption without support). The self-other distinction has disappeared.

Meditation is, of course, the science of attention training, and you may wish to pursue it further. We discuss it more below, in Chapters 8 and 9 particularly, and there is a list of contacts in the appendix at the end of the book.

Conclusions

Attention – only recently becoming a matter of investigation in therapy – has long been a source of interest amongst meditators. The key insight is that it is *not* a given. Just as we discovered that there is little point in trying to control thoughts, so we can give up on that one, so with attention we have seen that precisely the reverse is true: we probably thought that our attention 'bloweth where it listeth' and that we just had to put up with that. Actually, with practice we *can* gain a measure of control over how we focus.

We identified different dimensions of attention we can learn to operate:

1. Narrow-to-wide (or near-to-far)
2. Inside-looking-out to outside-looking-in
3. Detached-from to absorbed-in

Good luck in learning how to operate your own dial!

CHAPTER 7: SCHEMAS AND RULES

Prejudice – Formulation – Making a plan – Challenging core beliefs – The department store – Assumptions and rules – New core beliefs – Old model/new model – Positive log

Hopefully by now you've had a bit of a play with the ABC or other CBT techniques. From doing this you may have begun to notice that certain kinds of things tend to upset you, while there are other kinds of situations which you probably take in your stride. That is, there are certain patterns to your problems. (*Schema* means *pattern*, and it can refer to complexes of habitual thought and behaviour and/or neural pathways.) You may also have noticed that you tend to slip into certain thinking errors, but not others.

Sometimes the patterns that show up indicate the presence of certain life-rules or assumptions, which in turn relate to deeply held underlying or 'core' beliefs. Both of these are products of learning. In our early lives we have to make sense of what is going on, especially if it is not pleasant. The child's view of what happened forms the foundations of our (learned) beliefs. No wonder we sometimes don't have it quite right! At a deeper, more ancient level than that are the programs installed in the species by evolution like fight-or-flight – we could call them *instinctual* schemas – some of which even predate the existence of humanity, never mind your individual existence.

Before we start work on all of these, there are a few points we need to note about this kind of work:

1. Just thinking about this stuff can bring up a lot of emotion, some of which you might be reluctant to feel or even look at. So be easy on yourself – don't try to do everything at once. Access compassionate mind (see Chapter 10) just to work on this process, and once you've decided how much time (per day? Per week?) you're going to spend working on it,

be sure to balance it at other times of the day or week with pleasurable activities.

2. This is not a project that is going to take place entirely within the rational sphere. If it did, it wouldn't work. We need to try to bring some degree of rationality – and more importantly, acceptance – to this deep material, but if we're not touching the 'gut' level, we've hardly started.

3. Tackling schemas is like working with a prejudice. A prejudice, like a schema, is a deeply held pre-existent belief that comes into play and may prevent us responding appropriately to the situation. Take a moment and think of someone you know who holds a prejudice you *don't* hold. What happens if you try to argue rationally about it with them? They may argue from a narrow range of experience; dismiss more rational views; get angry; change the subject; discount any evidence against their position as 'the exception that proves the rule' and so on. So how do people overcome prejudice (when they do)? Usually by having *a number of experiences* that contradict their prejudice, and not discounting those experiences. So it is with the schemas. They have been with us for so long that they have come to seem like part of us. It is true that they give us trouble – rather like an old pair of shoes which were comfortable once even if they let the rain in now – but somehow we'd rather live with the memory of that old comfort than endure the real but temporary discomfort that would come with trying out a new pattern that might work better. So now we need to get to a place where we are prepared to break in the new 'shoes'.

In summary, we need to be prepared to be upset by strange and forgotten emotions coming to the surface; we need to be kind to ourselves to help cope with that and we need to be prepared for the long haul, which will not just be about what's rational, but will be about having different experiences.

When we are in 'schema mode' – that is, when a schema has been activated, it is like a button has been pressed and Program 37b has been set in motion. Actually, we no longer know what's going on. The person in front of us is no longer our boss or friend or lover, but is once more our father, mother or teacher from a previous era, or perhaps a predator from evolutionary time! Somehow, in the present, the person we were with has acted in such a way as to make this situation resemble

– just enough – a previous situation which was a threat to us, and the program was activated.

You will remember Robert Winston's cornfield analogy – how an old behaviour or habit is like a wide and easy path, while a new pattern is like fighting through the jungle. That describes both the problem of working with schemas and how it is trying to do something different. Once a schema gets activated, it seems to 'just happen'. If the situation has enough 'marks' that resemble that childhood situation, we are programmed, and no longer acting from choice: the robot has taken over. Or the dinosaur!

And this is no small point: although many of the programs that give us trouble, and most of those we will be investigating in this chapter, come from a misperception of early events in our life history, there are many other layers of patterning that predate our existence as an individual. The earliest of these derive from the oldest part of the brain; the fight-flight programs that are located in the *amygdala*, and which haven't evolved that much since we were dinosaurs. So when those powerful programs kick off, you're operating on lizard-brain. We'll look at that again under panic (Chapter 16).

Second, we are not born into a cultural vacuum. From the earliest days we are inducted into a set of beliefs and rules for living that are a product of our specific culture. Some of this is quite sophisticated, obviously, but some of it is much more primitive, and is a form of tribalism. Often, the second masquerades as the first, but that's another story...

Depending on which cultural milieu you find yourself in, there may be a belief that this is not the first time you have been here, which, if true, would constitute another level of patterning, which Hindus and Buddhists call *karma* – literally, *action*, but also the fruits of past action including any previous lives.

Furthermore, we underestimate the effects of our *perinatal* (in-the-womb) environment at our peril: Frank Lake's school of psychotherapy (Clinical Theology) emphasised that environment and the effects of birth trauma.

Finally, and what we will mostly focus on here, is our personal-historical material: what happened as we were growing up and what we made of it. But all of these layers may and will be affecting us in how we live our lives, and the more unconscious we are, the more we are simply a programmed robot.

So the first step in reclaiming our humanity is to try to recognise these programs and begin to unpick them. To do so, it will help if you understand how you came to develop the rules and beliefs that form the cognitive aspect of these programs. And it is always incumbent on us to accept that we can never know the whole story – there are just too many influences operating at any given time. But what we can get to know are some of the things that we remember, and more subtly, to learn to taste the flavour of programmed versus unprogrammed experience. When we look at mindfulness below, we will see that this is possible!

But for the moment we will be looking at different ways of accessing and re-evaluating our personal-historical material. You can work from the present backwards (see *Working backwards from safety behaviours* in Chapter 21) or from the past forwards. Doing the latter, we start by remembering any significant memories from our early experiences, with parents or early carers, brothers and sisters, or perhaps from our schooldays. The question to ask yourself is, "What did I make of that at the time?" It may not seem rational with hindsight – that doesn't matter, you were only a kid. You may have drawn some negative conclusions from these experiences – about yourself, about the world or about other people in general – and you may still be acting as though these conclusions were still true, just because you have never questioned them. Write them in here:

Early experiences	What I made of them (self, world, others)

Early experiences and core beliefs

When you are looking at beliefs about yourself, you may notice that many of them are unreservedly negative. Yet when you think back, it may seem that it was other people who acted negatively toward you. This is probably because we are hardwired for attachment. Or to put it another way, our parents or carers were our sources of nourishment and protection when we were too young to fend for ourselves, so it would have been much too dangerous to blame them – they might have abandoned us! So who else could we blame if things went wrong? Unfortunately, there's nobody left but ourselves. *That still doesn't mean that our negative core beliefs about ourselves are true!* In fact, from a thinking error point of view all core beliefs belong to the 'Black-and-White' complex: All or Nothing; Overgeneralisation or Labelling.

Core beliefs, assumptions and rules
So, as well as some positive beliefs – let's not forget those! – we've ended up with a whole package of negative beliefs about ourselves, the world and other people. These are usually much too painful to carry around all day in the forefront of our minds, so we have to find a way of 'fixing' or at least hiding them on a daily basis. This is where the so-called dysfunctional assumptions come in. I say so-called because in the beginning they weren't dysfunctional at all – they were the only way we could make sense of and manage our world. We could, as Christine Padesky does, rename them 'rules that protect'. Here are some examples:

- If my core belief about myself is telling me that "I'm unlovable", then maybe "If I can please everybody, then somebody will love me" (rule).

- If it registers that "I'm a failure", then "I have to succeed at everything I do and come top of the class, or there's no point in trying."

- If "I'm worthless", then perhaps "I really have to achieve something big."

- If my core belief is about the world or life in general, like: "Anger is dangerous", then "I must always avoid confrontation or I might get hurt."

- If someone close to me got sick and died and therefore "Life is precarious", then "I must always take extra special care of my health or I might die before my time."

- Perhaps if I was hurt by someone, I might think "I'm vulnerable" (core belief). So therefore "I must always predict what will happen in any situation, so nothing unpleasant can surprise me ever again" (rule) or alternatively "I'm going to attack first at the first sign of hostility, so no one can put one over on me" (rule).

Try formulating your own fix-it assumptions as 'if.../then...' statements, where the second part contains the core belief, e.g. "If I can please everyone, then that would show I'm not unlovable." (Core belief: "I'm unlovable.")

ASSUMPTIONS

If... *(strategy)*	Then... *(prevents or modifies core belief)*

If.../then...assumptions

The problem with trying to get rid of these assumptions is that they usually have a payoff. Initially that was in protecting you from being tormented by your core belief; but it probably also had some genuine positives. In the examples above, coming top of the class might have given you a really successful career; pleasing others may have led to some good friendships; avoiding confrontations, or finding ways of sidestepping them, may have got you a reputation for diplomacy, and so on.

Unfortunately, the very act of living by this assumption confirms at a deeper level (metamessage) that the core belief is true'. To turn the statements around:

- "I must be worthless or I wouldn't have to keep on proving my worth through achievement."
- "I must be unlovable or I wouldn't have to keep pleasing others all the time."
- "I must be vulnerable or I wouldn't have to keep organising my own protection."
- "I must be really bad if I always have to focus on being good."

Of course this is topsy-turvy logic, *actually* it is:

- Focusing on achievement (plus the memory based on the *misinterpretation* of historical events) that keeps us believing we're worthless.
- Focusing on people-pleasing that keeps us believing we're unlovable.
- Focusing on protection that keeps reminding us of vulnerability.

- Focusing on being good that keeps us believing we're bad, etc.

On the other hand, as we said, each assumption has a payoff. We therefore need not to throw the baby out with the bathwater. So one of the most helpful ways of working at the assumption level is the cost-benefit, which we will look at later. For now, we need to try to put it all together.

Sometimes we are aware of the rules or assumptions, but not of the core beliefs: you may have found it hard to do the exercise at the beginning of this chapter. Another way of getting to the same material is to start from the rules that you daren't break. First write the rule in the left-hand column of the table below. Then write down how you would feel, or what you think would happen if you didn't follow the rule, on the right.

Rule: (I must...)	Consequence of not doing it: (or...)
e.g. I must always please others	Or no one will like/love me (therefore I'm unlovable?)

Deriving underlying 'core' beliefs from rules

So now we can start to undermine this schema process. The order you do it in doesn't matter very much, but there is a certain logic in attacking things the way I have outlined here:

- Step 1: as above, work out the *formulation* of the schema, particularly the relationship between early experiences, core beliefs and assumptions (aka 'rules that protect').

- Step 2: look at, and re-evaluate, the *evidence from history* that seems to say that your core beliefs are true: use the three column sheet on page 85, and if you need to, work with a therapist to revisit the experiences that fixed the beliefs in your mind.

- Step 3: use the *continuum method*, and *department store* (see below) if appropriate, to discover whether your core beliefs are 100% true.

- Step 4: having discovered theoretically that the evidence in favour of your core beliefs is at the very least patchy, you may be prepared to start *questioning the assumptions/rules* which are helping to keep them in place. Look again at the formulation, and do a cost-benefit analysis on each assumption.

- Step 5: assuming that these rules are not really serving you after all, devise a *possibility goal* – something you really want to do that the old rule wouldn't let you do – and really go for it. If you need to, work up to it with a series of behavioural experiments. You are now beginning to act against your core beliefs. What is the new rule that supports you in achieving this possibility goal? Does it have any disadvantages?

- Step 6: now start to create an *alternative core belief* to provide a folder in which to place all the positive experiences that you've been ignoring all these years. Be careful with the language!

- Step 7: fill out the *old model/new model* formulation, putting in the new beliefs and rules.

- Step 8: do a *positive log* to reinforce the new model.

Now, to take these steps in more detail:

Step 1: formulation – we've just done that, but it will be useful for you to put it together in a diagram (see chart overleaf):

Step 2: re-evaluating evidence from history
When we become aware of our core beliefs, particularly about the self, we may know on a rational level that they are not true, but still we 'feel' them, in our guts, as it were. Sometimes it seems puzzling that they still have such a hold over us. In fact we are probably carrying around various memories from childhood – unconscious, most of the time – which we are still interpreting in a way that supports the core belief. Some of the following examples may ring true for you:

- "My own needs were never met, so I must be worthless."

- "They were always beating me up, so I must be a bad person."

- "I only ever got affection when I did well at school, so they didn't really love me for who I am – I'm unlovable."

Early experiences

....
....
....
....

Core beliefs (what as a child I made of those early experiences)

I am..
....
....
Other people are.............................
....
The world is.......................................
....

Assumptions, Rules & Strategies (what we do because of the core beliefs –
whatever we do to keep them (and painful early experiences) out of consciousness)

If..then..
& therefore I should always...

If..then..
& therefore I should always...

Critical incident(s) (whatever happened to stop you carrying out your rules or
compensatory strategies):

....
....

Hot cross bun(s)

Remember the first law of core beliefs: **they aren't true!** Let that sink in...

Again, they aren't true...

They *still* aren't true!

Also, as we noticed above, as relatively powerless children we didn't dare to blame our parents or carers for what went wrong. So who else did that leave to blame? That just leaves us, doesn't it – hence the negative core beliefs about the self.

There are basically two ways of undermining the evidence for the old core belief:

1. To look in, in our imagination, on the situation where the core belief originated or was reinforced, from the vantage point of a (compassionate!) family therapist or child psychologist, and ask the question, "Do I think that the way the grown-ups are treating this child means s/he's worthless/unlovable/bad?" The answer will of course be "No, but the parents/carers are certainly making him or her feel like that by their abuse/neglect/misguided help and advice/poor parenting skills."

This can be done on a three-column form like the one below; you may notice that it is the table from page 79 with another column added:

Early experience(s)	What I made it mean then (core belief)	What I think it means now: objective view

Challenging historical evidence for core beliefs

2. Sometimes, however, the core belief is so ingrained that even though you can see that the old view is not rational, the memories supporting it are so vivid and emotionally charged that we need to restructure those memories and images by using *experiential* techniques like 'empty chair', 'imagery rescripting' or even 'reliving' if there is a problem accepting that what happened actually happened. These are done on a one-to-one basis with your therapist, and only when you feel ready to have those sorts of experiences. For a description of

some of these techniques, see Chapter 10: *Different selves.*
The objective of these techniques is to transform the memory into something you can live with, even if unpleasant, rather than something you feel you have to suppress.

Step 3: using continua and the 'department store' to challenge negative core beliefs

As core beliefs, particularly about the self, are based on an all-or-nothing way of thinking, the best way to undermine them is to bring out the gradations, or shades of grey. So if you say you are bad, we need to point out that what you are saying, in effect, is that you = bad, or to put it another way, that you are 100% bad, and there is no goodness in you whatsoever. So if there were such a thing as a goodness scale or continuum, you would score 0% on it.

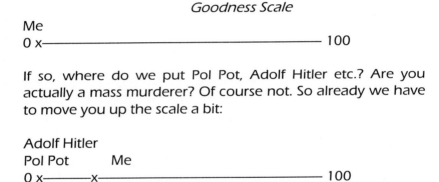

Goodness Scale

Me
0 x——————————————————————— 100

If so, where do we put Pol Pot, Adolf Hitler etc.? Are you actually a mass murderer? Of course not. So already we have to move you up the scale a bit:

Adolf Hitler
Pol Pot   Me
0 x————x————————————————— 100

But what about minor villains, politicians you really hate etc.? Again maybe we have to move you up the scale a bit more. And what about the good things you may have done, even by accident? Surely they must count for something? But to quibble about a percentage point or so is perhaps to miss the point, which is that you are, like the rest of us, a mixture of good and bad, lovable and unlovable, worthy and worthless and so on. In fact, as we see elsewhere, it is futile to try to measure the self as a whole anyway. Have *you* ever seen a selfometer?

Sometimes, though, it is good to expose just how unbalanced our estimation of ourselves really is. One way of doing this, which is really a development of the continuum idea, is the 'department store' technique. Because *the more globally we estimate ourselves, the more likely our estimation is to be influenced by mood*, So in the department store technique, the trick is to break our life down into its different parts. These may vary from person to person, but what are the important bits of *your* life? Here is a fictional example:

Joe's Department Store

Relationship	Children	Work
Social life	Church	Sport
Fishing	Gardening	Holidays

As you see, Joe has quite a balanced life. Supposing he thinks he's 'worthless', or if he's already done some continuum work, perhaps he gives himself a score of only 20% worthy. So we ask him how worthy he is in each department. How worthy are you as a husband? Or a father? Or as a gardener, or churchgoer? What often happens is that people give themselves much higher scores for specific areas than for their overall score. So I suggest a different way of coming to an overall score: simply add up the scores from the different departments and divide by the number of departments.

Joe's Department Store ('Worthiness' scores)

Relationship 60%	Children 85%	Work 90%
Social life 40%	Church 80%	Sport 50%
Fishing 70%	Gardening 90%	Holidays 65%

So if we added these scores up and divide by the number of departments, we would get 630 ÷ 9 = 70%. Seventy per cent is the cut-off point for a first class honours degree in most universities, and a lot higher than the 20% he rated himself overall. Of course his worthiness as husband, father or worker is probably more significant than his worthiness as a holidaymaker or fisherman, but it gives some illustration. Notice that Joe gives himself a much lower score in the 'social life' department, which seems to be where the main problem is that he's overgeneralising to mean that he's 'worthless' overall.

So try it for yourself. First identify the negative core belief about yourself, and give yourself an overall rating on the positive alternative (worthy, lovable, good). Bear in mind also what the optimum score is for you; sometimes people have a belief like "I don't matter" or "I'm not important." But how important do you want to be? (Think of the responsibility!) Now fill in a department store chart: I've put nine boxes in but you may want more or fewer.

Core belief about self:

Positive alternative (other end of the scale):

Overall rating:

My Department Store

Fill in the different bits of your life and rate the opposite quality from your core belief (your goodness or worthiness, lovability etc.) in each one. Now add up the total and divide by the number of departments. Make sure you aren't discounting the positive!
What are your conclusions? Does the core belief still really hold water?

Step 4: challenging dysfunctional assumptions or 'rules that protect'

There are two main ways to work with these unhealthy guidelines: one is to look at generally held unhelpful assumptions, note whether your own resemble these in any way, and review them for (in)accuracy and (un)helpfulness. Another is to do a cost-benefit analysis on your own assumptions, using such criteria as advantages/disadvantages, reasonable/unreasonable and realistic/unrealistic, and if you find they are not really serving you, then to devise new ones that work better.

David Burns (1980) lists ten common self-defeating beliefs/rules:

1. **"I should always feel happy, confident and in control of my emotions."** (Emotional perfectionism.)
2. **"I must never fail or make a mistake."** (Performance perfectionism.)
3. **"People will not love and accept me as a flawed and vulnerable human being."** (Perceived perfectionism.)
4. **"I need everybody's approval to be a worthwhile person."** (Fear of disapproval or criticism.)
5. **"If I am not loved, then life is not worth living."** (Fear of rejection.)
6. **"If I am alone, then I'm bound to feel miserable and unfulfilled."** (Fear of being alone.)

7. **"My worth depends on my achievement (or intelligence/ status/attractiveness)."** (Fear of failure.)
8. **"People who love each other should not fight."** (Fear of conflict.)
9. **"I should not feel angry, anxious, inadequate, jealous or vulnerable."** (Fear of emotions – emotophobia.)
10. **"People should always be the way that I expect them to be."** (Entitlement.)

With each of these rules – or at least any that apply to you – we can ask a number of questions that will help us establish whether they serve us or not. I suggest four:

1. Is this rule logical (does it make sense)?
2. Is this rule realistic (does the world work like this)?
3. Does it have more advantages than disadvantages for me?
4. Would I recommend it as a life-rule for someone I cared about (children, partner, close friend)?

If the answer to these questions is no, then clearly continuing to follow these rules is unlikely to be a good idea. So now choose the three rules which most closely correspond to the ones you are running, ask the questions, write down the answers and see what you find.

In fact, this leads us to the next way of working: the *cost-benefit analysis*, which follows:

Rule or assumption you wish to question (write here):

....

....

....

How much do I believe it? (0–100%)

Cost-benefit Analysis

In what ways does this rule make sense?	In what ways is this rule illogical?
How realistic is it to follow this rule?	How unrealistic is this rule?
What advantages are there for me or those I care about in following this rule?	What disadvantages are there for me and those I care about in following this rule?
Why would I recommend this rule as a guideline to those I care about?	Why wouldn't I recommend this rule as a guideline to those I care about?

Cost-benefit analysis

Note: one 'advantage' of your rule is likely to be that it *guards against activation of the core belief*. This is not to be underestimated, as it means that dropping this rule will mean that the core belief comes to the surface in all its unhinged glory. So we need to be prepared for that!

OK...what happened to your evaluation of the assumption? Do you still think it's a useful guideline?

Step 5: possibility goals and coming up with new guidelines
If it seems to you that the balance of your evaluation lies *against* continuing to follow the old rule, then we need a way of coming up with a new one. Try this: think of something you'd really, really like to do that your old rule won't allow. We call this a *possibility goal*. So for example, if you were running a perfectionist program (like example 2 above), yet you wanted to try something completely new – maybe you had always fancied learning a musical instrument – that would be difficult, because we all make mistakes when we're learning. Write your possibility goal below:

My Possibility Goal:
(e.g. take up playing the mandolin – make it clear and behavioural)

....
....
....

So what would be a different sort of guideline that would help you reach your possibility goal? In the example above it might be something like: "It's OK to make mistakes when I'm trying to learn something; it doesn't make me worthless/a failure/unlovable." Write your new guideline here:

New Guideline:

....
....
....

It may be that your possibility goal is now something you can do straight away – in which case, get on with it! Hooray!

On the other hand, it may be something you need to build up to, in which case construct a hierarchy of tasks that lead up to it. So rather than committing yourself to taking up the mandolin straight away, you might want to have a go on a friend's instrument, or try something else new that is less of a commitment to start with. These are behavioural experiments, which you will have come across in Chapter 5. You might find it useful to use the behavioural experiment record form.

Of course, you will have noticed that your old guideline did have advantages, or you wouldn't have been doing it all these years. Likewise it may be that your new guideline has disadvantages, especially in *not protecting you against the core belief that it was built to protect you from.*

Results

Now you have re-evaluated your rules and come up with alternatives, how much do you believe in the old rule/assumption?
Write here: 0–100%:

How much in the new one?
Write here: 0–100%:

If you have decided to adopt the new rule, what could you put on a flashcard (a small piece of card with a message on it that you can carry around with you) to remind you to use it?
Write here:

Step 6: coming up with new core beliefs
Now that, hopefully, you've at least started to act differently in the world – you're no longer entirely living by the rules that you developed to protect yourself against your core belief – you may be ready to think about devising some kind of new core belief that will be a) more accurate and b) more helpful.

Up to now, because of your old core belief, only evidence that seems to confirm it has been retained. It is like a computer program that can only retain information within certain parameters. In thinking error terms, this is Mental Filtering. So we need – at the very least – a new program which does not exclude evidence that contradicts the old core belief. Or to put it more simply, a new filing cabinet to store the positive evidence which you have been losing or discounting for lack of somewhere to store it.

However, there is a problem with what label we put on the front of the new 'filing cabinet'. If, for example our old core belief is 'failure', then we might be tempted to put 'success' on the front of the new one, like this:

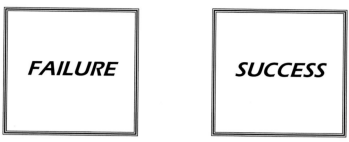

Unfortunately this has two negative consequences:
1. It reinforces the black-and-white approach that we are trying to get away from.
2. If you do anything that is less than 100% successful, it ends up putting more evidence in the failure box.

If less than 100% successful

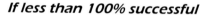

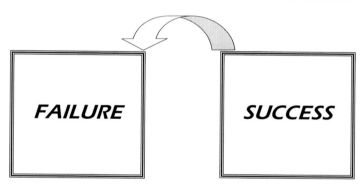

So instead we need to make the new cabinet/program less black-and-white, and more hard evidence-based. To do this we need to focus on things we have actually done, rather than global appraisals of ourselves.

So instead of 'success' we can use 'I have successes' e.g. passing my driving test; getting a job; even something like making a good cup of tea or putting your trousers on the right way round! Because if someone were to be a failure, they would have to be a *total* failure, which is to have *no* successes at all.

Some other examples of new filing cabinets/programs might be:

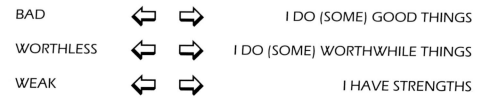

INADEQUATE		I DO (SOME) THINGS AS WELL OR BETTER THAN OTHERS
STUPID		I DO (SOME) INTELLIGENT THINGS

SPECIAL CASES

Some core beliefs, however, are special cases, and to find alternatives we need to follow a different procedure. Four that can give us trouble are:

- I don't matter
- I'm different
- I'm useless
- I'm unlovable

"I don't matter" seems to be quite common in people who suffer from obsessive compulsive disorder (OCD). (That is not to say that all who have OCD will necessarily have this core belief.) It is sometimes learned in a family situation where one is overlooked in favour of another sibling. Of course the opposite end of the scale would be "I'm the most important" which wouldn't be healthy either! In this case, a simple opposite: "I matter (as much as the next person)" is probably the most helpful.

Likewise, with "I'm different" the other end of the scale ("I'm a clone") probably doesn't work either. In fact, "I'm unique (like everybody else)" may be the best alternative, although the positive log (page 98) may be mostly about the ways in which you *share* characteristics with other members of the human race.

"I'm useless" is, to my mind, what the philosophers call a category mistake. Useful/useless is a way of talking about appliances or tools. Tools are things; we are not things. On the other hand one could follow the formula above and say, "I do some useful things." Perhaps the most useful contribution on the subject is that of Chuang Tzu, the Taoist sage.

The Useless Tree

Two characters were talking about a particular tree; one was commenting how useless it was – it didn't give fruit, it was all twisted and so was no good for timber, and so on... His wiser friend pointed out that if it gave fruit, someone would have put a fence round it and claimed it as their own; if it had been good for timber, someone would have chopped it down, but as it was, they could both sit under this 'useless' tree and have this conversation in the shade!

'Useful' things can be exploited!

"I'm unlovable" is a special case because we might all have differing views as to what lovability is, and we often confuse being lovable with being loved, or even being in a relationship or getting laid. As you only have to look around you to see, there are some very nice people who are alone and maybe lonely, while some veritable rogues appear to be getting all the goodies. And interestingly, the ones who appear to be popular don't seem to give a stuff what others think! So if we want to rediscover our lovability, we need to find that part of ourselves that is no longer so concerned about others' wishes.

On the other hand, what is it we find lovable in others? If 'unlovable' is (one of) your core belief(s), make a list of which qualities *you* find lovable in others:

....

....

And *that* is what lovable is for you, so if you exhibit any of these qualities, you're showing lovability! Do a positive log (see below) noting whenever you show these lovable qualities.

So now that we have identified some (potential) new core beliefs about the self, we need new core beliefs about the world and other people. These are usually easier to come up with, as it is easier to recognise unhelpful beliefs about the world and others as childish (egocentric) or irrational: "It's not fair" (of course it isn't); "They're all out to get me" etc. When devising alternatives, avoid *all-or-nothing thinking* and *overgeneralisation*.

Write your core beliefs about the world and other people here, and the new alternatives by the side:

Core beliefs about the world and other people

Old (unhelpful) core belief	New (adaptive) core belief
The world is. . .	The world is. . .
Other people are. . .	Other people are. . .

We are now ready for the next step:

Step 7: old model/new model

We now have the makings of a complete formulation, which you can continue to use, possibly for the rest of your life! We can map out the old operating system, which is what you were using before you started therapy, and put the new operating system alongside it. That way, whenever you hit what might be a *critical incident* for you, you can at first notice which system you are using, and with practice, choose the new one. (If you want to, you could say "choose to choose" the new one.)

Old model/New model

Early experiences:	
Old core beliefs Self: World: Others:	**New core beliefs** Self: World: Others:
Rules/Assumptions/Strategies:	**New rules/guidelines:**
Critical incident(s):	
Thoughts: Feelings: Body sensations: Behaviours:	Thoughts: Feelings: Body sensations: Behaviours:

Now you can fill it in. If it seems a bit daunting, here's an example:

Old model/New model

Early experiences: *Parents neglectful, distant. Bullied at school, picked on by teachers. Had a few friends, but we moved and I lost touch.*	
Old core beliefs Self: *I'm unlovable* *There's something wrong with me* World: *It's a hostile place* Others: *Can't be trusted*	**New core beliefs** Self: *I have some lovable qualities* *I'm basically OK* World: *Can be affected by how I act* Others: *Vary enormously; you don't know how they're going to be in advance*
Rules/Assumptions/Strategies: *If I please others, they won't leave me* *You have to test people's loyalty* *If they find out what I'm really like, they'll leave me*	**New rules/guidelines:** *If I do what I feel is good, then the right ones will stay* *You can push people away by testing them* *If they leave me when they find out who I am, then I don't need them*
Critical incident(s): *Relationship breakdown (maybe partner got fed up with alternating 'tests' and gifts)*	
Thoughts: *No one will ever love me* Feelings: *Depressed* Body sensations: *Sluggish, tense* Behaviours: *Stay indoors, withdraw*	Thoughts: *This has come to an end* Feelings: *Sad* Body Sensations: *Tearful* Behaviours: *Grieve for a while, then go out and mix with others again*

Now go back and fill in yours. Of course this is always work in progress, and you may want to revise it from time to time (particularly the new model) in the light of experience.

Step 8: the positive log
Well done, you're nearly there! This is the finishing strait. Unfortunately it goes on for a long way, because this is the homework that it will serve you to continue maybe for the rest of your life. Remember the prejudice model? These deep-seated beliefs can remain influential, especially at times of stress. Actually the positive log is just a not-very-detailed diary

which records examples of when you act in a way that accords with your new operating system, and particularly the new core beliefs.

At the end of each day record (in a nice, beautifully bound notebook) times when you *were* successful, lovable, showed strength or whatever it is. Don't worry about it being an unbalanced account – you've been screening out the positive for years, now it's time to right the balance!

Positive Log

Examples of things I did or ways I behaved today or at any time in the past that show evidence that support my new belief that ... ...

Monday:
Tuesday:
Wednesday:
Thursday:
Friday:
Saturday:
Sunday:

(Photocopy this page as a master for future use. or the larger blank at the back of the book)

Wow! That was quite an endeavour! And again it's important to emphasise that you can't do it all at once. Especially if you had a fairly torrid childhood, this may need coming back to again and again.

But please don't be discouraged – after all, we're all working on *something!*

And it's unlikely that long-held patterns will change in an instant, although people usually find that when their mood improves they no longer really believe their core beliefs to be true any more. (That is, they finally *get* the first law of core beliefs!) Actually there's some controversy about this: while some researchers have found this (that once you're recovered, you no longer believe the core beliefs), others of a more neurophysiological persuasion (like Professor Joseph LeDoux, for example) have found that the memories are still there, but dormant.

Perhaps a helpful way of thinking about this is to use the metaphor of railway points: if you're not (e.g.) depressed, the train (that's you, the person) goes by the core belief turning and doesn't take it (core beliefs don't exist). But if the person relapses into depression, then the points switch and the core beliefs reappear (underlying phenomena idea).

In the meantime, anyhow, it's helpful to take a leaf out of the famous schema therapist Jeff Young's book and keep an eye on your schemas as they kick off. There is a schema awareness form at the back of the book to help you (Appendix 2).

CHAPTER 8: THE ROLE OF THE BODY

In the body but not of it – Making friends with it – Therapeutic bodywork – Taking care of the body (exercise, food, appearance) – Gratitude – Connecting – Dealing with the anxious animal

An increased emphasis on the role of the body in therapy is one of the hallmarks of fourth wave CBT. In a trend that started with the work of John Teasdale, it was recognised that just thinking in a better way about your problems, while definitely a good idea, would not by itself necessarily make you feel better. It was necessary for you to be 'touched' emotionally in the process, so that therapy was not just an intellectual exercise. What we noticed about emotions as opposed to thoughts was that they had accompanying body sensations, hence we talk about *feeling* them. So just as it is possible to 'get into' your emotions via the thoughts which may trigger them, so also we can go via another 'arm' of the hot cross bun, and by connecting directly with the body sensations, we can also access both thoughts and feelings.

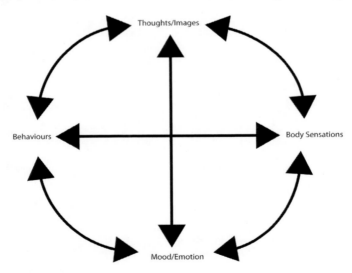

Hot cross bun

A difference in how we view the body in fourth wave CBT is revealed if we go back to the technique we used to help us see that we are not our thoughts (or feelings). You remember we proposed that "If I can be aware of it, then I am not it" to help us identify with that *which is aware*, rather than the *objects of our awareness*? Or to put it another way, I am the one who is aware of (whatever it is), rather than the (whatever it is). So can you be aware of your body? I would certainly hope so. Does that mean you are not your body? From a consciousness point of view, I would say you are not your body. Rather, you are the one who is aware of it. But it is certainly the vehicle – or the animal – in which you are travelling at the moment, so it is a good idea to make friends with it and to take care of it, because it is impossible for you to be here without it! And when you do that, you notice it has secrets to reveal about your emotions.

The essential technique for the discovery of these secrets when they manifest bodily is simply to breathe into whichever part of the body contains the tension or discomfort. It seems sometimes as though the body has a separate 'mind' from our conscious mind. When it is not possible for us to process what is happening to us, either because it is too intense, or because there is too much going on, or because for some other reason we simply cannot accept it, somehow this event is stored in the body, in the reaction we know as *stress*, or more severely *trauma*. By breathing into the place where the stress is held, sometimes we can access the unprocessed material, feel the feeling and relieve the stress. One client of mine who had experienced a series of traumatic events found that while she had completely dissociated at the time – her mind had gone AWOL – she could access a 'body-mind' which still remembered what had happened, and as long as it felt safe, would tell us about it.

Sometimes if there is a lot of stored unprocessed material, this can be felt as tension, odd aches and pains or restricted movement. This creates an unhealthy feedback loop as the body becomes an uncomfortable place to be, and one tends then to live more 'in one's head', and be less in touch with the body, and so less likely to connect with any unprocessed stuff.

This is emphatically *not* to say that all physical conditions are a result of emotional disorder. But the less one is plugged into body awareness, the harder it is to connect with and resolve emotional problems that seem to have become locked in the body. And on the other side of the same coin, the *less* one is in one's body, the *more seriously* one is likely to take the contents of one's head, i.e. thoughts, the over-valuing of which we know to be a characteristic of various emotional problems such as Generalised Anxiety Disorder (GAD) and Obsessive Compulsive Disorder (OCD).

THERAPEUTIC BODYWORK

Sometimes, with the aid of a therapist who is appropriately trained, it may be that some physical manipulation can help release something that appears to have become trapped in a particular part of the body. A client who had been very constrained during her childhood got in touch with the resentment and anger she felt. I invited her to have the long-overdue tantrum that she had been waiting to have for thirty-odd years. She lay down and kicked her feet and banged her legs on the floor. I invited her to say what she wanted to say to her parents, which she did a bit, but then looked at me and said, "There really aren't any words – it's in my body."
"Where?" I asked.
"In my leg," she said, pointing to the place. I gently massaged the place, with movements that went towards and beyond the feet. She shook slightly, not dramatically, and was still.
"I feel calmer," she said.

This resembles in some ways the Reichian-type treatments that prevailed in the 'progressive' therapy world of the 1970s, which is when I learned it. I am not endorsing a wholesale return to a philosophy of catharsis or discharge. But *when* the material is pre-verbal, and *if* the relationship is strong enough for the trust to be there (and there is no danger of exploitation), then I think this way of working can add something that is missing in conventional CBT or other purely cognitive approaches[7].

TAKING CARE OF THE BODY

In the next chapter we will look at the eight-week mindfulness programme. The originator of the clinical use of mindfulness, Jon Kabat-Zinn, talks about "coming to our senses". Another mindfulness teacher, Nigel Mills, talks of mindfulness as "putting the mind where the body is". So mindfulness and body awareness are intimately interconnected. I have sometimes thought that mindfulness ought really to be called 'bodyfulness'.

---

7 But bodywork and insight need to *both* be there – in 1970s bodywork the discharge might happen, but if the person didn't change the way they lived, the old patterns became re-established in the body pretty quickly, while in current CBT the constricting body patterns sometimes prevent the person from changing on a more-than-intellectual level. The heart, so to speak, is in the body. And even in bodywork, the first line of approach should be the client's breath, so it stays in their/your control.

If we recognise that the body is an important avenue for emotional work, then we may wake up to the fact that the body has its own needs, and is more likely to respond helpfully to our investigations if these needs are met. This may require some attention to diet, or exercise, or rest. If possible, it is a good idea to be kind to animals, and this is *your* animal we're talking about. Are we treating our bodies as though they are slaves to the all-powerful brain-dictator? Even if we exercise, are we really giving the body what it needs or likes? (Clue: it should feel good, at least afterwards, and preferably during.) And do we feel good during or after eating whatever we eat, or are we stuffed or bloated? Or are we perhaps using food, either by under- or overeating, to try to cut off from or stuff down any feelings which may be trying to manifest?

Exercise

To take these two issues in turn: exercise *is* essential. But it is much more likely that you will carry it on if it is fun, and closer to play. Most people can find a form of exercise that they enjoy if they try enough different things. But a lot of people go to the gym as a penance, and distract themselves while they are doing the exercise so they don't have to feel what is going on. This is called bullying your body, and is not a good way to make friends with it. If you want to do some more vigorous endeavour, fine, but *try to stay conscious during the process*. And stop *before* you break something! You are more likely to notice the warning signs if you are 'in there' – your consciousness is present, and not distracted – at the time!

On the other hand, some people stop at the first sign of discomfort. This is really the mind, not the body. It can be very useful simply to stay at the discomfort place, without either retreating from or pushing forward beyond discomfort into pain – what we call 'working the edge'. Gradually the limits on what you can do will expand.

Food

It is entirely understandable that some people comfort-eat, stuffing in sugar or other sorts of excess carbohydrate. For one thing, in terms of our evolutionary background, that's a useful program: extra fat will keep us through the lean times. In our personal beginnings, food and love came together in our mothers' milk. So when we're feeling a bit empty emotionally and lacking in love, it's not surprising if we try to fill our hearts by filling our bellies. The effect is usually to numb the emptiness temporarily, and again to disconnect us from our feelings. Some do it with food, others with cigarettes (a substitute nipple to fill the emptiness?)or booze or drugs and so on. I am not making any moral comment here. What these things have in common is the drive to fill up the empty hole inside. The question is, is this the best thing to do about this emptiness?

What anyone who has allowed themselves to experience this will tell you is that the *empty hole inside is in fact bottomless.* All attempts to fill it up simply cut ourselves off from it temporarily. This is tough stuff! But there may be a solution...

The Wrong Kind of Emptiness

Some kinds of emptiness are useful. If you are sitting in a room as you read this, think how uncomfortable you would be if it was crammed to the ceiling with boxes. Rooms definitely work better if there is more emptiness than stuff. And what about music? If there were no space between the notes, you would have a cacophony. But if you feel a bit down, and you become aware of this emptiness, you think you have to fill it up. Physicists tell us that at the heart of matter at a sub-atomic level, there is vast space with just a few 'bits' whizzing about. Maybe you are just feeling how it really is at a deeper level. Yes, it is empty, and that's just how it's supposed to be.

So try sitting in this emptiness: is it like a cave? Look at the edges if there are any. Sit on the bottom if there is a bottom, or just float, or allow whatever happens. Notice whatever arises in your mind as you explore this new territory. Is this really what you've been running from all this time? Did you really need to?

While some people are desperately trying to put too much stuff in, others are restricting input in a different sort of attempt to get away from their feelings. By increasing control over what they eat, they hope to gain a sense of control which is missing in how they are living their lives. Getting in touch with body sensation and emotion is much too painful, they think, but if you stay in your head, you can stay cut off from it – the body is numb and you get to control how you look, or at least one aspect of it.

There is instead a sort of pseudo-feeling – "I feel fat" – which is actually a distorted appraisal of shape which drives us towards ever-reduced intake, and if untreated, eventually starvation and death. Or bouncing between the two as in bulimia – over-input and then forced output, or the slave-driving exercise. Specialist treatment should definitely be sought if this is your problem area.

Appearance
This aspect of the body is unfortunately over-emphasised in our culture, so glamorous young things who seem impossibly thin, yet have unbounded energy, are used to sell us products to make us like them,

while (unwittingly or not) presenting themselves as a model of how we are supposed to be. If we are fooled by this, we can fall into eating disorders, or that much under-diagnosed condition body dysmorphic disorder (BDD), wherein our appearance (or some aspect of it) becomes the most important thing in our lives, to the point where we cannot get out of the house because our hair/nose/face etc. is not quite right, or is indeed repulsive to us to the extent that we think we cannot bear to be seen by others. (See more on this in Chapter 22.) Again, specialist treatment should be sought if you have this condition.

The body, then, can be a source of trouble or a source of healing. The difference, fundamentally, lies in the mode of attention employed and the attitude taken towards the body. The attitude needs to be one of friendship and gratitude – after all, this creature has got you this far! And, apart from Saturday night just before you go on a date, the beneficial mode of attention is more often going to be inside-looking-out, or inside-looking-in, which is not the same as looking *down* on it from the head while scanning for multiple defects or sicknesses. 'Being easy in your own skin' is a brilliant everyday expression of mental health. We could describe this as self-awareness rather than self-consciousness, or having 'awareness-in-self' rather than 'awareness-of-self' as the desirable *default* position, only moving towards the other pole when necessary.

In addition to using increased body-awareness (awareness-in-self) for direct therapeutic work, it is also helpful to develop your new-found friendship with your body by doing what is often referred to as energy work. This is where one is performing gentle exercise or meditative techniques which are not only, or even primarily, about physical exercise. While it is not the place of this book to try to establish the truth or otherwise of the claims made by, for example, various schools of yoga or tai chi/chi gong, it is clear that practitioners of these arts definitely claim – and in their own eyes, experience – greater health and well-being than most of us. What is happening here is mysterious, but proponents usually explain it in terms of subtle (i.e. not physically measurable) energy. In my experience trying to analyse what is happening *while* one is practising one of these arts prevents one from fully having the experience – thinking mind gets in the way – so pragmatically it makes sense simply to try the practice wholeheartedly in the session or class, and save the analysis for later. What definitely happens as a by-product of these sorts of practices is that one becomes more settled and at ease in this body-vehicle, and more likely to be able to stay in inside-looking-out or inside-looking-in as one goes about one's life.

In the spirit of CBT it is obviously not my place to determine what you should experience if you try one or more of these subtle energy practices. My own experience is mostly in the Far Eastern techniques: aikido, tai chi and chi gong. Bruce Frantzis, a well-known teacher and practitioner of these arts who has also explored Indian (kundalini) yoga, considers that the Far Eastern (Taoist/Buddhist) techniques tend to facilitate a constant, smooth flow of energy around the body, while the Indian systems tend more towards a build-up and release of energy. Be that as it may, there is, from our point of view, a more obvious yet more profound insight to be had from the practice of any of these disciplines. That is the discovery that, in feeling this energy (whether the *chi* of chi gong or the *prana* of yoga) one is *tapping into an impersonal network that transcends the individual*. Of course this has to be discovered for oneself, and approached with an experimental attitude. Some people, in my experience, feel it straight away; more often others will feel it after a few sessions; and some never feel it at all. Of the last group, some continue to practise anyway because they enjoy the exercise or feel the benefits in a more general way. Although I cannot be sure, it seems that some kinds of medication may interfere with the ability to sense this energy. But please don't make that a reason to stop any medication you may be taking, at least not without talking to your GP first And of course, sadly, there are many teachers of these arts who do not teach them well enough for the students to feel the energy directly, or who do not consider that experience to be important.

Assuming for the moment that you are one of the people who is lucky enough to be able, initially or after a few sessions of practice, to feel such an energy (and this is to some extent a combination of luck, good teaching and some kind of predisposition – it doesn't make you a 'better' person), then it is important to get the psychological benefits from such an experience. What does it mean that you feel this tingly, gently buzzing, quasi-electrical sensation? Well that, of course, is up to you! But the conventional explanation is that you are sensing what we are, and what the world is made of. Now this, if true, is a tremendous corrective to the identification of self with this 'skin bag' or only what's inside it. On an electrical analogy, it is the discovery that we are not battery-powered after all, but plugged into the (trans-) national grid:

After all,
just the (completely unique)
you-shaped bit of the
ultimately undivided universe.

No longer cut off from everything else! This has implications for how we are with ourselves and others, which can be illustrated with the following series of drawings.

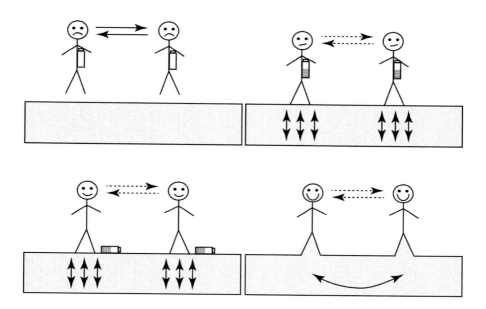

Much of our suffering comes from the idea that we are separate. We long for fulfilment; we feel empty; not enough, and so try to get fulfilment through another. Unfortunately they are empty too, and trying to get their 'juice' from us. If we are fortunate enough to discover some energy techniques, we find we can fill up independently from the earth (or, the Taoists would say, from heaven-and-earth), and no longer need to try and drain it out of others. It didn't work anyway! And I am not suggesting that it is only through energy techniques that one can find independent fulfilment – it may be through music or being with nature etc.

Eventually we put aside our 'batteries' and learn to trust our ability to plug in when we need to – actually, *we were never separate*. By and by, and perhaps with more meditation, we may discover that 'interbeing' more fully, and be content that there was nothing missing in the first place.

But there is an interesting question that comes up when we think about this: the drive to get our satisfaction or 'juice' from relationships of course echoes the attempt to be satisfied through mother's milk (and the love that, when all is going well, is indistinguishable to the infant from the milk itself); and there is a subtle tendency to get 'down on ourselves' if we feel this 'neediness' at a later time in our lives. Yet we all get lonely sometimes. How would it be if we thought about this 'neediness' as the misplaced desire for reunification with the whole? Not realising that actually, as we said, we were never separate...

THE BODY AND DEALING WITH ANXIETY

Being in touch with the body as 'my friend the animal' gives us a great guideline for how far to push when doing exposures. In general we use the guideline 'challenging, but not overwhelming'. But if we think of learning to deal with anxiety as learning to retrain a frightened animal, we get a much clearer idea of what this might mean in practice.

Bear in mind that when panic gets fired up, it is very much the animal side that has been awakened (see the section on the 'panic lizard' in Chapter 16). And rationalising with a lizard is pretty futile (have you ever tried to persuade a lizard?). Even if you think about trying to take a dog who has been maltreated into a situation that reminds him of that experience, you'll see why 'flooding', or just dumping your animal in the worst-case scenario, can be counterproductive. The dog may never go near whatever it is again.

So we have to become 'lizard-whisperers', gently persuading the animal that nothing terrible is going to happen as we cajole them towards the edge of the fear (see *working the edge* below in Chapter 9). Or like taking a young child to see that there really isn't a crocodile/tiger/monster under the bed – it's fine and necessary to hold their hand to start with. Suddenly the apparent contradiction between the principles of exposure and using safety measures disappears! All you have to ask yourself is this: "Is the safety measure that I am taking necessary to get the animal to stay in or enter the feared situation?" If the answer is yes, then it's OK – indeed, it may be necessary to use that safety measure. Unhelpful, safety-seeking behaviours are those which *prevent* you from finding out whether what you fear is true or not, not the things you do to *help* you find out.

BODYWORK IN FOURTH WAVE CBT: CONCLUSIONS

To sum up, there are four ways in which we can work with the body in fourth wave CBT:

1. Taking care of the animal: this means, coming from an awareness that, at the very least, we are not just our bodies, that we need to be kind to them and give them what they need (which may

not be the same as what they think they want – chocolate, alcohol etc.). Retraining them needs to be done with kindness, and gives us a good guide as to how far to 'push' in exposure and response prevention.

2. Many memories become 'locked' in the body in the case of stress and trauma. 'Mindful breathing into' (see more on this in the next chapter) can provide a way into this; if appropriate, and you are confident in and trust your therapist, some physically manipulative techniques may also be a way in.

3. Using attention in relation to the body – learning to be in it but not of it – can be helpful in any body-related condition. Eating mindfully (whatever the head is saying) makes binge-eating very difficult; being inside-looking-out means you are less likely to get caught up in appearance-related issues like BDD; and really settling *in* your body can prove more fruitful than scanning it 'from above' in questions of health anxiety, though it may take you a while to learn the difference.

4. In addition to the therapeutic work with the body, we can go some way towards overcoming our attachment issues through the practice of certain 'subtle energy' disciplines like chi gong or yoga, as we discover what it feels like to be connected again.

CHAPTER 9: MINDFULNESS TRAINING

Mindfulness and concentration – Mindfulness and therapy – The eight-week programme – Homework – Mindfulness or bodyfulness – Mistrusting thinking mind – Sitting meditation – Stress – Reacting and responding – Acceptance in the body – Minds in place and Big Mind – Metta practice

THE MINDFULNESS PROGRAMME — MINDFULNESS AND CONCENTRATION

Many years ago I was on a short retreat with Nancy Amphoux (Nan Shin) a late lamented female Zen master in the Deshimaru tradition, at the end of which, as is often the custom, there was a little party. So I walked down to the off-licence with her to get a few beers. She was wearing her full, formal, flowing robes, which caused some astonishment in the shop. One gentleman, who looked as though he was no stranger to a few beers himself, asked, "Is that some kind of martial art you're doing there?"
"Sort of," she replied, "only we don't move."
"Oh," he said, somewhat at a loss.

Why I like that story is that it links mindfulness to the body disciplines we were just discussing. Nigel Mills, at a British Association for Behavioural and Cognitive Psychotherapies spring conference workshop, offered the definition of mindfulness as "putting the mind where the body is". While that doesn't capture the whole of it (unsurprisingly – words cannot fully capture the meaning of the term), it is really helpful in distinguishing mindfulness from any kind of thinking or intellectual exercise. As Jon Kabat-Zinn says in *Coming to our Senses* "Mindfulness, it's not what you think." If you inhabit your body consciously, you *are* in the here-and-now, because that's where your body lives. And this leads to a much richer experience.

When we are looking at structured clinical mindfulness programmes, whether the original Mindfulness-Based Stress Reduction (MBSR) or derivatives like Mindfulness-Based Cognitive Therapy (MBCT), it is important to acknowledge that there are some important differences between these programmes and mindfulness as conventionally viewed within, say, the Theravada Buddhist tradition. 'Mindfulness' in the therapy world has become a sort of umbrella term for the clinical use of Buddhist meditation. In fact, the early stages of meditation involve more *concentration* than they do mindfulness – one needs a sort of bed of concentration, sometimes called 'access concentration', in which the seed of mindfulness can sprout. So although Jon Kabat-Zinn's original definition of mindfulness as "paying attention, on purpose, in the present moment without judgement" has pragmatic usefulness as that *is* what you do, in a way that is more about concentration. The Pali word *sati*, the word usually translated as mindfulness, literally means 'remembering'.

With continued practice of concentration and mindfulness, one develops the insight –'remembers', if you like – that "This am I not, this is not me, this is not myself." In other words the *insight* (another parallel term) is that I am not my mind-contents. But it is not just about having an *intellectual* understanding that this is the case, rather an *experiential* one. You *know* it all the way down to your socks – at least sometimes!

The eight-week programmes, described in detail in *Full Catastrophe Living* (MBSR) and *Mindfulness-Based Cognitive Therapy for Depression* (MBCT), have transformed the world of psychological interventions. I do not need to describe them fully here as they are clearly better portrayed by their authors. As well as these two programmes, a number of other variants have emerged, including other treatment systems involving mindfulness as an important element like Dialectical Behaviour Therapy (DBT) and Acceptance and Commitment Therapy (ACT).

However, what I can usefully do here is give something of an idea of the processes that are worked through in the particular eight-session version that I run, in the overall context of fourth wave CBT. In many ways it is not so different from MBSR or MBCT – indeed, it is really a re-synthesis of them – although the addition of a Big Mind element does add a different dimension.

MINDFULNESS DISTINGUISHED FROM THERAPY

At the beginning of any course, there is always some work on what is to follow – the rationale for what we are going to be doing. As I tend to run these courses in a mental health context, we need to make the distinction between mindfulness and therapy.

The VW Story

There's a story about a young couple who live in the desert in California. The husband goes off to work every day in the city; the wife looks after their young child. To get about, she has an old VW bus. One day, she is out with her child in the bus on the way to buy some groceries at a small town which is still some way from where they live. The bus breaks down. Being a resourceful woman, she gets out her toolbox and starts taking it apart, the carburettor and eventually the engine. She cleans it all up and puts it back together, but there's a problem. She's got a few little bits left over. What to do?

"Ah, well," she thinks, "let's try starting it up and see what happens".

So she does, and it works. She shrugs her shoulders, puts the few bits in her top shirt pocket, and drives to the small town where the grocery store is. First she calls in at the garage, and explains what has happened to the mechanic.

"Oh, yes," she remembers, "there were these few bits left over" and she hands him the components from her pocket.

"But..." says the mechanic, "you couldn't have got here without these parts!"

"Oh" she says. "Well, I guess that's your problem."

Now, as I wasn't there, and not being someone with any kind of mechanical aptitude, I don't know if that story is true or even possible. I don't know if you can make cars go without all the bits. But I *do* know that it's true of human beings. We don't have to have all our aspects functioning 100% in order to enjoy life and be fulfilled. The difference between mindfulness and therapy may be this: therapy is about finding what's not working and taking steps to deal with that problem. Mindfulness is about noticing what is already working (that we hadn't noticed before), despite whatever might not be! So I tell this story, and then invite people to introduce themselves to the group and tell us two positive things they like about themselves. And because it's not a therapy group, but a journey we're all on, I join in too.

COMING TO OUR SENSES

One of Jon Kabat-Zinn's wonderful books is called *Coming to our Senses*, and there probably couldn't be a better summary of what the whole course is about. We want people to begin to really *taste* life, rather than just thinking about it. So we then move to the famous raisin exercise, where we eat raisins, individually and very slowly in order to savour the experience. I ask people to give this a try, even if they think they don't like raisins. One of the funny things about this is that often, when they really pay attention, people who thought they didn't like raisins actually enjoy the experience. Sometimes the reverse happens: people who have been chugging back raisins for years eat some mindfully and discover they don't really like them at all! Either way, a gap is exposed between what we think and what is actually, sensually, the case. And again, that is a great metaphor for the whole course. We get much fuller and more accurate information when we pay attention. Around that point I usually introduce the first definition of mindfulness, from *The Mindful Way Through Depression* (Williams et al. 2007): "...the awareness that emerges through paying attention, on purpose, in the present moment and non-judgementally, to things as they are". As we said, this may not strictly be the best translation of the Pali word *sati* (remembering), but it definitely serves the purpose at this point.

We then move on to doing the *bodyscan*, an imaginal trip through the body from the inside, using the breath as a focusing device. You could say that we're tasting the breath in the body. It's very relaxing, usually, and most people's difficulty with it is staying awake. In fact some people have been referred into the course for insomnia, and I'm sure it's the bodyscan that is the main curative agent in that case. But what it definitely does is get you inside your body like no other technique I know.

'HOMEWORK'

The eight-week course is not just about what happens in the sessions. At the end of each session – just like in CBT – we give out tasks to do between classes. Amongst the mindfulness fraternity there is a great deal of debate about how much or how enthusiastically to encourage participants to 'do their home practice'. I think we are offering people a very precious opportunity to develop a practice which has the potential to enhance their lives – possibly more than anything else they may do. So *not* to be as encouraging as possible would be to deprive them of a wonderful opportunity – in short, it would be ripping them off. For when are you most likely to develop a steady practice? On your own without support, or during a course, with a structure and opportunities for feedback and troubleshooting?

Of course if people are for whatever reason having trouble doing all that is asked of them (because of childcare, irregular work schedules or just a very low week), it is not about being punitive! People do the best they can with what they know and the resources available. But just to give the idea that it doesn't matter whether they do the regular practice or not might be to miss the turning: "Hey, this way!"

The tasks during the early stages of the course are to do the bodyscan daily, to do some everyday tasks mindfully – including eating – and to notice *moments*.

We explore pleasant moments and discuss what makes them pleasant, and the following week, do the same with unpleasant moments. I'm not going to give it away here, but people usually come up with similar understandings, course after course.

MINDFULNESS OR BODYFULNESS?

Coming back to our senses means reconnecting with our bodies ("putting the mind where the body is"). That is a great reminder (remembering) because, as I keep on saying, our sense-experience *is* in the here-and-now. To help us do this, we introduce gentle bodywork. If you do a course, you may find the instructor uses chi gong or yoga, or perhaps a mixture of both as I do. Some people have a developed practice before they come on the course and want to stick with that. Others want to try something new. Great either way. The point is to really be *in* the body as you do whatever it is, rather than directing the body like a slave from 'above' in the head. For some, mindful walking may be the best version of that. Others may want to dance or run instead of what is being offered. There are particular benefits to be had, energy-wise, from learning a discipline like yoga or chi gong, but that is not the main purpose of this course, and if it feels like a mountain to climb, or "yet another thing I've got to do", then some mindful walking (running, dancing, swimming) may be an altogether better option.

MISTRUSTING 'THINKING MIND'

As well as learning to trust our senses through deliberately paying attention (to the breath, to our bodies and to everyday activities), we also have to learn to *mistrust* our thinking minds. Of course, those who have already done some CBT will have had a start on this. We look at different ways in which the thinking mind, by its very nature, narrows down our perception and makes itself even more partial, and how most of the time we don't even know that we are seeing a restricted view. The nine-dot puzzle is probably the best-known device for exposing this, but there is a whole range of optical illusions which also make the point.

The understanding we are coming to at this stage is the one so beloved of the Acceptance and Commitment Therapy (ACT) people, namely that a thought is not a thing. I sometimes draw a picture of a cup – which, despite my very limited artistic abilities, is usually recognisable – and make a pantomime of trying to drink out of it. "Why can't I do this?" I say, looking puzzled. "Because it's a picture!" my long-suffering clients remind me. And so with our thoughts: they are *representations* of stuff, **not the stuff**. But what I am trying to get across at this stage is that we are living through our heads – never mind computer-generated virtual reality, we are *already* in a sort of virtual reality. We stuff a handful of raisins down our necks, and provided the experience conforms roughly to the conceptual box marked *raisin*, we barely notice it. The box has been ticked, and we move on to the next thing. As with raisins, so with the rest of our lives.

Quite apart from the thinness of experience that you get from living your life like that, there is another problem: your experience has to fit the program/picture of it that you have created – even, strangely, when the picture isn't very nice. Things have to turn out a certain way, and if they don't, we get upset or angry because our *demands* (thinking error) aren't met. On the other hand, it is also important not to get too down on your thinking mind. It also has a good and useful job to do, as we saw in Chapter I.

The most helpful alternative is to try to see things as they really are – what in Buddhist meditation texts is called *yathabhutam*. This means stepping away from our programming and being in the moment with whatever it is. This is called *acceptance*. Even if we cannot stop creating representations of things (as Zen master Robert Aitken once said, "The mind secretes thoughts the way the stomach secretes pepsin"), at least we can make the representation fit what is actually happening, irrespective of our programs or schemas or whether we like it or not. But this fit – which in a way is what acceptance constitutes – is only ever temporary, because the world is always changing, and so are we.

Of course, sometimes our programming is so strong that the cost of accepting whatever it is seems too great. We think it would mean something terrible about us or the world or other people. But that's just an idea too, although of course ideas do have the power to affect us emotionally.

Somewhere around here, if the participants are not already familiar with them, I introduce the metaphors/exercises of: "I am not that chair", "the fridge", and "sky and clouds" (see Chapter 3). The chapter titled

Your suffering is not you, in *Full Catastrophe Living* (Jon Kabat-Zinn's original mindfulness handbook), makes the same point.

So we have three insights – or from a CBT point of view, hypotheses to be tested – that form the basis of the rest of the course:

1. My mind-contents are not real, but a (more or less) accurate representation of reality.
2. My mind-contents are not me; I am the one who is aware of them.
3. Acceptance means that one's representation – one's 'inner working model' of what has happened – fits what has actually happened. (We don't have to like it, or be resigned to it continuing that way.) The fit will always be temporary.

The second one is a provisional understanding, for reasons which will become clear.

If that seems a little challenging, you may like to contemplate the three 'terrible oaths' of Dorje Drolo, in *Tibetan Buddhism: An Incarnation of Padmasambhava*:

1. Whatever happens, may it happen.
2. Whichever way it goes, may it go that way.
3. There is no purpose.

Possibly *that* medicine is too strong at the moment!

There is one further area of exploration to which the foregoing leads us: that is, the continuing effect of our pre-existing programs. So even though we can now see in theory how to experience reality directly, that doesn't mean we can necessarily do it! So our practice now moves to an experiential exploration of how our schemas are continuing to operate in us. More on this below.

SITTING MEDITATION

By the fourth week of the course, we have already had three weeks of practising sitting meditation, as well as alternating the bodyscan with some mindful bodywork. As we learn the discipline of sitting still (physically only at first), and see the operation of our monkey-minds as they stray incessantly from the breath, we get an awareness of just how chaotic it is in there/here. But we can begin to learn, at least some of the time, to watch it.

Toddler Mind

You have just started to sit. So don't expect to be good at it from the off! Your mind has been used to going wherever it wants, and it won't take kindly –at first – to being directed. Like a two-year-old. Imagine you are sitting and chatting with a friend, and you have a toddler with you. It is quite a cold day, but unfortunately you only have an electric-bar fire to keep yourselves warm. The toddler sees the warm orange glow and is inevitably drawn towards it. There is no point in telling her off, or being cross with her. Without even needing to interrupt your conversation, you gently pick her up and take her back to her bricks that she was playing with before she became distracted by the fire. In a very little while you will need to do it again, probably every few minutes. You don't mind, because you see that this is just how it is at this stage in the toddler's development. So the fire is whatever distracts you from *your* object of meditation (the breath = the bricks), and the way you treat the toddler is the (gentle, patient) way you need to treat your own mind! Please!

Sitting, although it may be the technique that group participants like least to start with, often becomes the mainstay of people's mindfulness practice in the long term. We start with what is basically an exercise in *concentration* – that is, focusing our attention on the breath. It isn't an attempt to control the breath, however; more about hitching your awareness to the breath as it travels in and out of the nose, or up and down to the lower abdomen. That said, there is some benefit to be had from learning to breathe so that the main movement is in the abdomen rather than the chest. In western terms this means that the diaphragm is drawn down further on the inbreath, thus creating more space in the lungs. To the Japanese, you are breathing into the *hara* or *tanden* (or *dantien* in Chinese), which is our centre of power, gravity and energy, and focusing on it is the way to generate *joriki* – concentration power.

One way to start is to practise following the breath, which means tracking it from its point of entrance in the nose, down to wherever it goes – probably somewhere in the lower belly area – and then back up again on the outbreath. This is a perfectly valid practice in its own right, but after some time we usually shift to focusing directly on the *dantien*, a point traditionally described as being three finger-widths below the navel. So you just focus on the movement that happens there as you breathe in and out; expanding and contracting. I sometimes find it helpful to reflect that this very basic pulsation is one of the things we have in common with all living things!

We sit every day, for about ten minutes to begin with, and expanding by five or ten minutes a week. By the third week of sitting (the fourth week of the course) we are ready for another expansion – to a sense of the body as a whole. Again, that is not to say that there is anything lacking as a practice in just monitoring the breathing at *dantien*. But this new practice gives a sense of spaciousness that can be helpful. There is a saying in Zen: "The true human body is this whole universe"...

Of course, when we focus on the body as a whole, various things may happen. For a start, our bodies have probably already started to rebel against this forced stillness; any residual aches and pains are bound to come to the surface! If we have a tendency towards health anxiety, we are sure to engage in some monitoring of a less-than-helpful kind. But as we learn to just be with minor discomfort, we are learning an invaluable lesson in our bodies that we can hopefully generalise later: the ability to *be comfortable with discomfort.*

It is also here that we learn the basic skill of how to access our schemas, in the now anyway, as a felt-sense: to "walk the razor's edge" as Charlotte Joko Beck puts it. I quote from her at length here because she shows the process through which we can, through sitting (*zazen*), potentially shrink the schemas to nothing, or almost nothing, by becoming one with them:

> First, we need to know we're upset. Many people don't even know this when it happens. So step number one is, be aware that upset is taking place. When we do zazen and begin to know our minds and our reactions, we begin to be aware that yes, we are upset.
>
> That's the first step, but it's not the razor's edge. We're still separate, but now we know it. How do we bring our separated life together? To walk the razor's edge is to do that; we have once again to be what we basically are, which is seeing, touching, hearing, smelling; we have to experience whatever our life is, right this second. If we're upset we have to experience being upset. If we're frightened, we have to experience being frightened. If we're jealous we have to experience being jealous. And such experiencing is physical; it has nothing to do with the thoughts going on about the upset.
>
> When we are experiencing nonverbally we are walking the razor's edge – we are the present moment. When we walk the edge the agonising states of separateness are pulled together, and we experience perhaps not happiness but joy. Understanding the razor's edge (and not just understanding it, but doing it) is what Zen practice is. The reason it's difficult is that we don't want to do it. We know we don't want to do it. We want to escape from it.

If I feel I've been hurt by you, I want to stay with my thoughts about the hurt. I want to increase my separation; it feels good to be consumed by those fiery, self-righteous thoughts. By thinking, I try to avoid feeling the pain. The more sophisticated my practice becomes, the more quickly I see this trap and return to experiencing the pain, the razor's edge. And where I might once have stayed upset for two years, the upset shrinks to two months, two weeks, two minutes. Eventually I can experience an upset as it happens and stay right on the razor's edge.

In fact the enlightened life is simply being able to walk that edge all the time. And while I don't know of anyone who can always do this, certainly after years of practice we can do it much of the time. It is joy to walk that edge.
(Charlotte Joko Beck, **Everyday Zen**, p146–7)

Learning to stay with the physical sensations non-judgmentally becomes the key tool in coming to terms with our personal histories, which have somehow been remembered in the body.

While each of these practices (concentrating on the breath either following or in the abdomen, or concentrating on the breath in the whole body) is a complete and helpful practice by and in itself, there is also a sense in which each development builds on the last, so that in each sitting one spends some time at the *dantien*, then some time at the level of the whole body. We then get to another, very interesting, stage. For the time being we leave focusing on the breath altogether and concentrate on sound. This is interesting because for the first time the object of our awareness extends beyond the physical body – this 'skin bag' as Zen masters sometimes call it. These are the first intimations that what I call 'me' might not be entirely restricted to what is normally thought of as 'inside'. As you're practising listening to whatever sounds arise, see if you can *feel* the sensations of that seagull crying; that lorry going by...

We then move to viewing thoughts. This seems strange – after all, thoughts were the things that at first were getting in the way of our concentrating on the breath. As you sit waiting for them to arise, like a cat at a mousehole, they might not appear – until you get the one that says, "I'm not having any thoughts."

Oh, there you are!

The final stage in this sequence that we have been building up (following the one on Jon Kabat-Zinn's 'Guided Mindfulness Meditation, Series 1 sitting CD) is not to focus on anything in particular at all, but simply to be aware of whatever arises. This is sometimes known as choiceless awareness, or 'just sitting'.

Any of these practices, bar perhaps sitting with thoughts, could be undertaken on their own and not as part of a sequence. Sitting with thoughts is very difficult to do for more than a short period. Outside of or after the eight-week course it is advisable to seek a meditation teacher who will advise on which practice is most suitable for you.

So much for *what* you focus on; what is also important is *how* you sit. Although for some of us a straight-backed chair is the only option (and that's fine), it is still important to sit up straight if you can. If you can sit on one of those small, round cushions (called a *zafu*) or a meditation stool, so much the better. The easiest posture for those of us not yogically inclined is probably *seiza*, which is kneeling with one's behind on a stool or an upended cushion. This naturally puts one's back into a helpful position. The other one (at the easier end of the spectrum) is the posture called *Burmese*: one sits cross-legged, with one heel pulled in towards the groin and the other in front of it. Knees should be resting on the floor or mat, or supported by cushions. The so-called 'tailor's position', which is what we normally think of as cross-legged, is murder on the back over any length of time, and is not advised! Yogis and yoginis can of course do full- or half-lotus. I recall Zen master Genno Roshi, many years ago, telling us how she found it much easier to face difficult emotions that came up in sitting if she had a really solid posture – "sitting like a mountain" as it is sometimes called.

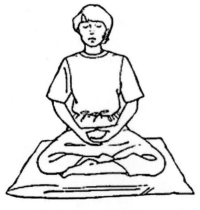

Burmese position

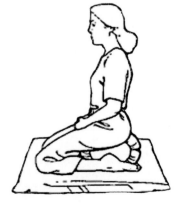

Seiza position

In Buddhist meditation the hands are usually placed one on top of the other, with palms facing up and the tips of the thumbs just touching, as though holding a thin sheet of paper. Alternatively you may choose to rest them on your thighs. On a workshop with a Taoist master many years ago, hands-on-thighs was described as *warrior*, hands together as above was *monk*. Take your pick!

Different meditation schools give different advice on whether the eyes should be closed or half-open. Most Indian schools advise the first; Zen usually advises the second. I suggest that you experiment. If you find you are the sort of person who tends to be more distracted by outside stimuli, then sit with your eyes closed. But if you find yourself more distracted by what's going on *inside*, then just let your eyelids drop a little, let the eyes defocus and rest your gaze about a yard in front of you. That way, you stay in the room!

Sometimes people report that they feel quite calm and relaxed during their sitting, but they find it hard to bring that kind of awareness to their daily life in the 'real world'. To help with this, the originators of the MBCT course devised the three-minute breathing space, the instructions for which I reproduce here:

> ### *The Three-minute Breathing Space: basic instructions*
>
> 1.   AWARENESS:
> Bring yourself into the present moment by deliberately adopting an erect and dignified posture. If possible, close your eyes. Then ask:
> "What is my experience right now ... in thoughts ... in feelings ... and in bodily sensations?
> Acknowledge and register your experience, even if it is unwanted.
>
> 2.   GATHERING:
> Then, gently redirect full attention to breathing, to each inbreath and to each outbreath as they follow, one after the other.
> Your breath can function as an anchor to bring you into the present and help you tune into a state of awareness and stillness.
>
> 3.   EXPANDING:
> Expand the field of your awareness around your breathing, so that it includes a sense of the body as a whole, your posture, and facial expression.
> The breathing space provides a way to step out of automatic pilot mode and reconnect with the present moment.
> The key skill in using MBCT is to maintain awareness in the present moment. Nothing else.
> From Segal, Williams & Teasdale (2002). Copyright by the Guilford Press.

"The key skill in using MBCT is to maintain awareness in the present moment." And while this is undoubtedly true, this statement, like many of the other hints and tips I have tried to reproduce in this chapter, still makes it sound as though meditation is something you do. I want to say that it's somewhere you go to hang out – yes, with concentration and awareness, but as the Zen teacher Baker Roshi (1997) puts it in *Seeing and Observing Karma*, Zen meditation – even with distractions – is a kind of re-parenting. So just get your backside onto a cushion *and let the practice work on you.*

STRESS

This term, coined by Hans Selye, refers primarily to a bodily state. Commonly, people use the term both for the state (or as a more acceptable alternative to *depressed* or *anxious*) and for the pressure they feel in certain kinds of situations. It is more helpful to think of these situations as *stressors*. These are whatever we can't deal with at the time. So *stress* is what occurs when we can't process what has happened or is happening to us at the time it is happening. The body saves it for later. The mindfulness hypothesis on this is that one has a much better chance of processing whatever it is if one is consciously *there in the moment.* If we are on a schema-driven program, or any other kind of automatic pilot, our attention is unlikely to be present. As it is not present, we will miss more. We may be in the wrong box, thinking about what's for tea. If we are more mindful, at least we have a chance of not picking up any more garbage! Of course, there are some situations that are so full-on, for whatever reason, that no one can be expected to process what is happening at the time. These are the situations that may give rise to Post Traumatic Stress Disorder (PTSD). See Chapter 24 for how to work with these.

As we have seen, when we start to sit and explore how it is 'inside' we find all kinds of stress-residues of greater or lesser import (often in the form of bodily tension) from previous unprocessed events, sometimes stretching all the way back to childhood. This is much of what we feel when we walk the razor's edge. It may not be much fun, but can be very liberating.

REACTING AND RESPONDING

Two contrasted concepts in the eight-week MBSR programme are *reacting* and *responding* to stress(ors). We know intuitively what reacting is – as in 'knee-jerk'. In terms of what we were talking about before, it is when we are operating through our computer programs or schemas/modes – unconscious, but not necessarily 'bad'. Whatever the trigger, Program 37b is activated and off we go, completely out of control until the course of action is complete. Most of our lives are lived like that for most of the time. It is akin to instinctual behaviour in animals. Our programs may have been (wholly or partly) learned, but they are just as automatic.

The alternative is to develop 'standbackability' and think about what we are doing, in the sense of paying attention both to what is without and what is within. We can then act – respond – in the way that is most helpful (or fun!) at the time, and paradoxically, spontaneity is reborn.

As we saw in the section on schemas in Chapter 7, rules may not be all bad! But there is a difference between choosing to do something that happens to conform to a rule because it is the genuine best call you can make under the circumstances, and doing it because it conforms to (or goes against) a particular rule. We are trying to learn to take responsibility for our actions, thereby coming closer to a 'demand-free' life.

ACCEPTANCE IN THE BODY

As we develop the discipline of sitting and other mindfulness practices, and learn to step out of automatic pilot more often, we find ourselves more in our bodies and in our senses. This has three consequences: first, life is richer as we taste it more. The second is that we notice more when we slip out of conscious awareness and back into automatic pilot. In the programme we encourage participants to deliberately notice what kinds of situations or triggers have this effect. Third, we become aware of the tensions and areas of holding in our bodies – the stress-residues that we talked about earlier. So while generally we can say that our bodies are always in the present, we also notice that *the past is also in our bodies*. Various theories have been put forward as to why and how this is so, of which the most famous is probably Wilhelm Reich's 'character armouring'. All I would like to say at this point is that *somehow* the body remembers. But what this means is that we can access and bring to consciousness the unprocessed material from the past by using the breath to connect with it inside our bodies. As we become more mindful, we can ask ourselves: "What is this particular tension? Does it have something to say to me? What happens; what do I become aware of if I try breathing into it, taking the inbreath to the centre of the tension and noticing what I become aware of then and as I breathe out?"

Now this is a very different approach from the one that says: "I shouldn't be feeling like this" and tries to somehow root it out and get rid of it altogether, or alternatively tries to intellectually unpick whatever the program is ("Why am I feeling like this? There must be something really wrong with me.") with the aim of making it better but the actual outcome being to plunge the person even further into rumination. Mark Williams et al. describe this as "when critical thinking volunteers for a job it can't do". The more we ruminate, the worse it gets. The 'cosmic law' underlying this is "What we resist, persists." Or to put the same thing in a slightly different way:

Pain x Resistance =Suffering

So rather than trying to somehow *fix* whatever program it is that we don't like by dissecting it with our minds, we try instead to *connect* with it non-judgementally in our bodies, using the sense of tension and holding as a guide as to where to focus our attention. This goes back to the idea we touched on under *Thoughts and feelings as my children*. You may not always do what your children say, but it's a good idea to connect with them and hear it!

Often people describe the centre of their tension as a place in their chest or belly that feels like a ball or closed fist. If you have had this tension for a long time, 'it' may not feel like opening up immediately.

The Reluctant Child-in-the-Body

If you have ever been with children who have not been looked after properly or who haven't been listened to, you won't be surprised that when you do offer them attention, they are reluctant at first to speak to you. They don't know what you might do, or if they can trust you not to misuse the information they give you. You may have to spend a long time just being with them, gaining their confidence, before they can tell you what's on their minds.

It is like this with the residues in our bodies. Indeed they may have been laid down at a time when you were a child, sometimes even before you could speak. So they may not just come to the surface the first time you ask them to! Sometimes we need to sit with whatever it is, patiently somehow allowing that sense of safety to permeate to that closed-up place, until 'it' feels OK about opening and revealing its contents; there are no guarantees. Sometimes people describe it as being like a closed-up fist that only gradually unfurls... You just have to be comfortable waiting for the internal phone to ring, and it may be very quiet. And it may not tell you everything at once. People talk about areas of closedness, heaviness, tension gradually shrinking during treatment as more things come to the surface. Be patient, let the small child talk when s/he is ready...

So we are now developing acceptance in two ways:

1. We are learning to respond more in the moment to what is actually happening, whether we like it or not and irrespective of how much it fits with our pre-existing ideas or programs about how it should be.

2. We are becoming aware of where at least some of these programs are located or held in our bodies, and are beginning to relate to them in a more helpful way, so that their influence over us decreases.

As with all mindfulness practices, the key thing here is noticing what is going on. And although it may not always be appropriate or useful to teach Buddhism in these courses, there are some traditional stories which fit the bill beautifully:

The Story of Mara

In traditional Buddhist mythology, there existed a demon called Mara. In typical demon fashion he attempted to undermine the Buddha's journey to enlightenment, but despite all his efforts the Buddha succeeded. Even afterwards when the Buddha was teaching he did not give up, but would turn up in disguise and try to undermine proceedings there too. However, the Buddha, with his all-seeing eye, would realise what was happening, and would call out, "I see you Mara" at which Mara was compelled to return to his true form and thus could no longer continue his mischief-making.

There is even a story that at some point Mara asked for a private audience with the Buddha, which was granted. Mara complained that it really was no fun because the Buddha always won. The Buddha replied that he realised it was very difficult for Mara but that he appreciated Mara's efforts and encouraged him to carry on because it was so useful in propagating the teachings!

We can learn a lot from this story. One, if we can unmask a process, then it has much less power over us. In fact, at the end of week four I tell this story, and people use it as a way to help them notice schemas being activated ("I see you, Mara"). How clever Mara is to have discovered this new psychological form! Even if you can't immediately see *which* pattern has been triggered, it is still tremendously useful to see *that* a pattern has been triggered, which you can usually tell by the excessive upsurge of emotion that accompanies the event.

The other thing is that the Buddha doesn't tell Mara to stop: our schemas arose out of events in the past (see Chapter 7) and were the best we could do at the time, and the process of uncovering them is profoundly healing, if sometimes painful.

MINDS-IN-PLACE AND THE BIG MIND PROCESS

Another way of talking about these different programs is as aspects of ourselves or 'minds-in-place' (to borrow Robert Ornstein's helpful term). When we look at what we normally call the self in this way, we get another perspective on how our minds work, or we could say a different kind of *metaperspective*.

Up to now we have been working on what we can call a *horizontal* perspective – that is, we look at the different parts of our minds: thoughts, feelings, body sensations etc. as though they were parts laid out on a workbench. But as we started to ask the body sensations what they contained, we were beginning to look at ourselves in a different way – looking at different parts as particular subpersonalities, if you like. We can call this way of working *vertical*, in that each part may have its own thoughts, feelings and body sensations (stacked up on each other, so to speak).

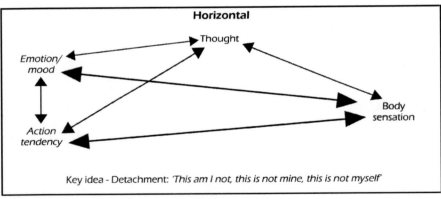

Horizontal

Thought

Emotion/mood

Body sensation

Action tendency

Key idea - Detachment: *'This am I not, this is not mine, this is not myself'*

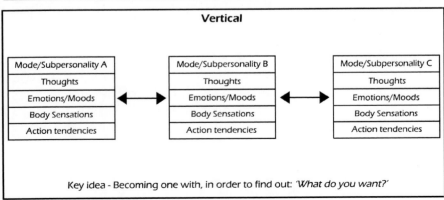

Vertical

Mode/Subpersonality A	Mode/Subpersonality B	Mode/Subpersonality C
Thoughts	Thoughts	Thoughts
Emotions/Moods	Emotions/Moods	Emotions/Moods
Body Sensations	Body Sensations	Body Sensations
Action tendencies	Action tendencies	Action tendencies

Key idea - Becoming one with, in order to find out: *'What do you want?'*

While the horizontal mindfulness (or CBT) approach is expressed in the maxim, "This am I not, this is not mine, this is not myself" (to use the Buddhist version), working with particular parts may involve *identifying* with them, albeit in a temporary way. Even if we start off dialoguing with a part, some techniques (like 'empty chair' from Gestalt therapy) involve us also becoming that part in order to find out its point of view.

A more general discussion of vertical metaperspective techniques follows in the next chapter, but of relevance here is D. Genpo Merzel's technique known as the Big Mind Process, which I introduce right after the session on reacting to stress (Session 4) in mindfulness programmes that I run. In that process, we can directly access the different subpersonalities which have been driving our patterned ways of interacting with life since our earliest times. And as we are becoming aware of our long-standing patterns of reactivity, whether we call them schemas, minds-in-place or just conditioning, wouldn't it be nice to speak to them directly and have them tell us what they want? And wouldn't it be even nicer to be able to access ways of seeing and experiencing that were not limited in the ways that these patterns are bound to be? These are the states, aspects or voices that are *non-dual*, and not normally accessed until one has done meditation for some years.

Some people initially find it hard to let go sufficiently to experience the non-dual voices, but almost everyone values the process anyway for the direct experience of the dualistic or 'ordinary' voices which seems inexorably to bring the awareness that *all parts have their value*. A few people dislike the process if they feel they are already having difficulty 'keeping it all together', although that is unusual by this stage of the course. If they do not like it, then the great thing is that all the other mindfulness techniques they have learned are still available to them and are entirely sufficient.

After the Big Mind session, any participants who would like to are encouraged to do what D. Genpo Merzel has called a modern mindfulness technique, which is to become aware at any given time of which aspect is dominant, or "Who's holding the microphone?"

METTA PRACTICE AND COMPASSIONATE MIND

There has been some controversy between different practitioners of the eight-week programmes about whether the practice known to Buddhists as *metta* (lovingkindness) should be included. The practice, in its most basic form, simply involves wishing oneself and others well, usually in some prescribed formulation like "May I be well and happy and free from suffering", which one then, when ready, extends to others in a particular order. In one version you choose to extend this good feeling to, in succession, somebody you like, somebody you don't like and then somebody you don't feel anything towards. In another version, you still start with the self, but simply extend, as it were, concentrically, to others in the room, the house, the street, the town and so on until you get to 'all beings'.

In most forms of Buddhism, *metta* practice of some form is considered essential to prevent the meditation becoming a dry intellectual exercise. The reason, as I understand it, why *metta* practice is not routinely taught in, for example, MBCT, is because it seems to imply that "I am not OK as I am" which is perhaps the key idea about the self in depression. While this is understandable theoretically, it is outweighed in my view by the need to engender *compassionate mind*, which we touched on previously in Chapter 7 and will come back to below.

Compassionate mind training allows more than the intellect to become involved in the process of change. Of course, from an absolute point of view you are completely OK as you are! But you may not be aware of that fact. The question is, does wishing yourself well highlight your inadequacies or make you feel better? It is of course up to you to see what works. I would formulate it like this: we are all OK 'underneath it all', but have become so detached from this awareness that we need to give ourselves encouragement and warmth to help us realise this fact experientially and moment-to-moment.

In the version of the programme that I lead, we bring in compassionate mind explicitly alongside acceptance, using Paul Gilbert's formulation of compassion as, to paraphrase him, a way of feeling secure enough that you don't need to *do* anything. In a way, feeling safe enough is a precondition for stopping the frantic drive to achieve, and in doing a practice of this kind we are attempting to recreate the sense we hopefully had as babies in our mother's arms of everything being absolutely OK. Chemically, we are then triggering our inner opiates, and not surprisingly, feel relaxed. Remember 'teapot compassion'?

RESPONDING TO STRESS

Having really got inside the different minds or aspects, and begun to allow ourselves to be compassionate both to ourselves and to the parts and emotions that we come across, we can begin to do something different. To start with, of course, we only notice a particular pattern kicking off when it's already activated and we've already acted, perhaps in ways we don't like. But that's a start. Then maybe we see it sooner, but just too late to stop ourselves falling into the hole. But by and by, at least with our lesser unhelpful tendencies, we can begin to see the pattern at an earlier stage of proceedings. Taking regular three-minute breathing spaces helps! From them, we have three choices, if we want to go a little deeper:

1. we can go into bodily exploration (the body door) to notice what's arising,
2. the 'thought door' which takes us, if you like, back into CBT, to check out the helpfulness or not of our ideas about what's going on; or
3. the 'door of skilful action' which – once you've checked out the other two if you need to – is discovering the option that you would like to take in terms of behaviour.

Jon Kabat-Zinn talks about problem-focused and emotion-focused coping. Having seen what is our own 'stuff' and acknowledged and accepted it, we can then move to appropriate action.

MINDFULNESS, INTER- AND INTRAPERSONALLY

Having introduced the experience of 'being' different parts, we then move to exploring using mindfulness with other people. How can we be more mindful in our interactions?

This is prefaced by doing the stressful communication calendar as homework the week before, so that we find out where we have difficulty (Sartre: 'Hell is other people'). We follow feeding back about the calendar with a bodily exploration of the four different styles of behaviour according to the assertiveness model (passive, aggressive, indirect or passive-aggressive and assertive). The exercise is derived from aikido, the Japanese internal martial art, although nobody gets hurt! Essentially, after modelling the three 'unhealthy' options, participants have to learn to *blend* with their 'attackers'. This means allowing your body to turn so that you are facing in the same direction as the person trying to attack you, without collapsing and going too floppy! So you are seeing the world in the same way, and from the same (or at least an adjacent) perspective. This is a great physical metaphor for helpful communication: it is much easier to be assertive with someone if you can see what *they* want.

Communication

A chap had got into a negative loop with his teenage daughters. He said black, they said white. They asked for something, he said no. He asked them to do something, they refused. You know how it is.

He did the aikido exercise and came back the next week with a look of astonishment on his face.

"You know, Donna asked me if she could go shopping. Normally I'd just have said no, because she hasn't been that good recently. But after the exercise I thought 'Why not?' and let her go. You know, the next day she'd tidied her room without being asked, something I've been trying to get her to do for months!"

So if we can adopt the same perspective – at least temporarily – as the person we're having difficulty with, we may have a better chance of coming to some resolution. But what about what's going on inside? Sometimes we don't like parts of *ourselves* that emerge – spiteful parts, perhaps, or excessively horny ones. If we are trying to get rid of them, in the Big Mind process we call that *disowning* voices. Sometimes they are so disowned we don't know they're there (what the psychoanalysts call *repressed* parts); other aspects we try to *suppress* consciously. Either way, if we don't let them come up, they can cause trouble. So how can we *blend* with these internal 'opponents'? Rumi, the eighth-century Persian Sufi poet and mystic, has a good suggestion:

The Guest House

This human being is a guest house.
Every morning a new arrival.
A joy, a depression, a meanness,
Some momentary awareness comes
as an unexpected visitor.
Welcome and entertain them all!
Even if they're a crowd of sorrows,
who violently sweep your house
Empty of its furniture,
Still, treat each guest honourably.
He may be clearing you out
for some new delight.
The dark thought, the shame, the malice.
Meet them at the door laughing,
And invite them in.
Be grateful for whoever comes,
Because each has been sent
as a guide from beyond.

From Barks and Moyne *The Essential Rumi*. Copyright 1995 by Coleman Barks and John Moyne. Originally published by Threshold Books. Reprinted by permission of Threshold Books

A practical way of applying this is provided by the extended version of the three-minute breathing space. In this we notice our thoughts, feelings and bodily sensations as before, pull them together on the breath and expand to a sense of the whole body, again as before, but now we deliberately turn *towards* areas of tension in the body and say to ourselves: "Whatever it is, it's OK; let me feel it." So we are back to walking the razor's edge!

SUMMARY OF THE MINDFULNESS PROGRAMME

This has given perhaps an indication of what the main processes are that you might go through if you did the eight-week course, though what it cannot convey is the experience of continuing to work at these techniques over time. We hope that people's skills in being able to sit, and in the practice of whichever form of bodywork they have chosen, will improve, as well as the course giving them a useful educational experience. In introducing such a variety of techniques over a short space of time, I sometimes liken it to being in a sweet shop: if you keep practising these different techniques, sooner or later you are going to find one or more that you like, which will be more likely to keep you practising. While during the course you may have had certain experiences that might profoundly change the way you look at things, it is keeping on practising that is going to maintain that openness. Therapeutically speaking, that will hopefully mean that you are more aware of your programs or tendencies when they kick off, less likely to act on or from them, and are more appreciative of your life in the present moment.

Jon Kabat-Zinn discusses the difference between mindfulness the state and mindfulness practices, which he calls the 'scaffolding'. Of course, in *mindfulness the state* there is nothing to achieve, but we can certainly learn how to become better at putting up scaffolding, most simply through practice. And although again we could see mindfulness as being a goal-free state, nonetheless it is useful to think about goals in relation to meditation: how to develop and nurture our practice, where we want to take it next, and so on. In some versions of the course there is a whole-day retreat to get a feeling of what it is like to practise silently for a day. If you do a course that does not have one of these, it is great to find a retreat that you can go on to have the experience of more intensive practice; not to 'get enlightened' but to go a little deeper, to clarify your understanding, and yes, perhaps to be open to the *possibility* of a 'sudden clash of thunder'.

It is also great to experiment by sitting with different groups; to get a feel of what suits you. Instructors of the clinical programme are great for helping you start the journey, but they are not usually experienced in taking you much further in your unfolding, and you probably need to read a bit and check out some local meditation groups to see what's next. Trust your intuition to help guide you into what is a good group for you.

For a deeper exploration of using mindfulness in this way, see my forthcoming book *Learning to Play Your Mind II - The Mindfulness Handbook.*

Further reading:

Jan Chozen Bays (2009) *Mindful Eating*, Shambhala
Charlotte Joko Beck (1997) *Everyday Zen: Love and Work*, Harper
Tara Brach (2003) *Radical Acceptance*, Bantam Dell
Christopher Germer (2009) *The Mindful Path to Self Compassion*, Guilford
Jonty Heaversedge and Ed Halliwell (2010) *The Mindful Manifesto*, Hay House
Jon Kabat-Zinn (1990) *Full Catastrophe Living*, Dell and (2005) *Coming to our Senses*, Hyperion
Jack Kornfield (2008) *The Wise Heart*, Bantam Dell
Dennis Genpo Merzel (2007) *Big Mind, Big Heart, Finding Your Way*, Big Mind Publishing
Thich Nhat Hanh (1976) *The Miracle of Mindfulness*, Beacon and (1996) *The Long Road Turns to Joy: A Guide to Walking Meditation*, Parallax Press
Mark Williams, Zindel Segal, John Teasdale and Jon Kabat-Zinn (2007) *The Mindful Way Through Depression*, Guilford

CHAPTER 10: DIFFERENT SELVES

*Vertical and Horizontal metaperspective – Big I, Little I – Empty chair –
Imagery rescripting – Unhooking the glitch – Compassionate mind and
the perfect nurturer – The Big Mind process*

We had a brief introduction to the Big Mind process in the previous
chapter because of its use in my modified version of the mindfulness
programme. In the introduction I introduced the idea of vertical and
horizontal *metaperspective. Horizontal* being what we have used in
most cases up to now – that is, dividing up what we normally think
of as the self into its different components (body, behaviour, emotion,
thoughts and feelings) to see how they interact. *Vertical* divides up the
self in a different way: each sub-personality or mind-in-place having its
own thoughts, feelings, associated body sensations and behavioural
tendencies. One of the aims of fourth wave CBT is to provide an
integration of these two avenues to understanding so that you can see
when you need to use which approach.

In western psychotherapy, that which I am calling *vertical*
metaperspective was in fact there first. Indeed, the very name
psychodynamic, an umbrella term for things psychoanalytical (or similar),
implies examining the interaction between different parts. For Sigmund
Freud, it was a battle between ego, id and superego; by bringing that
battle to light, as a sort of impartial referee, the psychoanalyst could
set up a process of negotiation that was more civil and thereby, to use
Freud's famous phrase, turn depression into "ordinary unhappiness".
But we could look even further back, to the world of shamans who
worked (and still work) to access parts of the mind not normally seen as
being *within* the self, but who nonetheless could bring about healing
by – in their terms – accessing the spirit world, sometimes with the aid
of naturally occurring psychoactive plants. More modern therapeutic
versions of the vertical or sub-personality route include the Gestalt
'Empty Chair' technique and Hal and Sidra Stone's Voice Dialogue.

Horizontal metaperspective in the west may be seen to start with the Stoics, encapsulated in Epictetus' well-known saying: "Men are disturbed not by things but by the views they take of them" (from *The Enchiridion*), which Aaron T. Beck quotes as a primary inspiration in his (1979) *Cognitive Therapy of Depression*. Similar detachment comes in the repeated refrain in the Hindu Upanishads: "*neti, neti*" or "not this, not that". And we have already cited the similar Buddhist reminder: "This am I not, this is not mine, this is not myself."

A modern therapeutic version is 'classic' CBT, wherein we break down a psychological problem into its component parts – thoughts, mood or emotion, body sensation and behaviour – and analyse each separately and in interaction.

"So why do I need to know all this theory?" I hear you ask. Well, I reply, each way of working has its own set of tools, and by learning how to use both sets according to the nature of the problem, you are doubly empowered. Let us not forget that the aim of CBT is for you to become your own therapist, and fourth wave CBT is no different in that. But what we do need to establish is when to use which set, and we can perhaps lay down some tentative principles here:

- Where the problem is that the emotion is too intense and you feel overwhelmed by it, it is useful as a first step to learn to step back and see what is happening ('standbackability'). What are these thoughts and feelings, and how do they fit together? This is working with *horizontal metaperspective*.

- Where the problem is that you have become cut off from some emotion, and you wish to re-engage with it in order for some overdue processing to happen, then you need not so much to stand back as to speak directly to the part itself, and then *become* the part and answer your own question. This is *vertical metaperspective*.

- Often you may wish to move from one to the other: horizontal first, to get an overview of what is happening from a detached perspective, then vertical as you enter the part that needs to process. I call this 'unhooking the glitch' in trauma reliving.

- As a rule, horizontal metaperspective, as in mindfulness, is a good default option, although we aim for the flexibility to be able to move from one to the other instantly according to what we need or want.

Theoretically, as already mentioned, CBT works mostly in the horizontal style, although the lack of a vertical option led CBT practitioners from quite early days of cognitive therapy to borrow from Gestalt therapy[8]. Other cognitive therapists have moved towards identifying and working with parts – A. T. Beck himself clusters schemas together into *modes*, while John Teasdale distinguishes between *propositional* (head) and *implicational* (heart) ways of thinking, with the major insight that if we don't touch the heart we're not going to make any significant changes. He also refers to Robert Ornstein's notion of 'mind-in-place', which may be the most useful term for a part or sub-personality. But in my view, the most helpful presentation on this overall in the world of the cognitive and behavioural therapies is Windy Dryden's (1997) answer to the self-esteem problem: Big I, Little I.

When people talk about low self-esteem, that means, literally, that they have a low esteem of themselves. Or to put it another way, that they 'esteem' (measure) themselves lowly. We have seen from the section on thinking errors in Chapter 4 that this constitutes *labelling*, an extreme form of overgeneralising whereby the self is reduced to one quality; or we could say to one (negative) end of one continuum. So if I deem myself 'unlovable' then I am giving myself a zero score on the continuum of lovability; ditto 'worthless', 'bad', 'weak' etc. Rather than measure the self as a whole, Dryden proposes we see the self as a multi-faceted organism, with lots of little Is making up the whole:

```
IIIIIIIIIIII
  IIIIIIII
  IIIIIIII
  IIIIIIII
  IIIIIIII
  IIIIIIII
  IIIIIIII
  IIIIIIII
IIIIIIIIIIII
```

Big I Little I'
There are a number of points of interest about this: one, that there is no single I that can be called a self. Two, that although the little Is are arranged in a pattern that looks like a big I, it is *our minds that are doing that*. In fact there is no boundary line that goes around the outside of the figure.

---

8 David J. A. Edwards (1989) *Cognitive Restructuring through Guided Imagery – Lessons from Gestalt Therapy*

There are of course parts that we would like to work on, but if we do not mistake our 'faults' for the whole of who we are, then they are just that – projects for development. If we want to be able to run faster, we can train to do that. Does that make us a better person? No – just someone who can run faster. If someone is disabled and cannot run, are they a lesser person? No – just someone who cannot run.

In the Voice Dialogue and Big Mind approaches, if a voice (mind-in-place, mode, sub-personality) has been suppressed or repressed it is called 'disowned'. The idea is that if it has not been allowed to speak, it will cause trouble, and somehow make itself known. Often you may find that, using mindfulness, you become aware that there are certain bodily tensions and stresses that do not appear to have a physical explanation. Here we can shift from horizontal to vertical:

The Intercom

A young couple were worried about their toddler, who had been waking in the evening in some distress. They decided to fit an intercom so they could reassure him. One end they attached to the wall by his bed, and the other downstairs where it could be heard from the kitchen or living room. The first evening after they had installed it, they put little Johnny to bed in the usual way, but omitted to tell him about the intercom.

Later, he started to grizzle; Dad came to the intercom and spoke to his son, "What's the matter Johnny, do you need anything?"

Terrified, the young boy looked toward where the mysterious voice was coming from, "What do you want, wall?" he quavered...

And in a way that is what we need to do: "What do you want, tight place in my chest?" We talked above about the 'reluctant child-in-the-body' and how to sit with him/her until ready to open, and it is often the body sensations that give us the best indication that there is something held, rather than just having an idea that there is something we need to work on. But of course there are lots of other routes – you may have been doing ABCs or schema work, which have given you an awareness that significant others from past or present may be having an undue influence on the way you are interacting with the world.

If the voice of the self-critic sounds loud in your ears, it is worth asking yourself: "Whose voice is this?", not just in what is said, but in the tone of voice. Sometimes the way to distance yourself helpfully from critical voices if they do sound like a parent or other critical adult is just to say,

"Hello Mum/Dad/Mr Bloggs" and in that simple step recognising that *what is being said is not your freely chosen opinion of your own worth or ability.*

EMPTY CHAIR

Of course, this can be the beginning of a conversation. In 'empty chair', a technique originally taken from Gestalt therapy, you take it further by placing Mum, Dad or Mr Bloggs in a chair facing yours and say what you need to say to them. Then it can be interesting to sit in their chair, become them, and talk back to the self from their perspective.

What is always emphasised in this kind of work is that whether it is Mum, Dad, Mr or Mrs Bloggs we are working with, they are not really those people but our *inner working models* of them – that is, another part of the self. After all, the original person who may have caused you the grief may no longer still be alive, but it is the *internalised memory* of them and what they did or said that is continuing to trouble you. So while we cannot change other people, we can certainly work on different parts of the self, or little Is.

This can be used in a number of ways, usually with a therapist to help; the most common are probably to give expression to and let go of long unfelt feelings from past events (as in Leslie Greenberg's Emotion Focused Therapy) and to resolve inner conflicts that are still playing out in the psyche.

IMAGERY RESCRIPTING

Sometimes we need to do something a little more elaborate to resolve such conflicts by creating *alternative possibilities* around past events. Some people object to this on the grounds that we are trying to rewrite history, but we are not trying to do this. We are only helping to generate a sense that what happened was not the *only* possibility (although it was the one that actually took place), and this can help to reduce any sense of self-blame for incidents that were not your fault.
It is perhaps more important to stay with the recognition that what is *continuing* to trouble you is not the event itself, but *your stored memory* of that event – which is part of 'you'. Then it is entirely permissible to create alternative neural pathways in your brain so that you are less troubled.

Honestly, it is hard to understand really why imagery rescripting works. Part of its efficacy is its compassionate side: you beat yourself up less if you can see that in an only-slightly-different parallel universe, you might have been rescued. Another way of seeing it is as a little I, which certainly had something bad happen to it (you) in a previous time, but by creating another version where it doesn't happen now, you are at least preventing the eternal replaying of that incident. And of course your original memory of the event may have been distorted by your sense of powerlessness at the time, and if you can have it happen again in a different way, that may enable you to see the players in a different light – all-powerful parents are reduced to ordinary flawed human beings, for example.

Imagery rescripting: instructions

So how do we do it? For a start, I would say don't try this at home! (Or at least not unless you have done it with a therapist once or twice before, and they have agreed that you are OK to do it.) That said, the first thing is to create a *safe space*, a visualisation of somewhere that you can return to; a vision of somewhere nice where you've felt relaxed and safe. Now be in that space, and remember that you can return to it whenever you need to.

The next bit is to remember the attention dial – you recall that one dimension of attention was from *standing back* to *becoming absorbed in*? You may want to practise this a bit a few times with a *harmless* incident first. One way of doing this is to imagine you are watching a movie; even visualise the edges of the screen, so you are *outside* what is going on. Now practise zooming in to the movie and becoming part of it; a character for a little while as the story unfolds. Now zoom back out till you are watching the movie again. I repeat, do this with a harmless incident first, so you are comfortable doing this attention-manipulation. When you are happy that you can do this – and if you get freaked out by anything, you can go back to the safe space to recoup – only then do the actual imagery rescripting with a difficult memory.

So, **stage 1:** create a safe space.

Stage 2: run the whole incident as a movie, staying as an objective observer. See yourself, in the original incident, as though you are somebody else – not you, but (e.g.) a vulnerable child in that situation. At any time you need to, 'pause' it and go into your safe space.

Stage 3: now review the situation and ask yourself two questions:
1) At what point did something need to happen to prevent or avert what actually happened? and

2) Who needed to come into the situation to change it so that it didn't happen like that?

You will need to discuss this with your therapist. The choice of 'rescuer' is important. Sometimes it can be you, *but as you are now.* If you still feel you would be overwhelmed by the perpetrator/bully/parent then you have three options – go with whichever you think will work best:

a) Give yourself some added powers – this is an exercise of imagination; you don't have to be limited in the way you were when it happened.

b) Think of somebody whom the perpetrator/bully/parent would have taken notice of at the time, and have them enter the situation at the crucial point and intervene to save you.

c) Bring in anyone you like who would be powerful in the appropriate way – it can be a fictional character. Sometimes Clint Eastwood as the man with no name or Dirty Harry might be your best option! But somebody whose intervention would have left you (the victim) feeling very differently at the end from how it happened first time around.

Stage 4: now rerun the situation, and at the crucial point have whoever needs to come in, come in. If it is you as an adult, zoom in to the movie and confront the perpetrator. See their astonishment. If you like, explain the consequences of their actions to them (if you think they would care) – be assertive. Reassure your younger self. If you are bringing in help, it is up to you whether you enter the movie or stay as an observer and just watch what happens to the perpetrator and your younger self as the rescuer does his or her stuff – stay safe, and know you can pause and withdraw to the safe space. After the confrontation has finished, you may want to lead your younger self out of the situation to somewhere nice. 'They' may seem a little bewildered, so you can explain what has just happened.

Stage 5: reflect on how the whole exercise has left you feeling. In particular, how is the 'younger you' feeling? Maybe s/he needs to go through it again from his or her own point of view, with lots of compassionate input (see below)?

Are there any changes in your beliefs about what happened? Are you ready to do some experiments where you approach situations you may have been avoiding because of this? If not, what else needs to happen?

Classroom Incident

Wilbert's social phobia started when he was ridiculed publicly at work. Even though he could see that it was his manager who had behaved badly, and his colleagues sympathised with him after the incident, none of the work he did with his therapist connected to what happened or the exposure work focussed on going out seemed to really hit the spot.

After some discussion, along with breathing into the place in the body where he felt most tense when anxious, it turned out that the humiliation situation at work reminded him – carried some 'markers' – of a situation at primary school where he had been ridiculed by a teacher for wetting his pants, even though he had asked to go to the toilet and been refused.

Wilbert felt strong enough to re-enter the situation as an adult and spoke his mind assertively to the teacher, who (he said) looked 'very surprised' at being given a lesson in how to treat children.

Then Wilbert visualised himself taking the young Wilbert out to play on the swings, "I think you've been in that classroom long enough," he told him.

UNHOOKING THE GLITCH

Hopefully the above has the effect of either preventing the occurrence of, or reducing the 'charge' on, the intrusive memory which pops up whenever a situation happens which resembles the original situation.

This is one method of 'unhooking the glitch' – by making what happened acceptable, the mind/brain can put it away. The lack of a believable or acceptable story for the mind/brain seems to lie behind many examples of Post-Traumatic Stress Disorder (see Part Two: Applications). Sometimes we just have to find and bring to consciousness whatever it is that is stopping the mind/brain putting it away. Often this is a passing thought at the time of the incident such as, "This can't be happening to me" or "I can't believe it", or even an awareness that you might have died in that situation so you 'shouldn't' be here. And of course flashbacks are most likely to be triggered when there is enough about the current incident that reminds you of an early one – even if you're not initially aware of the connection.

From a metaperspective view, we can see that little Is may be from the past as well as the present, and we may have to dialogue with them or temporarily 'become' them and/or important others from our past in order to resolve whatever it is from our personal history that's coming in and disturbing us.

However, even seeing that what is happening *is an intrusion from the past* (rather than "Me going mad", for example) can itself be really helpful in letting ourselves off the hook.

COMPASSIONATE MIND AND THE PERFECT NURTURER

However, letting ourselves of the hook is not always as easy as it sounds. We may be running a program like "I don't deserve it", or in some other way blaming ourselves for our plight, even if it is not (or only partly) our 'fault'. In terms of the little Is, we could say that the one called the 'self-critic' has been activated. S/he is often very loud during depression.

The self-critic probably learned how to do his or her job from an expert – perhaps a critical parent, or another carping voice from the past. Yet another part of ourselves, perhaps the 'victim' or the 'damaged self', is on the receiving end of all this criticism, and it hurts! You can do the empty chair exercise to open up this unpleasant dialogue and see what is going on.

Apart from anything else, one of the things that happens when the self-critic gets going is that 'we' (on the receiving end) feel more anxious. The criticism is experienced as a threat. The primitive part of our brain that still pretty much functions like it did when we were dinosaurs gets triggered – *it* doesn't know where the attack is coming from – and we get the same physiological sensations as we would if we were being attacked physically: hello physical symptoms of a panic attack. And that's not going to make us feel very good about ourselves! So the victim part needs an ally, but as we're thinking we don't deserve it, or that we're worthless or unlovable or bad, that help has to come from 'outside'.

Fortunately, there is a system in the brain – a 'wiring' – for compassion. We could say that it is there because (in evolutionary terms) we are not solitary animals. So while it is 'good' to be selfish in terms of the survival of the individual, for the species to survive we need to be able to co-operate. At the most basic level that means looking out for the family, but of course it can extend much further outwards. But it can also be turned inwards, which is what we need to do here.

To come at the same problem another way, when we are under threat one set of chemicals is activated (adrenaline etc.) and that prompts us to action to deal with the threat. Now if we really have to fight off a sabre-toothed tiger or its modern equivalent, that's great. Essentially we can divide threats into two: the kind it's good to do something about and the kind that trying to do something about only makes worse. Because if you try to do something and it fails, guess who's just there ready to get on your case? Hello self-critic! And that's experienced as a threat, which triggers the adrenaline, and off you go again. So we need to discover whether the threat is immediate and real (in which case, act!) or not. And if not, then we need to get out of that loop that is making us feel so bad.

The First Law of Holes

If you're in one, stop digging

We need to access a different voice here, which comes (wouldn't you know it?) with a different chemical. This is the way a baby feels in its mother's arms when everything's just fine. Completely held; secure; loved. Feeling that way is thought to activate our inner opiates, and this takes away the pain of 'failure'. But if our self-critic is very strong and loud, it's hard to get this mechanism going. So what we have to do is activate a compassion satellite, to create or connect with something 'outside' that will beam compassion back to us. Deborah Lee calls this a 'perfect nurturer'.

There are many ways to do this, but essentially they boil down to three:

1. History. Look for someone in your past (or present) who always has or had your best interests at heart. Sometimes a grandparent or uncle or aunt, or a teacher who always seemed to believe in you; it doesn't really matter what their relationship to you was if *when you think of them, that triggers the right feeling*. Warm; secure; encouraged; supported.

2. Religious. Devotional religions in particular have developed this to a fine art, although most religions have a devotional aspect. In Christianity, the notion of the guardian angel is exactly what we're talking about, although the Catholic attitude to the Virgin Mary is also apposite. In fact the female version of godhood is, not surprisingly, a source of compassion for many religious practitioners. The Japanese version of the *bodhisattva* ('enlightenment-being') of compassion has as one of her names *Kanzeon*, which translates as "She who hears the cries of the world." Of course it's up to you whether you feel happier accessing a figure like that, or a more personalised version like the guardian angel.

3. Customised. I think of this as the *Blue Peter* version – here's one I made earlier. You may not be happy to work with anything that feels religious, and it may be that your childhood was unfortunately lacking in supportive people whom you can draw on to help. Don't despair! What we are trying to access is a state of mind (or better, a state of heart), and this can again be assisted by imagination. The process is similar to that of finding someone powerful to help us in the traumatic situation we explored above. Who would you like to back you up here? S/he can be a character from fiction or a famous figure you never met – it doesn't matter! Just imagine what it would be like if you asked them for support in this matter, whatever it is. Having seen him on television talking and listening attentively with ordinary people, I like to think, "What would Nelson Mandela say about this, if I had his ear for half an hour?" and visualise that wonderful smile he has. So use whoever is your hero, heroine or role model – even fictional characters are fine.

So you've identified your 'perfect nurturer' who can be your compassionate helper. If you like, you can have more than one, according perhaps to whether the situation requires a coach, mentor, or spiritual guide! How do we use him or her? It's important that this is not just an intellectual exercise; if it stays intellectual, it stays dualistic. We need to be held completely, and the more we feel that, the more intensely the proper chemicals will be activated. So don't just think about *what* your compassionate figure would say, also think about *how* they would say it, what they would *look* like, how they would *sound*, even how it would *feel* to be held or cuddled by them if that's appropriate for you. The more representational systems in the brain we can activate, the better the *invocation*. That is, the more completely we can allow ourselves to be affected by our perfect nurturer, the better...

The key thing, whoever you 'adopt', is to be clear that they would always be in your corner, backing you unconditionally and advising you well by telling you the truth in a way that you could hear it. See them, hear them, smell them, be touched by them if you like. And let them influence you. In that way you have created a compassion satellite, whereby your own hidden wisdom and compassion can come back to you.

Perfect nurturer

Who is it?	
Appearance, clothing, complexion	
Tone of voice and other sounds	
Touch?	
Perfume?	
What are their particular qualities?	
What do they say?	

FROM EMPTY CHAIR TO VOICE DIALOGUE: REINTEGRATING THE COMMITTEE

The self-critic and the perfect nurturer are two different minds-in-place or little Is. Empty chair techniques provide a way for one little I to talk to another. A kind of therapy called 'voice dialogue', invented by Hal and Sidra Stone, takes this a step further. Using a procedure whereby one can learn to shift at will from one mind-in-place to another by changing body position slightly in the chair, you can access *all* the different members of the committee. And although this is working 'vertically', the effect of this (and some would say the most important effect) is to make one aware that whichever 'voice' is talking, *it is not the (whole) self*. So one gets an *experiential* understanding that whoever is holding the microphone, so to speak, is just another committee member putting forward his or her point of view. So the self-critic is self-critical – that's her job! Anxiety is scared of what's going to happen – he's supposed to be!

Voice Dialogue is a separate and complete therapy in its own right, and interested readers can follow the references. From my point of view, its main significance is in its part as a stepping stone which allowed D. Genpo Merzel to invent or discover the Big Mind process.

BRIDGES TO THE BOUNDLESS: THE BIG MIND PROCESS

Let me say that in my opinion the Big Mind process is the most efficient means that I have come across of working 'vertically'. By speaking directly as the part or mind-in-place, you can cut out any interpretative layer which might obscure what the part wants to say. And, in this time of scarce resources, you only need one chair per person!

We usually start the process with some kind of introduction, reassuring participants that they won't be pushed into going anywhere they don't want to go, and that participation in the process as a whole or any part of it is entirely voluntary. We then explain the mechanics of it, shifting position in the chair when you want to shift 'voices', and speaking about the self in the third person when you are 'in voice'.

We then move on to the voices which we need to speak to in order to get the whole process underway, namely the Protector and the Controller; the first to reiterate that s/he can come in at any time if unhappy about where we are wanting to go, and the second in his or her function as gatekeeper for the other voices or parts, to keep the ones we are not talking to quiet (including him or herself) and to give us a clear channel to the voice we want to speak to at the time. This sequence can be heard on D. Genpo Merzel's DVDs and CDs on the Big Mind process. At first it seems a bit like acting or role-play, but after a surprisingly little while it takes on a life of its own, and people are moving fluidly from one voice to another. It is perfectly possible for you to practise this by obtaining one of the DVDs (which are recordings of live workshops), and simply shifting in your chair at home when Genpo Roshi asks the participants to shift.

It is customary, depending on the purpose of the session, to spend some time in (some of) the dualistic voices: the Fixer, the Sceptic, the Damaged Self, Fear, Anger, Desire, the Innocent and Vulnerable Child, the Self-Critic and so on. Also, sometimes, the voice of 'Don't Give a Shit' (especially in OCD!). It may be, especially in a therapeutic environment, that you work in these for some sessions. But even if you are working primarily with therapeutic (as opposed to spiritual) aims, going to the non-dual voices affords a much greater perspective, so at some point, provided you're OK with it, it's a good idea to make the shift into these.

The process is the same, except we usually encourage participants to sit upright, akin to a meditation posture, for the non-dual voices: the Way, Non-seeking Mind, Big Mind, Big Heart, Great Intimacy and so on. If the dualistic voices are the little Is in the Big I, Little I diagram, the non-dual voices are the spaces between and around the Is as well – and the paper the diagram is written on, and the writer, etc. etc.

Different Routes

In traditional Buddhism, in both the Theravada and Tibetan versions, it is acknowledged that there are two routes to enlightenment, according to personality type (although usually both are taken). One is the route of calm; this is the practice of *samatha* meditation, whereby the desires are quelled in increasingly deep states of concentration and absorption (*jhanas*). In fact, there are clear parallels for this in the practice of yoga – not the exercise system but the meditation system described in the Yoga Sutras of Patanjali. It is thought that when the young prince Gautama left home seeking to find himself, *samatha* was one of the practices available that he learned from teachers. The other route – which the Buddha is considered to have discovered for himself – is the route of insight, gained through the practice of *vipassana* meditation, in which ignorance is dispelled, and the truth of no abiding self is discovered experientially.

Many people practising the Big Mind process seem to find some non-dual voices easier to access than others. The more one can let go of the belief that one has to know what a state is going to be like before one enters it, the easier they will all be! But I suggest there may be a parallel with the calm/ insight routes; some people seem to find it OK to follow the route Sceptic/Doubt →Controller →Big Mind (insight). Others struggle with this (typical dialogue: "I can't get my head around Big Mind"..."That's right, you can't")

But they find it OK to shift from Desire → Seeking Mind →Non-Seeking Mind (calm). It may be that these channels reiterate those ancient channels in Buddhism.

WORKING WITH NON-DUAL VOICES

Sooner or (occasionally) later, people usually find their way into Big Mind. If the personal self is like the unique formation of a wave (which doesn't know it's the ocean!), Big Mind is the experience of being the ocean; it is, however, completely detached emotionally (although it includes all emotions) – as Genpo Roshi says, "Big Mind doesn't feel, it just is."

When we take the next step and move into Big Heart, the boundlessness is the same but there is *feeling*. The Japanese Buddhist personification of this state is *Kanzeon*, literally: "She who hears the cries of the world."

Although compassion can be directed, basically it is a non-preferential, infinite capacity extending in all directions in time and space. There are other non-dual voices, which, as you might expect, weave in and out of each other, and as you work in these you find ways to transcend seemingly impossible dichotomies, using what Genpo refers to as 'triangles'. These pairs (at the bottom of the triangle) can involve a dualistic and a non-dualistic voice, two non-dualistic voices, or two dualistic voices along the base of the triangle. At the apex will be the voice which includes and transcends the two at the bottom.

A problem which has plagued mystics through the ages has been the attachment to non-dual states. So if we move from the 'small self' on one side of the triangle to the 'Big Mind' state itself on the other side, we may initially be reluctant to re-enter the ordinary world because we have become attached to being in Big Mind. We may mistake it for the goal of our practice (because, in a way, it is). In this state there is no beginning, no end, no birth and death, and everything seems perfect. Yet a Zen *koan* (puzzle) tells of a Zen teacher who was reborn for 500 lives as a fox for saying that the enlightened man is not subject to the laws of causation!

To avoid such a long time in the animal realms, we need to reintegrate our awakening into ordinary life. As Jack Kornfield has it, "After the ecstasy, the laundry." So the path after awakening needs to include both the dualistic and the non-dual.

The next stage, then, is to find a way of transcending these opposites. It's a bit like sets in Maths: you have the set of even numbers, and the set of odd numbers, which are opposites. But the set of *numbers* includes both and there is no contradiction between them! We can represent this as a triangle, with one opposite at bottom left, and one at bottom right, with, at the apex the quality that includes and transcends the opposites.

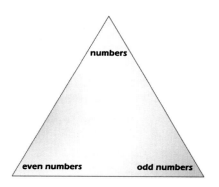

The first triangle, then, can have the small self and Big Mind at the bottom, and the True Self – which includes and transcends both the dual and the non-dual – at the apex. Another triangle has the self = ordinary mind on one bottom corner, no self = the Way at the other, and at the apex, Zen legend Joshu's famous dictum "Ordinary Mind is the Way."

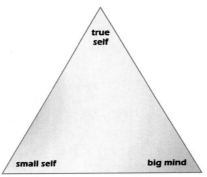

WORKING THERAPEUTICALLY

At a more prosaic level, we can have simple Caring at bottom left, Don't Give a Shit at bottom right, and what we could call Objective Caring at the apex. This particular one has been really useful for those with problems around excessive responsibility, e.g. people suffering from OCD. Even accessing Don't Give a Shit has enabled them to try levels of exposure previously unthinkable!

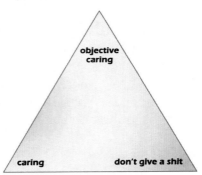

Another development of this process has been working with immature and mature voices. So, for example, the immature Damaged Self is very similar to the Victim ('poor me'), who has to pick up all the crap but doesn't know why, while the more mature version sees that it has an invaluable function for the organism as a whole (akin to the role of the toilet in a house – without one, all the rooms get dirty!) and as such is actually an arm of Compassion. Yet as Big Mind extends in all directions in time as well as space, both versions are accessible at any given time.

Immature and Mature Protectors (for example) both have distinct and valuable roles.

The mystical nature of this work may seem to obscure the very real therapeutic possibilities of working in this way; the chance to get what the real nature of the problem is 'from the horse's mouth' can save enormous time and suffering. Here are some examples:

I was working once with someone who was suffering with Obsessive Compulsive Disorder, Body Dysmorphic Disorder and low self-esteem. She understood the process but asked me, "But what if what the Self-Critic is saying is true?"

I said, "Well, I don't know, let's find out. Can I please speak to the voice of the Self-Critic?"

So I spoke to the Self-Critic, who duly obliged with some blisteringly negative appraisals of the person's appearance. I then thanked her, and said, "Can I please speak to the voice of Truth?"

"Hello," she said.

"Can I ask you, are you the same as the Self-Critic?"

"No," she said, "I'm not so negative!"

Another consideration when working this way is how not to be limited in the range of possibilities that we think are available. For example, someone I was working with was having problems in his relationship with his dog. So (through him) I asked to speak to the dog to find out what was going wrong. Information came up that the owner *hadn't been aware of* before we did this process, which then made it possible for him to change some ways he was behaving with the dog. It also confirmed that the dog was utterly devoted to him!

Another example was where – and I know this may sound unbelievable – I spoke to the voice of someone's lithium, the mood-stabilising drug often used in the treatment of bipolar affective disorder. It said something like this: "I feel really sad, you know. All these years I've been helping her keep roughly on the level, but she despises me and is always looking for ways to get rid of me. But without me she'd have been away with the fairies and getting into all kinds of trouble. A little recognition would be nice." The person was astonished, and much reconciled to continuing to take her medication.

Perhaps the clearest example of how using the Big Mind process can short-cut (potentially) years of schema-focused work is provided in the following case example:

'Gwen', a successful account manager for a large firm, was in her 40s when she had a crisis brought on by multiple stressors in both her work and personal life, which led her to come for group CBT. She also chose to take the mindfulness programme, and engaged well with both processes. Gradually she began to take care of herself better, and to recognise her negative thoughts for what they were. What emerged was a lifelong history of being unable to set or hold boundaries in her personal life, although she was much more able to be assertive in some aspects of her work life. To this end we devised 'Gwen & Co.', as a way of thinking about herself so that she could begin to be as forthright in looking after herself in her personal life as she would be for her customers. What also emerged was that her father had committed suicide when she was nine, although she did not know this until much later on, when she was in her thirties.

We were doing the Big Mind process in a small group, all of whom had been working together for a while, and got on well. We visited Protector, Controller, Desire, Seeking Mind, Non-Seeking Mind, Big Mind and Big Heart. All went smoothly. Then we did 'Feminine' Compassion (the nurturing aspect) and 'Masculine' Compassion (the more active, directive, boundary-setting part). As we went into Integrated Compassion, Gwen piped up, "You know, there's a hole where my Male Compassion ought to be. It's not there."

I explained about disowned voices, and got permission from the group to work just with Gwen for a bit. I asked to speak to disowned Male Compassion, and asked when it had been "shoved in the cellar".

"When Father left," she said.

"In that case," I asked, "what would it take for you (disowned Male Compassion) to become re-owned, i.e. to be let out of the cellar?"

"Father would have to be forgiven," she replied.

"And who would need to forgive him?"

"The child," she said.

So I asked to speak to the child, who was very angry. "He didn't even leave us a note," she raged. "He never told us he loved us!"

So I decided to ask to speak to the father directly. Interestingly, the first part to speak was the child again, "He's very sorry," she said, but you could sense his presence in the room.

Wanting to speak directly, I asked, "And who is this speaking?"

"The child," said the child.

"So can I speak to the father please?" I said.

So Gwen shifted position again and spoke as the father: "I'm very sorry. I was very ill. I do love you, and please also tell your sister." I thanked him.

After a little while I checked out how Gwen was feeling. She said she *could* fall apart at this point, but the Controller was keeping a close eye on things, and (with a laugh), she added that there was 'Gwen & Co.' too. In the week after this session, Gwen quite naturally started to put boundaries in place, which surprised some people who had got used to being able to dominate her. This for me confirmed the effectiveness of our session.

Once you have begun to explore the possibilities of working like this, it can be helpful to get the assistance of the expert. And where is s/he to be found? That's right: within *you*. Traditionally known as the voice of the Master, this has unpleasant cultural overtones for some people (particularly gender- and authority-wise), when in fact it only implies Zen Master. So we sometimes use the Adept as a more neutral name for this part, and of course the Adept is good at using the appropriate voice.

> Master Zuigan Shigen used to go out from his temple every morning, sit on a rock and say, "Master, are you there?"
>
> And he would answer himself:
>
> "Yes"
>
> "Are you awake?"
>
> "Yes"
>
> "Do not be deceived by anything or anyone, any time"
>
> "No, I will not"
>
> One of the earliest examples of doing the Big Mind process!

As you can see from these vignettes, the limitations of working with the Big Mind process are mostly those which we impose. On the other hand, people whose personality structures are very fragile sometimes find this too much. Basically, "Protector says 'no'!" And that's fine; that doesn't mean these people can't have access to boundless states, but they may need to build up some stability first through the regular CBT work, including working with schemas when they're ready, the cultivation of what the Japanese call *joriki* or 'concentration power' through sitting meditation, and (perhaps most importantly) compassionate mind training.

Others may benefit hugely from an exploration of the dualistic voices, but find some of the non-dual voices either inaccessible or too scary. Usually if I work one-to-one with them we can find out what or who is in the way and take care of it. In our local weekly meditation group, we have Big Mind once a month and sitting the rest of the time; some people make sure they're always there for the Big Mind, while others always come for the sitting, but not for the Big Mind.

Summary

It is hard to know how to conclude a section on working vertically, and even harder when the subject is working with a process like Big Mind/Big Heart. If you haven't experienced something like it and would like to, then please follow up the references and either get yourself to a workshop or purchase the book or DVDs and have a go. In providing a bridge to the boundless, infinite freedom is available, against which your personal problems may be put properly in perspective – which in my view is what CBT should be about anyway.

We should also not forget that this process is only one version of vertical working. But it may be the quickest – for example, as a way of accessing compassionate mind in one form or another. The main thing is the discovery that you are in control – to some extent – of the attention dial, and that by practice that control can be improved, once you understand something of the different ways you can use it – attention training, mindfulness, empty chair, imagery rescripting, compassionate mind training and Big Mind – and learning to experiment with whichever process seems most helpful for what you're dealing with. It can be fun.

CHAPTER 11: COMPASSION REVISITED: THE COMPASSION CYCLE

The six realms – Self-denial, teapot and hosepipe compassion – Free will?

Having now seen all the techniques which we have at our disposal, from ABCs all the way through to Big Mind, I want to come back to the question of self-care, receiving, giving and compassion, because this is an area in which we have so much trouble, in a way that would probably be incomprehensible to someone from Tibet or Thailand. So I am going to draw on some Buddhist ways of looking at this issue!

In a Buddhist way of understanding the world, there are different realms, similar to our views of Heaven and Hell. Some people understand these realms as literal places into which we are physically reborn; others see them more as states of mind. Being sophisticated and scientific westerners, we probably prefer to think of them in that way. The realms are: Animal (characterised by desire and fear); Hell (if you're reading this book, you probably know that one); Hungry Ghost (you almost certainly know that one too, but you may not know that you know it); God or *devas* (a place of long-lasting bliss and indulgence, which nonetheless comes to an end eventually); Angry, Fighting Deity or *asuras* (whose behaviour resembles the super-stressed corporate executive); and finally the Human Being realm, which was, traditionally, the only starting place from which one could become enlightened, and thus permanently liberated from the whole business.[9]

Without artificially attempting to superimpose another model onto the Buddhist picture of six realms, it is clear that we have different problems *vis-à-vis* giving and compassion depending on which realm we are inhabiting, bearing in mind that we shift between realms (as between

9 Until the arrival of the *bodhisattva* Kshitigarbha or Jizo, one of whose special powers is to be able to rescue beings from any or all realms, including hell. We could say that a Buddhistically-inclined psychotherapist teaching meditation is manifesting Jizo consciousness!

little Is) several times a day, if not several times an hour or even minute. The Animal state is relatively uncomplicated at least; unselfconsciously we go for what desire tells us to go for, except when fear pops up and propels us in the opposite direction. We just go for getting our needs met, which may include the needs of our offspring and so on.

In the *Hell* realms nothing works, and everything we do makes it worse. We become demons and suffer more, and cause suffering more. If we go anywhere from here, it is to the *Hungry Ghost* realm, which is that of unfulfilled and unfulfillable desire. The hungry ghosts are portrayed as having swollen, empty bellies with pinhole mouths too thin to be able to take anything in, and being present, unseen, at the meals of human beings. In Buddhist meal ceremonies food is put aside for them as an offering. Psychologically this is a problem of receiving; sometimes we are being offered love, but we cannot take it in. Perhaps we fear that it may be taken away again, and we think the loss would be too great. Or for whatever core belief-type reason, we think we don't deserve it. Yet if we do get some, it is never enough, and only serves to make us even more aware of that aching inner emptiness which we try to block off with yet more food, drugs, alcohol, sex or other distractions. Whatever we do, we can't fill it up, try as we might. Somehow the pit is truly bottomless. One route out of this state is sitting with the unfilled emptiness; making one's home in this cave.

It is, as we say, unsurprising that we desire to try to fill up this emptiness. From our earliest beginnings, the pangs of emptiness were soothed by that inimitable combination of food and love that came from mother's breast. So now if emptiness makes itself felt, we try to block it out somehow (food, drink, drugs etc.) in an imitation of that earliest action. But it doesn't reconnect to that love, or does so only temporarily, and then we feel emptier than ever. But what if our problem was actually that this is a *different kind of emptiness*? That just maybe, this is not the sort you have to fill up? Some kinds of emptiness are good. Our lungs, for example, need to be empty so they can take in air. Rooms need to be mostly empty so we can sit in them. And to take a slightly wider view, physicists tell us that at the sub-atomic level the reality that to us seems so solid is in fact vast space, with just a few little bits whizzing around. Just supposing that when you felt empty, that wasn't a sign of physical or emotional hunger, but just an awareness of a different level of existence? So why not try sitting with emptiness, or in emptiness, or being emptiness, and see what happens?

Of course, usually we don't think to react to emptiness in this way, but go on trying to fill it up, with more and better and stronger fillings. And it still doesn't work, but we don't notice, so caught up are we in the quest to get whatever it is. This leads us to anger and frustration, and the world of the *asuras*, where we get stuck in an endless loop of threat and achievement which just mimics the fear and anger of the animal realms, played out on a different level. Often the motivation may be compassionate (to create wealth, jobs, security etc.), even as one is hard put in practice to be anything other than an angry, deluded warrior in such a situation. This is another realm. To get out of it requires, in Buddhist terms, the discovery of *equanimity*, which we could define as "Freedom from attachment to results." In an instant we become a true warrior. Compassion for others is of course especially important here, too. Two stories illustrate:

The Aikido Grading

I had the good fortune to train for some years with the Aikido master Kanetsuka Sensei. We used to grade annually at the week-long summer school. I was going for a particular grade, and was making a pig's ear of it altogether. At some point I realised that I had messed it up pretty badly, and just thought, "What the hell, I'm just going to enjoy the practice." I relaxed and things started working properly. I ended up being awarded the grade, but with marks that were theoretically a fail! But I had again entered the spirit of aikido (harmony-energy-way).

Hakuin and the Samurai

There is a lovely story about the Rinzai Zen master Hakuin Ekaku's encounter with a samurai, who asked him about heaven and hell.
Hakuin is said to have replied, "Someone as dunderheaded as you couldn't get it if I spent all day telling you."
The samurai went to draw his sword.
Undeterred, Hakuin went on, "I bet your sword is as blunt as your intellect."
The warrior approached him, sword drawn.
"This," said Hakuin, "is the way to hell".
Impressed by Hakuin's imperturbability, the warrior re-sheathed his sword.
"And that," Hakuin continued, "is the way to heaven."

But to revert to the question of giving and receiving, we can see it as a cycle – perhaps starting in that awful hungry ghost realm, where we can neither give nor receive, but only look on piteously. Our awareness is of *lack*: the milk is not flowing, but even if it were, we couldn't take it in.

At first we cannot do anything, but somehow we manage to find a way of accessing some kind of compassionate figure externally or internally, and the juice begins to flow. We learn to let ourselves off the hook. Perhaps we practise *metta* or lovingkindness for ourselves: "May I be well and happy and free from suffering." We take, and appreciate, and in that very gratitude become more open and can receive it more. Perhaps this becomes the realm of the *devas*: the godlike existence where everything seems to fall into our laps.

By and by, we become aware of others' suffering. This is unbearable, reminding us of what it was like to be a hungry ghost ourselves. Yet we carry on indulging when others want! Out comes the self-critic again, and we feel so *bad*! So we give, not really because of the suffering of others, but because we have to shut the self-critic up, and instead get the approval of others for being a 'good person'. A lot of giving is like this, and it should be acknowledged that, for example, money given in this spirit still fills bellies. A more subtle version is the attempt to preserve the *deva*-like existence through giving – if I can make those around me happy and content, then my world will be a much better place to live in and the easy life can be eked out for a few years more. We could call this political giving.

We may in turn become disgusted with this; the self-critic starts up again with terms like 'selfish'. "You're only really doing this to make yourself feel better, you don't really care about others at all." This leads us to the next stop: the place of the martyr, of self-denial. It is your duty and only right to put yourself right at the bottom of the list. Parents, particularly mothers, often do this with their children and then feel guilty about the terrible resentment they feel, although of course parenthood is the one place where this style of giving is justified. Christian teachings are sometimes distorted in the service of this, while the commandment "Love thy neighbour *as thyself*" is forgotten.

Self-serving or not?

Mahatma Gandhi was one accosted by a critic.

"You are only really helping others to further your spiritual practice," he said.

Gandhi replied, "It is true that I help myself by helping others. But it is also true that I help others by helping myself."

The Gift

Someone gives you a gift; it is something you've always wanted. You are happy. Then you find out from an impeccable source that the person who gave it to you gave it because they thought they had to, that it was their duty. How do you feel about the gift now?

Someone else gives you a gift; you don't really like it, perhaps it's a bit tacky, not to your taste. If you'd bought it yourself in a moment of madness you'd probably throw it away. But you find out from the same reliable source that the person really gave it out of love, and so wanted you to be happy. How do you feel about this gift?

Sometimes self-denial is good and right, of course – particularly if it is an emergency. If firemen said, "I'm not going in there – it's too hot; I might get burnt", we would all be in trouble. But firemen need to take care of themselves – as much as they can in the emergency, and lots outside of it. It is understandable that people who have very dangerous jobs sometimes go a bit wild off-duty.

So here we can effect a complete reversal from how it was before, or at least take care of the provider of compassion. Instead of, or at least as well as, giving to others in order to make ourselves feel better, we can give to ourselves in order that we can give better to others. This is the *overflow* rather than the *self-denial* model of compassion. Our *metta* practice goes from "May I be well and happy and free from suffering" to "May those around me be well and happy and free from suffering", but only when we ourselves feel full up.

Teapot Compassion

I explained about self-denial and overflow compassion to a client who wasn't taking very good care of herself. She came back the next week in better spirits.
"That teapot compassion is really good," she said.
"I don't remember saying anything about teapots," I said. "What do you mean?"
"You know, you can't pour someone a cup of tea if you haven't got anything in your teapot, and you are the teapot."
That put it much better than I had!

To amplify this 'teapot' stage a little more, it is really about having no double standards: treat yourself as you would treat others, or be done by as you would do (to reverse a common saying). The spiritual aspect of this is to recognise the presence of the Buddha (or the Divine, or the simply human if you prefer) within. So if you really appreciate something – a beautiful sunset, or a cup of tea or whatever – you are making an offering to (feeding) the one inside. Ultimately, Buddhism rejects the self/other distinction, so why treat the one 'inside' any worse than the ones 'outside'?

That doesn't mean it is OK to ignore the ones outside either. Indeed, it is somewhere around here that we make the shift from sympathy ("Oh, poor you") to empathy ("Ouch!"). Taizan Maezumi Roshi talked about the difference before and after realisation: before, if you see somebody fall over and hurt his arm, you either ignore it or you think "Poor chap" and go and help. After realisation, you go to help because it hurts. It's your arm! For most of us, most of the time, that is not our awareness. But when empathy strikes, when we see ourselves in the position of the other and feel in our hearts what we would then feel, we are closer to that fundamental connection.

Up to now it is fair to say that we have been talking about caring: caring for others, caring for self, and seeing the connection between the two. The giving is definitely deliberate, and directed, and possibly effortful – though that disappears when it's *your arm!*

The next place on the cycle is – to follow our hydraulic metaphors – the shift from teapot to hosepipe compassion. Here is Genpo Roshi (in *Big Mind, Big Heart: Finding Your Way*) speaking as the voice of Generosity:

> *It's kind of like a garden hose. If both the spigot and the nozzle are closed, the water doesn't flow and the garden hose has just got what it's got. If it's got water in it, it's got that much... However, if you open both the spigot and the nozzle, it's a never-ending flow... The more I give and the more I allow myself to offer, to serve, the more the source continues to flow through me. I become more like a conduit than a bucket... I see that each of us is just a vessel, or you can say a conduit, for that source, that energy, for that which is greater than the self, whatever we want to call it...There's nothing more fulfilling than just being an open conduit, just letting the source flow through.*
> (p137–138)

Later on, in the same voice, Genpo Roshi also talks about *not* caring; how attachment to results, to what others do with the gift, is itself a limitation on generosity. In relation to the Big Mind process itself, he observes:

> When he (Genpo Roshi) first started doing Big Mind, he wanted people at least to appreciate it. I remember that if there were a hundred people in the room, and maybe five people went away not feeling they really got it, then of course he was disappointed, and they were disappointed...Now I notice close to a hundred per cent are getting it, and I think the difference is this not caring...They don't have to appreciate it, I give it freely. (p139)

Which brings us back to equanimity, the freedom from attachment to results, and the paradox that the less you are attached to outcomes, the better those outcomes are likely to be. This also makes sense in terms of mindfulness and the focus of our attention: if we are completely absorbed in what we are doing, 100% of our energy and attention is on the task; on the other hand, if a proportion of that energy is monitoring how well we are doing, that proportion is taken away from the task.

Hosepipe compassion is the manifestation of Big Heart in the world. Big Heart itself is not limited by plastic, or rubber, or human, or whatever the hosepipe is made of! As boundless compassion, it just radiates in all directions infinitely, but is also infinitely receptive (Kanzeon: *She who hears the cries of the world*). Big Heart feels, while Big Mind just is – and doesn't care.

As Bodhidharma said to the Chinese emperor when asked what was the nature of the teachings he had brought from India, "Vast emptiness; nothing holy." So we are back where we started, at emptiness. Yet when emptiness meets suffering, perhaps that's when Big Heart arises; the manifestation of which is perhaps the true potential of the human realm.

SELVES REVISITED...FREE WILL OR INSTINCT?

When we started to look at different parts of the self, or different selves, with the *Big I, Little I* diagram, the one that we normally call 'the self' was omitted – deliberately, because when it's present we tend to think of that as all we are, and then it's very hard to see the others! Ken Wilber (2000) talks about the 'proximate' and the 'distal' selves: the 'I' and the 'me'. In his scheme of things the proximate self is the navigator through stage development, which to Wilber is not just about growing up but about becoming more conscious – "from sub-conscious to self-conscious to super-conscious" (*Integral Psychology* p37) – i.e. to the unbounded.

I would suggest – and there is no necessary reason why you should follow me on this one – that here we have an interesting illustration of the relation between free will and instinct. To understand it we need to rewind a little to the notion of attachment. For children to survive, they are programmed to be attached to their parents, and as every parent who has ever heard their baby cry knows, parents are also strongly programmed to stay connected with their young offspring. We might use our intellect or ingenuity (free will) to help us deal with this problem (giving them a mobile phone when they're a little older, for example), but basically we're just acting from our instinctual programming.

What some may find unpalatable is that our journey to super-conscious that the proximate self is navigating may already be a kind of instinctual programming, which is known across various religious traditions as the 'return to the source'. For those with a theistic approach it is God or the Great Spirit calling His/Her children home; it is the moth to a flame, or the frogs returning year after year to their ancestral pond. So while the navigator *thinks* s/he is working out how best to get from where s/he is to where s/he wants to go, in fact it is just the *lila* (game) of life working itself out. As anyone who's just ended a relationship knows, the desire for attachment doesn't go away, because at bottom our desire is to merge back with the Whole, which is not just, in my view, about returning to the womb. But as I say, that just happens to be where I am with it, and I don't expect anyone necessarily to agree with me!

Summary

Most of us start out on this quest wanting to feel better; not remotely bothered about anyone else, but struggling with our own demons of emptiness, desire, hate, fear and so on. If we're in the realm of the *devas* we probably think we don't need to change. But even their satisfaction begins to pall after a while, and we fall back into another state of mind. Through therapy we may discover that we are as worthy of love as anyone else, and we can start to operate teapot compassion. Naturally that starts to flow into hosepipe compassion, as we forget the self without denying our needs. More and more the path seems to open up before us as we practise – not that we don't experience dilemmas or problems, but these perhaps become less troublesome the more we retain a sense of *inter-being*.

CHAPTER 12: CONCLUSION AND SUMMARY TO PART 1:

The 'fearless moral inventory' – Formulation revisited – Stages in the process

So we have travelled a way! We started out by looking at how to formulate our problems and come up with useful goals. We explored the nature and function of emotions and our cognitions – our thoughts and images about whatever was going on outside or inside our heads – and what to do or not do about them, including some ideas about our relationship to our mind-contents, which may be new to you. We looked at the schemas or underlying patterns of thought and behaviour. As well as the contents of our minds, we also discovered how we can work with our *attention*. We also emphasised the importance of the body and being in tune with it, both as a therapeutic tool and as a route into mindfulness. We did a tour of the mindfulness programme – and hopefully you had a go at one or more of the practices – and explored the Big Mind process both as a way of working with our 'parts' and also for deepening our meditative experiences. And we looked at compassionate mind training and the cycle of giving and compassion, and made a stab at thinking what the whole process is really about. Now that we have the tools on board, so to speak, we can take a voyage to the different places where they're needed.

There is only one more process that we need to address before completing Part 1, and then we will have something approaching a full range of tools available to us. This is what the 12-step people (Alcoholics Anonymous et al.) call the 'fearless moral inventory', which is a process that has to walk the tightrope between self-blame and not taking responsibility.

We don't want to slip into self-blame, because that can all too easily confirm the unhelpful belief that you are a 'bad person', which can make it more likely that you will slip back into the very behaviour(s) you are trying to put a stop to. On the other hand, *not* doing something like this can make you think that you are totally at the mercy of your 'habit energies', schemas or other personal programming, and that there is no hope for change.

What it amounts to is taking stock of how our habitual tendencies (whether prehistoric, inherited or learned) have landed us in the brown stuff and caused damage and destruction to others, while preventing us from having much in the way of genuine enjoyment. This is taking responsibility. On the other hand, noting also that *without awareness* we had no control, and that we did the best we could with what we knew and the resources available. However, it wasn't good enough (or you wouldn't be reading this book). So this is a paradox. You can think of it as having been taken over by your programming/conditioning/habits, so that you weren't really *conscious* of what you were doing. On the other hand, you were *responsible* for your actions – because whatever you did, nobody else did it!

So we need to note the effects of having lived in the unconscious way that we've lived. By now you'll be pretty familiar with your unhelpful rules and beliefs and their effects. Go back and have a look at Chapter 7 on schemas to remind yourself, and then fill in this form. In a way what you're doing here is reviewing your goals, but now from a place of (hopefully) much greater insight.

(Refer to chart on the next page.)

Now we see, perhaps for the first time, not only that living in the old way isn't the only option, but that it isn't really a workable option at all. OK, previously you weren't aware of what you were doing, but now you see the negative effects of living the programmed life. That *still* doesn't mean beating yourself up for your past! And some habits *are* certainly hard to let go of, but now you are in a position to make some kind of resolution to change these problem behaviours. Along with that, there needs to be some kind of acknowledgement that this is unlikely to happen using whatever methods or frame of reference you've used up to now (otherwise they'd already be fixed).

So we come back to Dogen Zenji:

> *To study the self is to forget the self.*
> *To forget the self is to be enlightened by all things.*

Kind of situation	Problem behaviour	Tendency or protective instinct it represents	Negative effects on self and others	What would be useful instead?
Driving	Road rage	Fear of being belittled	Family unhappy at being in the car with me; upset with self at lack of control	Not to take others' bad driving behaviour personally
Relationship	Staying in unhealthy relationships	Fear of abandonment	Not being true to myself; pretending love to others	To be honest; to be prepared to live alone

So to forget the self means, as both the 12-step and the ACT people have observed, a willingness to be open to that which is beyond ego; beyond selfish concerns; beyond protection of our small-self boundaries.

So when we (re)formulate our goals, they should be framed in terms of living a life that is open to this, and as free from our narrow, unhelpfully self-oriented programs as much as is humanly possible. And, in true CBT style, we should observe the results of the ongoing experiment: what happens when we stop trying to impose our will on the world, and instead try working with it?[10] We ought to put a rider to this, though, to add that this process isn't about denying this unique combination that is the integrated self (perhaps yet to be discovered or uncovered) or what

---

10 This is the message of the martial art *aikido* ('harmony-energy-way') – if you go with the way of the universe (which to Morihei Ueshiba, known to practitioners as Ō Sensei, meant the way of love) – then you are invincible. If you resist with force, you are easily defeated.

it/you want(s). You don't have to become somebody else, although once you have a better sense of who you really are, you may feel like somebody else in some ways. That sentence will become clearer a little further down the road, I expect.

Anyway, as you reflect on what you have read so far, and before we embark on its application to different problem areas, hopefully you can begin to see a pattern emerging, a sort of stage theory of treatment, which in slightly different forms will apply across the board to the different kinds of problem areas. Of course it doesn't have to happen in precisely this order, and there will be variation between both people and disorders.

Stage 1: *Formulation*

- Some or all of: hot cross bun; vicious daisy; individualised 'central heating diagram'. Historical formulation – this should also include a recognition of the programmed nature of the content. These can be prehistoric in origin – reptilian or early mammalian mind, like the limbic system – or from your upbringing, through the formation of schemas or even what in Buddhism is called *vashana*, which Thích Nhất Hạnh translates as "habit energies". Clearly, all of these three can and do overlap. What is particularly important here is to be *compassionate* with yourself about all this stuff. By the time you have a provisional formulation, you should be able to say something like: "No wonder I fell down that hole; given what happened to me at (.....), it couldn't have turned out any other way" or "It's not surprising I developed a tendency to (.......), it was the only way I could protect myself under those circumstances."

- And of course a formulation, however provisional, should include *goals*. "Now that I see that this program/schema was my (childish?) reaction to that (e.g. extreme situation), but that it has not been serving me well recently, how do I want to function *instead*?"

- We need to note clearly the effects on ourselves and others of having lived according to these old programs. But having discovered that the contents of our mind are not freely chosen, but are the product of all this history and prehistory over which we had no control, that leads us naturally to the next stage:

Stage 2: *Thought and attention*

- Mistrust thinking mind; *recognise* the automatic/intrusive nature of the thinking (clue: check for thinking errors).

- *Do* thought records or other reframing/ reattribution techniques if appropriate and/or necessary.

- Check if my *attention* is where I want it to be.

Stage 3: *Using mindful awareness*

- Remind yourself that *you are not your thoughts/feelings* ('fridge consciousness'); thereby discovering you can at least tolerate their existence (become comfortable with discomfort)!

- Similarly with the *body* – notice that "I am the one who lives in it"; seeing it as the *vehicle* or the *animal*, but one which can sometimes give me very useful messages!

- Be willing to be open to that which is beyond our egoistic concerns. If you don't like any of the religious or spiritual conceptions, just accepting that the world has its own dynamic; perhaps thinking more about what the world wants from me, rather than what I can get from it.

Stage 4: *Compassionate uncovering*

- Listen to thoughts, feelings and body *compassionately* to see what they want or are trying to tell you.

- See what the feelings remind you of, or which markers from previous situations are being activated that are giving them extra 'juice'. Relate to your formulation.

- Remember, or access for the first time, the decisions you made at the time (e.g. "I'm never going to let this happen again"); be kind to yourself about this activation, and if necessary, validate the decision *for then*, while re-evaluating it for now – is it interfering with your free functioning? Are you really living by the rules you want to live by?

- Uncover whatever unprocessed material is being stored in the body, which is making it uncomfortable and tense. Can you let it come to the surface? Listen to it kindly, like the suffering child that it is.

Stage 5: *Acting in your own best interests (AIYOBI!)*

- Whatever the thoughts or images are saying; remember that this is not just about what is good for me (self-centred), but what is good for everyone. Equally, it is not just about what is good for others (martyr)! Think teapot or hosepipe compassion instead.

- Test out new understandings using behavioural experiments.

Stage 6: *Maintenance*

- Rework the formulation as you go along: old model/new model (see Chapter 7). In future, use this as a benchmark for choosing a course of action.

- Learn to listen more closely, and on a regular basis, to what your body is trying to tell you. It is your friend – or if it isn't, make friends with it!

- Note what kinds of situations are most likely to trigger relapse (or collapse) for you, and what signals your body and mind are likely to give out under those circumstances (relapse signature). Do a blueprint (see appendix).

- Maintain your spiritual fitness practice, whatever that is (meditation, tai chi, dance etc.).

- Note how it is when you allow the universe to do what *it* wants to do (power with), as opposed to trying to impose *your* will on it (force).

Of course the process doesn't have to unfold in the order above; that is just a guide. In fact, we could pare it down even more:

1. Formulate compassionately.
2. Notice, but do not automatically believe, what thinking mind is saying.
3. Plug in and listen (to emotions, to body, to spirit).
4. Act in your own and others' best interests (teapot and hosepipe compassion).

PART 2: SOME APPLICATIONS

In looking at the specific kinds of problems, we will start with depression and then go to its close cousin, low self-esteem, before visiting the anxiety disorders and one or two body-related conditions. I am not attempting to deal with every known condition in this book, but if your problem area isn't described, there may be something on it in Chapter 26 and in any case the scheme above and the general principles outlined should (hopefully!) be of use

CHAPTER 13: DEPRESSION

Emotional shutdown – Evolutionary origins – Rumination – Depression FM – Activity scheduling – Turnip time – Doing and being – Shame

WHAT IS DEPRESSION? FORMULATION OF THE PROBLEM

"What's the point?" "I can't go on." "I don't deserve anything better anyway." "I feel like ending it all..."

If these are the sorts of things that are going through your mind, the chances are that you are suffering from depression. Sometimes people ask, "What is depression?" When we are doing ABCs or other kinds of thought records, we put depression in the *mood* or *emotion* column. But in a way it might be more helpful to think of it as a *non*-feeling; as what happens when we can't cope with feeling any more and *emotional shutdown* happens, rather like a fuse blowing when there's a surge of electricity that the wiring couldn't cope with. Too much sadness or grief leads to emotional overload, and depression kicks in.

Daniel Goleman, in his groundbreaking book *Emotional Intelligence*, suggests an evolutionary origin for depression in the hunting situation of our Stone-Age ancestors. He visualises the close-knit nature of the hunting group, and then imagines the consequences of how you feel when a close fellow member of the party (perhaps a brother) is killed in a hunt (maybe by one of the creatures you were trying to capture). Of course, bereft. Then how much use would you be on the next trip? More than likely, you'd be a liability to yourself and the rest of the group. So emotional shutdown kicks in and sends you to grieve in your cave until you're functioning again.

Another, more developmental version (though in the same vein) is provided by Paul Gilbert:

For many mammals, including humans, separation from the mother puts juveniles at risk from a variety of dangers. While she is present, she signals safeness and access to a source of support. She also provides food and comfort, and will help the infant calm down if it is anxious and upset. So she regulates her infant's threat/stress system with soothing and care because the infant cannot do this for itself...In the mother's absence, the world becomes threatening and the child shows a protest/despair reaction, which is part of a normal, evolved protection strategy. Protest involves distress, anxiety, crying and seeking to connect again with the mother. The infant is programmed to engage in urgent searching and to signal/communicate distress (e.g. distress calling and crying) to elicit help, protection and support via reunion with a caring 'other' – that is, the signal is designed to impact on others. This may be called yearning. This protection 'protest' strategy can be turned off when the infant is soothed or the mother herself arrives.

Things may not turn out so well, however. Suppose the efforts expended by crying and searching do not result in the return of the mother or in soothing signals from her. This is potentially very dangerous. For most mammals, a distressed/searching young individual on its own is in danger of attracting predators, or of becoming lost and/or exhausted and starved. In such contexts, sitting tight and waiting for the parent to return may be the best protection strategy for survival. Despair is a form of behavioural deactivation when protest does not work. Positive emotions and feelings of confidence and the desire to explore, search and seek out must be toned down because this aspect of the protection strategy is designed to stop the individual signalling and moving about in the environment when to do so is dangerous. It is saying: "Go to the back of the cave and stay there."

There are, in fact, many life events and situations, such as major defeats and setbacks or being bullied or rejected, that make our brain want to go into 'back of the cave' self-protect mode. It feels terrible because this self-protection strategy works by turning off our positive emotions and making us focus on bad things. It evolved long before we humans came along, able to think about ourselves and our futures. And it evolved long before we developed self-consciousness or self-awareness, which allows us to realise how unpleasant these feelings 'feel'.
(*The Compassionate Mind* p141–143)

So whether this is an evolutionary mechanism that predates humans or is a specific development dating from a common occurrence in the life of the cave human (actually, it would be easy to place the bereavement response as a specific example of the protest/despair reaction), what is clear is that these feelings are, in Gilbert's terms "innate and archetypal"

– the automatic reaction of our antique brains to a threat that is more severe than we can deal with. A difference between modern humans and our prehistoric ancestors is that we often can't (or feel we can't) escape. Earlier versions of life offered more opportunities to run away from threatening situations. But there may be greater perceived threats to us if we try to escape a soul-destroying job or a bad marriage, and so we stay because we think we ought to, and the older self-protection mechanism kicks in and we get depressed instead.

Another view of depression is the classic psychodynamic view that it is 'anger turned inwards'. While there is undoubtedly an element of self-attacking in depression, I think it makes more sense to see this as a *consequence* of depression – if we put depression or feeling depressed as an A (see Chapter 4 for an overview of the ABC model), and we think (unsurprisingly) that "It's not OK for me to feel like this" at B, *then* we feel angry with ourselves at C, and the behaviour is to attack ourselves; to try and whip ourselves into shape – what the psychologist Mark Williams calls "boot camp mind". This is **rumination**, the constant comparison of how it is now with how in our minds it 'ought' to be. But of course that makes us feel worse, more under threat, more battered, and we don't feel like we have the stuffing left in us to go on fighting.

John Teasdale has identified a core idea about the self that is at the heart of depression as "I'm not OK as I am." Most clients I have worked with agree with this, as though being depressed were some kind of character deficit. Of course, if you're not essentially OK as you are, then you (think you) have to somehow beat yourself into being someone else, or pretend to be someone else. Either way, it confirms the basic idea you're not OK as you are. We can show this simply in a diagram:

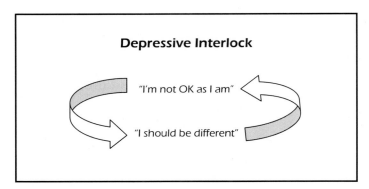

Depressive Interlock

"I'm not OK as I am"

"I should be different"

Everything we do to try and make ourselves different ends up confirming our basic inadequacy. Like the Chinese finger-trap, the harder we pull, the more stuck we get.

DEPRESSION FM

So what is the way out of this horrible trap? It is simple, if not easy. You need to recognise that you are suffering from an illness called depression, which f***s with your mind! If you had chickenpox, malaria, diabetes or a heart condition, you would be unlikely to say that meant, "I'm not OK as a person." You would be more likely to say, "I am OK as a person, but unfortunately suffering from this illness." Try this version on for size with depression! A tool to help you remember that depression is an illness that f***s with your mind is the idea of *Depression FM*. Depression FM is that nasty propaganda radio station that broadcasts in your brain when you're depressed, but because it is so loud and persistent when you are depressed, you end up believing what it says. **Don't!**

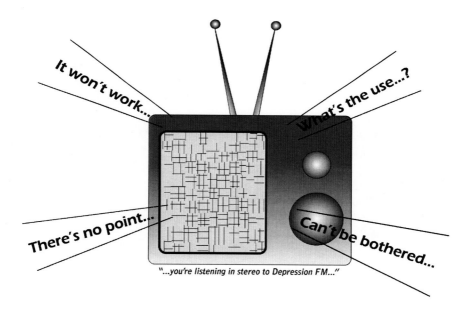

"*...you're listening in stereo to Depression FM...*"

Bearing in mind that *we are not our thoughts*, we can view any kind of mind-contents, including depression, as something we are passing through, or more accurately, that is passing through us. People often describe depression as a black cloud, yet still blame themselves for having it! Do you normally blame yourself for the weather?

Another way of thinking about it is as a *frequency*, which it probably is in terms of brain-stuff. Your brain has tuned into Depression FM as a familiar frequency – like a pair of old slippers, one client described it to me. Adopting a bigger perspective through (for example) Big Mind enables you to see it as just that: a particular bandwidth of black cloud, with the associated turbulence. Navigate an AIYOBI! (Act In Your Own Best Interests) direction, and sooner or later you will pass through it.

So instead of trying to beat yourself out of depression by ruminating, recognise instead that you have unwittingly steered into this condition, *and don't blame yourself*! Instead, invoke compassionate mind, whose comments often seem to start with something like, "Well, it's not surprising that you are feeling like this, given what happened to you..."

ACTIVITY SCHEDULING

Now, what would be helpful for you at this point? Almost certainly you will be doing too little, although some people soldier on for months and sometimes years, battling against the odds and not enjoying a moment of it. In which case it may be about the *type* of activity, rather than how much. Either way, we start with something called an Activity Schedule.

On the next page is Mr G's activity schedule. He is moderately depressed. We can see that on the one hand he takes care of himself (eats, cleans up etc.) but that he spends a lot of time alone. When he makes the effort to meet others, it's rewarding (Sunday), but he has a problem around looking for work. Notice that his overall mood rating changes according to what he does on different days – although there's usually some fluctuation anyway.

ACTIVITY SCHEDULE Week beginning: /   /

Rate each activity (0–10) for M (mastery/effort) and P (pleasure), according to how *challenging* or *pleasurable* the activity was for you.

Days→ Time	Monday	Tuesday	Wednesday	Thursday	Friday	Saturday	Sunday
6am–8am	Asleep	Restless, got up M6 P0	Asleep	Asleep	Asleep	Asleep	Asleep
8am–10am	Got up M5, P0 Made and ate breakfast M6, P4	Made and ate breakfast M5, P3	Slept in M0 P5 Had breakfast M6 P4	Had breakfast M6 P4 Took car to be serviced M8 P0	Got up late Made and ate breakfast M7 P3	Got up late Went to get papers and breakfast M4 P5	Got up Made and ate breakfast M6 P3
10am–12pm	Went back to bed M0, P3 Went shopping M7 P3	Went to see friend M8 P5	Went to supermarket M8 P2	Stayed in town, did window-shopping M4 P4	Read papers M6 P2 Did housework M5 P3	Had breakfast and read papers M2 P3	Went to friend's for day M9 P6
12pm–2pm	Had lunch out M6 P4	With friend M8 P5	Made and ate lunch M4 P4	Came home, made and ate lunch M3 P2	Had sandwich M3 P6	Went for a walk M8 P6	Lunch at friends' M9 P6
2pm–4pm	Came home, did garden M7 P6	With friend M8 P5	Read novel M6 P5	Phoned friend M7 P7 Read novel M6 P4	Went into town to collect car; not ready M8 P0	Came home, had lunch M3 P5 and then a nap M0 P0	Walk in country with friends M5 P8
4pm–6pm	Made dinner M7 P2	Came home, sat around M0 P0	Read novel M6 P5	Looked on internet for work options M9 P1	Browsed in bookshop M3 P7	Phoned children M7 P7	Walking M5 P8
6pm–8pm	Had dinner in front of TV M3 P3	Went swimming M6 P8	Went for a walk M7 P4	Felt depressed, went to bed M0 P0	Met friends down pub, ate out M4 P7	Went to a film M5 P8	Dinner with friends M4 P8
8pm–10pm	Watched more TV M0 P3	Came home, watched TV M0 P4 Had takeaway M0 P6	Had ready-made dinner M2 P2 Went to pub M6 P5	In bed	Out with friends M4 P7	Film M5 P8 Went to pub in town M8 P4	Came home, watched TV M0 P3
10pm–12am	Went to bed	Went to bed	Came home, went to bed	Watched TV M3 P3	Came home went to bed, couldn't sleep M6 P0	In pub M5 P6 Came home went to bed	Went to bed
12am–2am	Asleep	Asleep	Asleep	Went to bed late	Finally slept	Asleep	Asleep
Overall mood rating (0–10)	4	6	3	1	3	5	7

Following Mr G's version there is a blank for you to use in Appendix 2. If you're suffering from depression, I suggest you fill one in for a week. Don't worry about doing them perfectly, but try and get something in all the boxes (even if it's just 'asleep').

Usually activity schedules are done weekly (see Chapter 5), and to start with, you just record in a few words what you do every hour or two and rate it out of ten for *mastery* and *pleasure*. 'Pleasure' is fairly self-explanatory; of course you don't expect to get as much pleasure out of something when you're depressed as you did before, but if you don't do it at all you are guaranteed not to get any! 'Mastery' really means the amount of effort you have to put in to achieve whatever the task is.And it should relate to the amount of effort it takes you to do it – in the state you're in, not the amount you think it *ought to* take if you were well. So for most people who are depressed, it is a serious achievement to get out of bed before eight or nine o'clock in the morning. So if that is how it is for you, and you manage to do it, then that scores a 10, irrespective of the fact that when you're well you get up at seven without even thinking about it.

At the end of each day, give yourself an overall mood score for that day, where zero is really awful and ten is not depressed at all.

Now that you've filled the Activity Schedule in for a week, what do you notice? Is there a balance of mastery and pleasure? Was your overall mood rating the same every day? Was that affected by what you did? What sort of things seemed to make the most difference in lifting your mood, if anything?

Write them here:
....
....
....
....
....

After you've filled a schedule in for a week, then you need to review how it went. There are lots of things to notice here. One is the daily mood score – were there any differences? If there were, what did you do differently on the days when the score was higher? If there was any variation at all, then it shows your depression is not completely constant, even though that's often how it feels. Maybe I *can* affect my mood to some extent by what I do with my time...

The concepts of mastery and pleasure remind us – as does the attempt to balance them in the activity schedule – of the old saying "All work and no play makes Jack a dull boy." That applies to Jill, too, although she's probably a girl. And where this duality of work and play holds sway it is vital to make sure that play has enough space[11]. Because when people get depressed, they tend to stop doing the fun stuff, as they don't think it's going to be any fun (because they're depressed), and because everything's so much effort that it's all they can do to take care of the 'essential' stuff. Actually, where your mood's concerned, pleasure *is* essential.

So we need to build in what we're lacking – usually this will be pleasurable stuff, but sometimes, especially for you stressed-out executive types, the addiction to achievement will need feeding too!

If that's the case, how about mowing the lawn or (only if you fancy it) putting up that shelf you've been meaning to do for ages?

PLEASURABLE ACTIVITY AND THE ACTIVITY WINDOW

Think about what gives you pleasure. I know – at the moment, little or nothing. But what kinds of things used to 'float your boat' before? List them here:

```
┌─────────────────────────────────────────────────────────┐
│                                                           │
│             Things I used to enjoy                        │
│                                                           │
│  ........................................................ │
│  ........................................................ │
│  ........................................................ │
│  ........................................................ │
│  ........................................................ │
│  ........................................................ │
│                                                           │
└─────────────────────────────────────────────────────────┘
```

If you're struggling to remember, you might like to think of it this way: I asked a group of people who were attending a 'coping with depression' group, "What are the things you used to do before you became depressed, that you gave up when you became depressed (which then made you more depressed)?"

---

11 But when the poet composes her sonnet, or the musician just reaches that peak of performance, is that work? Certainly it may have taken much work to get there, but at that point? We say that we are 'playing' music. One of the old sayings of the hippies was that *work + love = play*.

I wrote their answers on the flipchart, and the activities seemed to fall quite naturally into four categories: social, physical, nature and creative.

We can represent that on something we call the 'activity window' like this:

SOCIAL	NATURE
CREATIVE	PHYSICAL

So when you're planning what to do to put in some pleasurable activities, and you can't initially think what to put in, try choosing one thing from each of these boxes. Of course often you don't feel like it, but just put that down to the *faulty feelometer*, which means that because you've got depression, your brain isn't giving you accurate readings. It is *depression* that doesn't feel like it; the real you that does and can feel is obscured underneath.

Often depression is linked to having overly high expectations – these sometimes get linked to the recovery process too. Doing something creative, for example, doesn't mean you've got to compose and play something that's better than a Mozart piano concerto, armed only with a kazoo and no previous knowledge of music.

Some activities fit in more than one box: dancing could be creative and also exercise (physical). Gardening combines creative, nature and physical – and social too, if you belong to an allotment club. No wonder gardeners can get very depressed if they stop gardening.

Other ways of connecting to the nature side don't have to involve giving up on civilisation altogether and living in the woods (although that might be fun); even stroking your cat or dog, if you have one, is connecting to nature.

Physical activity may be the most important of these four for antidoting depression, just because of the very physical sluggishness that is so often a symptom. You can quite literally burn it off by really going for it at the gym. But remember the realistic expectations thing – if you haven't exercised for twenty years and are four stone overweight, then talk to your doctor first about what is appropriate and be easy on yourself, at least to begin with. Don't make it into a punishment session. Actually doing the kind of exercise you enjoy will be what works best in the long term. And although the gym may have some great equipment, other types of exercise may have more of a social element – lots of sports clubs meet up for a drink and a chat after the session, or perhaps the nature of the game requires some interaction. ("Over here, on me head!")

Naturally, if you're feeling depressed, you probably don't feel much like socialising. ("They don't want to hear how depressed I am.") So it is helpful to meet with people where there is another focus for meeting, like a sports club. Or perhaps there is some political activity you care about, or you are involved in your local school's PTA. What, when you aren't depressed, do you care about? Focusing your attention outwards both distracts you from your depression and may do some good – which will make you feel better and begin to restore that sense of purpose. It depends how depressed you are – for some of you, a chat on the phone with a good friend will be the most you can manage. Great! Do it! And maybe next week, you could meet them for coffee somewhere...

Stuff that gets in the way and how to overcome it (AIYOBI!)
Again and again in depression we come back to what some would call *resistance*; statements which people say to justify not doing activity when they're depressed:

- "I don't feel like it."
- "I haven't got the energy."
- "I lack motivation."
- "I haven't got the confidence."
- "There's no point."
- "I won't enjoy it."

There are two aspects to these statements – we will deal with the content of each one in a moment, but more important perhaps is the question of who or what (which little I) is saying them. It has to be our old 'friend' Depression FM, and how much is it really going to help us to listen to *that* station? Well, you maybe can't help but listen to it at the moment, but you don't have to believe what it's saying.

"I don't feel like it."
Well, you wouldn't, would you? When you're suffering from depression, you don't feel like much. But is (whatever it is) a good idea? Is it possible or useful? Might it give you some benefit if you did it? If the answer to these questions is yes, then to do this activity is *in your own best interest*. And the solution to your not feeling like it (emotional reasoning fuelled

by depression) is to Act In Your Own Best Interests (or AIYOBI! for short) – whether you *feel* like it or not.

Think of it as a war cry to defeat depression. Remember, when you're depressed what you *feel* like will probably be giving you bogus information because your *feelometer* is faulty! That's why AIYOBI! is so helpful. Try shouting it out loud – though possibly not in the supermarket!

"I haven't got the energy."

This statement rests on a thinking error that we need to add to the main list: the 'battery-powered' thinking error. Especially, but not only, when we're depressed, we think we have a finite amount of energy, as though we were battery-operated. In addition, one of the clear biological symptoms of depression is that incredible tiredness, that utter lethargy.

So *of course* it is difficult to get up and get going; that's why we suggest setting lower, more manageable goals when you're suffering from depression. Let's look at it on a hot cross bun:

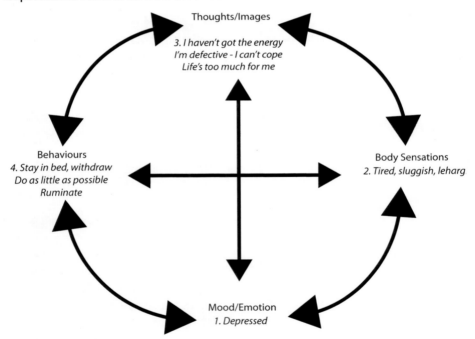

Low energy hot cross bun

If we start with the depression (1), this is the source of all that's going on here, but you don't need me to tell you that. This gives rise to the physical symptoms of tiredness and lethargy (2), which make you feel like you haven't got any energy, which is quite reasonably how you make sense of your physical sensations at (3). But being in a depressed state of mind, you probably go further and believe that this means that there's something intrinsically lacking in your character. This is a step or three too far, and it's just the depression that makes you feel like that. So let's look at it another way:

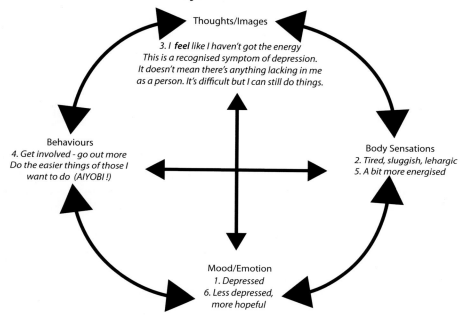

Thoughts/Images
*3. I **feel** like I haven't got the energy*
This is a recognised symptom of depression.
It doesn't mean there's anything lacking in me
as a person. It's difficult but I can still do things.

Behaviours
4. Get involved - go out more
Do the easier things of those I
want to do (AIYOBI !)

Body Sensations
2. Tired, sluggish, lehargic
5. A bit more energised

Mood/Emotion
1. Depressed
6. Less depressed,
more hopeful

Alternative energy hot cross bun

Here we start in the same place, with depressed mood (1). As before, this makes us feel tired, sluggish and lethargic at (2). But this time, we recognise it (3) as a symptom of the condition rather than the truth, and we don't assume that it means there's anything *lacking in me as a human being.*

Nonetheless, we acknowledge that it does make life more difficult. Even so, we can see that acting in our own best interests means (4) getting out and doing stuff as much as we can; but we don't expect ourselves to be firing on all cylinders just yet, so we just attempt the easier stuff to begin with. This in turn (5) makes us feel a bit more energised in our bodies and (6) a little more hopeful and less depressed.

What can we learn from this? In short, that doing stuff recharges our batteries – they've become flat from lack of use. And actually, we may be mains-powered after all if we can only learn how to plug in... and that is one of the functions of the 'nature' and 'creative' parts of the activity window.

Disciplines like chi gong are also about plugging in. More on this shortly, under *Doing and being*.

"I lack motivation."
'Motivation' is one of those strange concepts that you come across in self-help books, but almost nobody uses the term unless they're *struggling to do something they don't really want to do*.

Did you need motivation to eat your second chocolate ice cream (assuming you liked the first one)? If you're lacking motivation you need to ask yourself if you're really living the life you want. This may be causal in your depression (see below). But once depression has struck, *of course* you lack motivation. Motivation literally means 'moving power', and a lack of it is a symptom of depression, like the lack of energy above.

Motivation will increase *after* you do the thing that works for you (nature, social, creative, physical). This is particularly true of physical activity; most people find it hard to get themselves to the gym, but nearly everyone feels better afterwards from the production of endorphins that happens during physical exercise. So being put off activity by lack of motivation is one example of putting the cart before the horse – motivation increases *after* doing stuff, rather than being something you have to have in your pocket *before* you take part in the activity. So accept that because of Depression FM, you may and probably do *feel* unmotivated, and then, if you possibly can, do whatever it is anyway!

"I haven't got the confidence."
This is 'cart before horse #2'. Literally it means 'with faith' (*con* = *with*; *fidence* from Latin *fides*, meaning *faith*). With any new activity, of course you don't know whether you can do it or not. When you first learned to ride a bicycle, were you confident? No! How did you get to be confident? By doing it, and falling off sometimes. So again, confidence comes from doing, it's not something you have to have in your pocket beforehand.

If you've been depressed for a while, the chances are you've become used to 'duvet-diving', so everything 'out there' feels new. Also, *you* feel different; the body sensations that come with depression mean that you don't feel like the same person who used to feel confident about most things (if you did). So let's accept what has actually always been true: that you and the world do change from moment to moment; that no two situations are exactly alike, but that however you may be feeling, most routine tasks have enough in common for you to be able to cope with them well enough. And that your confidence *will* increase with activity.

"There's no point", and other ruminating

Are you a philosopher? If you are, then ignore this paragraph. But if you're not, when did you start asking about the point of things? This is another thinking error that didn't make it into the usually accepted list – I call it 'false geometry'. Why does everything have to have a point? What's wrong with circles or ovals? Or, as the Japanese have it, "You don't eat in order to shit."

Ruminating about the point of things is – yes, you guessed it – another symptom of depression; that's the propaganda radio station that's pumping this noxious stuff into your brain. Or to be more precise, **rumination is buying into and engaging with Depression FM as though it were a useful and intelligent source of information**. The branch of CBT known as Behavioural Activation correctly identifies ruminating as a behaviour. Like worrying, it's something you *do*. And, like worrying, it's something you can learn to *stop doing* (although, like other addictions, it can take some effort to free yourself from).

To do something 'for a point' is the opposite of doing something for its own sake. Yet, funnily enough, if we accuse someone of doing something for an ulterior motive, that's seen as a sign of insincerity! So how about the idea that to do something for its own sake, rather than for any 'point', is a *good* thing? Let's raise the flag for a more pointless life, at least some of the time; for appreciation of the taste and texture of whatever sensations are coming our way, and for the rediscovery of the life you had lost, perhaps years before you became depressed. When did you last dance? Or do anything else just for fun?[12]

"I won't enjoy the activity."

This is fortune-telling and all-or-nothing thinking. But you're right: you probably won't enjoy it *as much as* you used to before you got depressed. But how can we find out if you'll enjoy it at all? That's right – you've got to have a go, because you certainly won't get pleasure from it if you don't do it!

And there is another matter here, which is central to the problems we encounter in depression: this is the question of *how often we evaluate*. In depression, the tendency is not to be involved in the activity itself, but to be standing back from it, in our heads, trying to see if it's working.

---

12 In the traditional Christian story about creation, God creating the world in six days and then taking a day off sounds like a building project. In the present context, it might be more helpful instead to think of one of the Hindu versions: the unfolding, ever-changing universe *is* the continuing dance of Shiva Nataraja. Continuous play with no point except the joy of expression...

And in that mental stance, we cut ourselves off from having fun. What we need to do is the opposite: to stand back from the thoughts going through our minds and instead absorb ourselves; jump right into, the activity. The most obvious example I can think of is sex! Do we want to be, in the midst of all that activity, thinking, "Is this good enough? Am I having fun? What's the point of this?" Will thinking like this increase my pleasure, or that of my partner, come to that? I doubt it, although it might be a way of prolonging matters...

So decide, before doing an activity, when is the right time to evaluate how much enjoyment you got from it. Usually that will be immediately afterwards! And if you find your brain doing its automatic evaluation bit, just say to it, "Not now, I'll catch you later" and return your attention to your pleasurable activity, and particularly your *sensory* experience of it.

TURNIP TIME AND COMPASSIONATE MIND

You may be noticing a shift in emphasis towards mindfulness, putting your mind where the body is, getting absorbed in activity rather than thinking about it, and so on. And you'd be right, and we'll discuss this more in the section on doing and being. But first I just want to acknowledge the situation where the depression seems absolutely overwhelming, and despite reading all the previous tips, you still just can't get going today. When this happens, it's easy to start beating yourself up for not doing all the stuff I've said in the preceding paragraphs. Don't! Employ compassionate mind (see Chapter 10). If the depressive inertia is too much, it's too much! If you attack yourself about it, that will make it worse. You can have another go tomorrow, or later on today, but for now let's just sit quietly, somewhere peaceful. People sometimes give themselves a hard time about this: "just being a vegetable". Well, a client and I turned this around. On days when the depression was too bad, he did what we called 'turnip time': just sitting quietly – not ruminating, but watching his breathing. He couldn't find the energy sometimes to do stuff, but would sit with his dogs and practise being a 'conscious turnip', till the energy came back. And it always does come back, eventually...

DOING AND BEING – *recurrent depression and mindfulness*

On the behavioural side, we could see the treatment for depression as having two stages: stage one, which is what we have been talking about, could be summed up in the phrase "Don't just sit there; do something" (though certainly not in the punitive tone that seems to come with that statement).

Stage two is the opposite: once we're up and running again, we need to hear, "Don't just do something; sit there!" Because *doing* is only half the story. And in fact, as the authors of *The Mindful Way Through Depression* (Williams, Teasdale, Segal and Kabat-Zinn) have expressed so eloquently, it is this *doing* mode of mind that can actually make depression worse. In an effort to solve the problem of sadness or other emotions that we don't like – for perfectly understandable reasons – 'boot camp mind' by trying to beat us into a more 'desirable' state, ends up confirming the idea that I'm not OK as I am, and thus keeps the depression in place.

So doing mode is great when we are talking about real action in the world: genuine threats to be avoided on the one hand, and helpful experiences to be gained on the other. But the inner world is not like this, and we treat it so at our peril. To put it simply: if you're depressed, keep doing mode for physical actions in the world – exercising, making some food, cleaning up, going for a walk etc., and as much as possible, stick with being (or non-doing mode) when it comes to your mind, unless it's a really clear problem-solving situation, like planning a train journey.

Of course if our backgrounds contain serial memories of unpleasant emotion, it is not surprising that we have a tendency to *experiential avoidance*. In a metaphor reminiscent of Depression FM, Williams et al. remark, "Who wouldn't tune out feelings and body sensations if the news on this frequency had been too unpleasant too often?"

So (they ask), how can we tune back in without going even further down? Some of the things that may help us have been outlined in the generic part of the book. To recap, the first is to remember that we are *not* our thoughts – look back over the fridge, furniture and sky/cloud metaphors in Chapter 3. Because of this, we do not need to *buy into* their contents. Rather, we can treat them as unpleasant emotional weather – we don't have to *like* them, but there is nothing to be done about it; it's not in our control. Instead, it makes more sense to treat this unpleasant emotion as a sign of something that is hurting; an unhappy child in the nursery of our thoughts and feelings who needs comforting. Using the practice of mindful meditation, we can learn first to tolerate, and then to engage in a different way with these difficult parts.

Perhaps by focusing our breathing on, or even speaking directly (using the Big Mind process or the Gestalt empty chair technique) to these unheard, wailing 'painfulnesses', they can become reabsorbed into the society of our psyche. And in learning to turn towards the difficult (as there is no longer any good reason not to), we are changing the programming of a lifetime, and reducing the chances of relapsing.

In addition to awareness pure and simple, we have two further allies to make this turning towards easier: compassionate mind and our bodies. If we have been paralysed by depression and unable to do what we think we 'ought' to, we probably feel ashamed. This is a sign that the voice of the self-critic has started up. This is another version of the same loop we were just talking about. Paul Gilbert talks about this in terms of three different emotional systems in the brain, which we can paraphrase as threat, incentive and self-soothing.

If an unpleasant emotion starts up, we feel under attack, just as if we were being threatened by some predator from outside. In fact, the *amygdala*, the part of the old brain that is in charge of threat responses, doesn't know the difference between inside and outside threats. It just presses the button that sends us into fight-and-flight (see the 'panic lizard' in Chapter 16). Then we are on a war footing, trying to protect ourselves against the enemy. The critic starts up. But where is the enemy? *Inside.* Help! Of course if the enemy were outside it might be a different story. We could take some action and repel it. But we can't. This is where critical thinking has volunteered for a job it can't do. The critic becomes the *self-critic*. And the effect of the self-critic is to compound the original attack, and we wilt in shame underneath it.

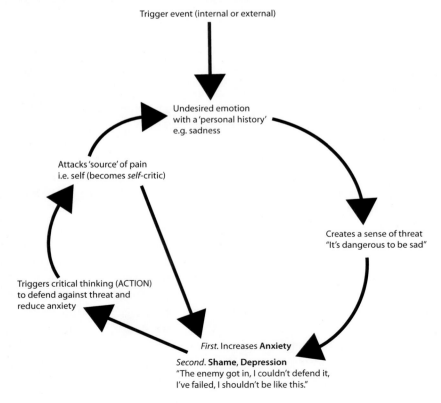

Trigger event (internal or external)

Undesired emotion with a 'personal history' e.g. sadness

Attacks 'source' of pain i.e. self (becomes *self*-critic)

Creates a sense of threat "It's dangerous to be sad"

Triggers critical thinking (ACTION) to defend against threat and reduce anxiety

First. Increases **Anxiety**

Second. **Shame, Depression** "The enemy got in, I couldn't defend it, I've failed, I shouldn't be like this."

This is a sign that the wrong system has been activated. In our society, unfortunately, we are mostly operating on two (*threat* and *incentive*) out of the three systems. We operate instinctually (*old mind/brain* in Gilbert's way of talking) in areas of anger and fear, while the learning (*new mind/brain*) is all about action and achievement. Of course, action is fine when there is a problem that can be solved by action, and as we have seen, that does have its part to play in combating depression (activity scheduling; activity window), but where the threat is not one that can be dealt with by doing, then any *attempt* at doing will simply exacerbate the problem, and as the strategy fails, the self-critic will get activated.

So while, to get out of depression, the organism needs to be activated (doing), that needs to be in the spirit of AIYOBI! And instead of self-critical thinking, the other ***self-soothing*** system needs to get activated. This is the way a baby feels in its mother's arms when absolutely everything is OK. Not surprisingly, those who didn't have this experience at all or very often as children may find it harder to access this state. Fortunately you can overcome these historical difficulties by employing the techniques we talked about in Chapter 10. So activate your perfect nurturer, tune in to your compassion satellite or Big Heart, and get it going – even if for the moment you don't believe you deserve it! It's OK – you're a fully paid-up member of the human race, and we're all allowed to activate our self-soothing systems.

Rights

An anarchist friend said to me long ago, "Dheeresh, do you know what you've got to do to claim your full human rights?"
"No," I answered.
"Breathe," he replied.

So now that your compassionate self, your individual version of boundless compassion, is at least somewhere in the picture, how are you going to be?

There are lots of techniques and systems available to help you with being. Because of our society's preoccupation with achievement, most of them come from other cultures further east (e.g. meditation, yoga, tai chi, chi gong), or sometimes further west (e.g. Native American shamanism). Occasionally, Christian traditions of contemplation (or *recollection* = remembering = mindfulness) have been maintained in the world, rather than just in the cloisters. Creative pursuits, another way into being mode, are more easily found.

When we do an exercise in the mindfulness programme[13] where people describe what they found pleasant in the preceding week, what almost always come out are not examples of achievement, but times of *connection*. Normally in depression we don't feel connected, because of the sense of threat. We are just cut off; isolated in our own seemingly endless suffering. We need to learn how to plug back in to the mains. No, not literally – that really would be unhelpful – but the 'mains' of life itself. In the Far East this is described as *chi*, the energy we're all made of; that everything is made of. *Élan vital*, 'life energy', is the western way of saying it. Most of us only get as far as trying to somehow satisfy ourselves (=fill ourselves up from others) in relationship, which of course rarely (if ever) works. Paradoxically, it is only when we discover that there is no scarcity of this 'juice'; that it is readily available to anyone who learns how to plug in (using meditation, chi gong, yoga etc.), that our relationships become less strained: "To those that have, shall it be given."

And of course in the end, or hopefully before, we discover that we are *nothing but* 'it'- identical with the universe, if you like. Still, the minds and bodies benefit from the practice of meditation, chi gong, yoga etc., even if there is no longer anything to 'get'.

The Daily Activity Diary is a way of helping you; reminding you to take time to reconnect, and scheduling in times and places to make sure it happens. It's like activity schedule meets pleasant events calendar, but the emphasis is straightforwardly on connection – doing what makes you feel connected, and trying to make sure you're there at the time!

WHAT ABOUT THE THERAPY? *What don't I want to look at (and not forcing yourself)*

So far, much of what we have covered in this chapter is not what people think of as psychotherapy for depression. In fact, some third wave CBT approaches (Behavioural Activation; Acceptance and Commitment Therapy) have thrown out dealing with the content altogether, and have some pretty convincing statistics to back up their case. But these approaches are new, and I suspect that while they may work well for some, in time we may notice a tendency to relapse if the problem that was at the heart of the onset of depression is not addressed.

For this reason, I think it is still helpful to do some work of a conventional CBT nature on the contents of the depression. However, this can only happen once the activity level is back up and running (or at least

13 The 'pleasant events calendar'.

walking). And it is important to do the work in the context of activity scheduling – this is serious mastery stuff, and needs to be balanced (I would say at least 2:1) in favour of pleasure through pleasurable or 'plugging-in' activities. So for every hour you spend on doing the ABCs or schema work, spend at least two doing good stuff for yourself.

Because otherwise, in ignoring the content of the depression altogether, we may be doing a disservice to our own intelligence. We did not *initially* become depressed for no reason. Something made the fuse blow, or sent us to the back of the cave. So it may be time to look again at the wiring, or whether we are overloading the circuits. And for this, we may need to rejig the rules – it's almost always about rules. So when your mood level is tolerable, look again at the cognitive work in the generic part of the book (Chapters 3–7), in particular taking a compassionate look at your own individual formulation.

If you don't have to keep disproving your core beliefs (unlovable/ worthless/bad/weak), then maybe you don't need to please others, or achieve hugely, or be an angel 24/7. So then, in the spirit of AIYOBI! you don't have to **run yourself ragged chasing unsustainable ways of being.**

You can be nice to others because you want to – not because you think you're unlovable and can't get your 'juice' any other way, but rather out of the natural overflowing of your teapot. Not because you think you'll be condemned to hell if you don't. (You were in hell, remember?) You can achieve because it's fun, but not achieving doesn't make you worthless.

If it seems helpful, see if you can identify (but *only if you can do it in a compassionate and self-forgiving way*) what the glitch was in your life that led to you becoming depressed in the first place – **but without ruminating!** It may not have been an external trigger, but some critical incident in terms of your own meaning system that meant you had failed in some way to live up to some misbegotten rule.

Actually, the rule wasn't really misbegotten. It probably worked very well when you were five, seven or whatever. So validate it for then, but when you're reflecting on whether or not to take a certain course of action in the present, look to see whether it is in accord with the old or the new model – and of course I suggest going with the new model – from now on. That new model which values being compassionate towards the self, and Acts In Your Own Best Interests, which of course involves naturally radiating out good stuff to others too! And it also means that sometimes you'll have the feelings of sad, angry, anxious, disgusted – they're all part of your emotional toolkit – *without that experience needing to drop you back into depression*, because you know that, as you're so much more than your mind-contents, you can *allow* yourself to feel those feelings, and won't need to flee from them in a wild frenzy of over-achievement, people-pleasing or whatever. So the short-circuit mechanism won't need to cut in and give you depression to stop you frying altogether.

And remember that living by the new model won't become the default option straight away – to start with, most of life will seem like a conscious behavioural experiment (or a series of them): rather effortful, 'unnatural' and deliberate.

Few people actually are glad they've had depression. But many have come as far as to admit that they couldn't have sustained the life they were leading, that depression was the necessary shutdown that *had to happen*, and that the combination of CBT and mindfulness and Big Mind techniques has led to them having a richer life than they ever thought possible. I hope that (perhaps with the help of this book) this happens for you too.

Further reading

Mark Williams, Zindel Segal, John Teasdale and Jon Kabat-Zinn (2007) *The Mindful Way Through Depression*, Guilford
Paul Gilbert (2009) *Overcoming Depression* (third edition), Constable Robinson
David Veale and Rob Willson (2007) *Manage Your Mood*, Constable Robinson
Dennis Greenberger and Christine Padesky (1995) *Mind Over Mood*, Guilford

Daily Activity Schedule and Presence Gauge
DAY:

Time	Event or Activity (What was I doing?)	Sense of mastery or achievement (M = 0-10)	Sense of pleasure (P = 0-10)	Which senses? Did I see, hear, smell, taste, touch or think about it?	Creative? Social? Physical? Nature? (C, P, S or N?)	Was I there in my body as it was happening? (yes, no, a bit)	What do I think or feel about it now?
4 - 7am							
7 - 9am							
9 -11am							
11am - 12noon							
12 noon - 2pm							
2 - 4pm							
4 - 6pm							
6 - 8pm							
8 -10pm							
10pm - 12midnight							
12midnight - 4am							

189

CHAPTER 14: LOW SELF-ESTEEM

Chariot story – Big I, Little I – The self-critic – The department store revisited – Self-concept inventory – Personal self, ego, no-self and Big Mind

Depression and low self-esteem are often bedfellows – they both induce us to stay under the covers sometimes. But it is of course possible to have low self-esteem without having depression. And to use Melanie Fennell's phrase, the person with low self-esteem just does whatever they have to do to avoid the 'bottom line' of worthlessness, unlovability or whatever. And if you can keep doing that, maybe you can stay out of major depression, although the ongoing, underlying low mood known to psychologists as *dysthymia* is probably no stranger to you. And how much fun do you have?

To me, the most helpful explanation of the problem is the one put forward by Windy Dryden (a Rational Emotive Behaviour Therapist) and mentioned in Chapter 10; namely that our problem stems largely from *trying to measure ourselves as a whole*. Or to put it another way, trying to measure our *self* as a whole.

In short, to esteem means to measure (think *estimate*). So we need to consider whether what we are dealing with is a measurable entity. But what are we dealing with?

The Chariot Story (paraphrased from 'The Questions of King Milinda')

Alexander the Great conquered lands far beyond his native Macedonia. In fact his empire extended East as far as North India. But Alexander – maybe feeling homesick – left one of his senior generals in charge of this portion of his realm. This general was Menander; we can deduce that he was an educated man, perhaps in the 'philosopher-king' mould. In the Buddhist records of the time, there is a record of a series of debates between Menander (known to the Buddhists as Milinda) and a Buddhist monk called Nagasena. Perhaps the most famous is the interaction regarding the nature and existence of the self, which went something like this:

Nagasena: "I see you came in a fine chariot today."
Menander: "This is true..."
N: "Will you do one thing for me...? Could you detach the horses from the chariot?"
(Menander complies.)
N: "Now tell me, are these horses the chariot?"
M: "No, they're the horses."
N: "Thank you. Let's put them over there to one side... now, can you take the wheels off?"
(Again Menander complies.)
N: "So, are these wheels the chariot?
M: "No, they're the wheels."
N: "OK, put them over there with the horses."
And so on with the axles, the yoke and all the other parts of the chariot, until there is nothing left.
Nagasena feigns puzzlement: "I don't understand, where is the chariot, there doesn't seem to be anything here?"
In frustration Menander replies: "The chariot is what you get when you put all those bits together, put the horses on the front, and use it to go somewhere!"
"Just so with the self," responds Nagasena, "it is no more than an assemblage of arms, legs, liver, spleen, thoughts, feelings and so on. You give the whole lot a name and then you have what you call 'a self' – merely a conventional designation. No such thing as a self actually exists..."

So, if we agree with Nagasena, we can see that perhaps there isn't such a thing as a self. But don't take his word for it – can *you* find one? Look and see.

Leaving aside for the moment whether there is a self or not, I asserted before that to esteem means to measure; like in the term 'estimate'. If I want to measure how fast a car is going, I look at the speedometer, or, to measure how high a plane is flying, an altimeter (from the Latin *alter*, meaning high or deep). If something really exists, somebody can usually find a way to measure it, but have you ever seen a *self*ometer? Surely one would have been devised if such a thing were possible? Perhaps Nagasena is right after all, and there is nothing real we can call a self.

But there are lots of things *about* the self that we can measure: particular qualities or aspects, like how tall you are, or how much you weigh, or how fast you can run 100 metres, or how good you are at solving crossword puzzles. And there are other parts which are difficult if not impossible to measure, like how kind you are, or how much you enjoy the feeling of the wind on your cheeks, or how affected you are emotionally by news items or changes in atmospheric pressure. So different parts can sometimes be measured, and sometimes not, which brings us back to Windy Dryden's 'Big I, Little I'. Let's have another look at it:

```
IIIIIIIIIII
 IIIIIIIII
 IIIIIIIII
 IIIIIIIII
 IIIIIIIII
 IIIIIIIII
 IIIIIIIII
 IIIIIIIII
 IIIIIIIII
 IIIIIIIII
IIIIIIIIIIII
```

We notice there are lots of little Is. Perhaps in reality there are as many as we have whims or notions. Bear in mind also what we said about the origin of these: some are positively prehistoric; some are human, but really genetic programs about which we can do nothing, while many more were laid down in infancy when we didn't really have any power or influence over how we developed.

And of course at any given time there are some which are to the fore and some which are dormant, depending on the situation, your mood and which psychological patterns (or *schemas* or *modes*) have been activated.

If we are suffering from what we have come to call low self-esteem, that means we are doing one (or both) of two things:

1. We are probably measuring the self *as a whole* in a way that makes us feel bad – calling ourselves 'bad' or 'weak' or 'worthless' or 'unlovable'. Do these labels (remember *thinking errors*) sound familiar? What we're probably doing

is overemphasising our 'negative' qualities to the (ridiculous) point where we can't see the positive ones or redeeming factors. We're probably back in the land of core beliefs (see Chapter 7), but in any case, when you think about how little we had to do with the construction of how this brain works (as Paul Gilbert says, "We all just find ourselves here"), it seems ridiculous to blame yourself for any deficiencies. Instead, we need to cut ourselves some slack about the current state of play, and only try and *esteem* that which is *estimable*.

2. Although we may recognise intellectually that we are more than our negative sides or little Is – i.e. we know that we do have some positive qualities – somehow we have trouble when we try to access them. This is a *competing memory* problem. Somehow the dominant bits in our minds are all the stories about how bad, worthless or unlovable we are.

SELF-ACCEPTANCE

But even recognising that this may be the case means we've now made one step in the right direction: we're thinking about measuring our qualities, rather than ourselves as a whole. This is definitely a step towards *self-acceptance*, which is at the heart, psychologically speaking, of being comfortable in your own skin. We may not be good at maths, but we can run fast. Or we may not be able to run fast, but we're good at maths. Either way, if we want to do something about the thing we're not good at, and because *it doesn't represent our value as a human being*, we can simply take care of it – go training, whether in evening classes in the case of maths, or running around the track. Does doing this make us a 'better' person? No, just better at maths or running.

But it is important to understand why we do this – this *mistaking the part for the whole*, which ends up causing us so much trouble. It is probably best understood by thinking about what happens if we have got injured physically: suppose we have fallen over and badly bruised our arm. Physically, the sore arm seems to occupy all of our consciousness. (I suppose this is so that we're careful not to bump into things and injure it further.) So the one-tenth or so of our physical mass occupies nine-tenths of our awareness, because there's something wrong and we need to prevent further injury. I suggest that it's just the same with mental stuff we're not happy about: because we perceive it as being wrong or damaged, it occupies more of our awareness, sometimes to the point where it seems to count as the whole.

COMPARISON

Even when we have let go of our tendency to measure our self as a whole, and only work on 'improving' particular skills or aspects of our lives, there is still another issue that can get in the way of us feeling OK about who we are, and that is the odious matter of *comparison:*

- "Even though I worked really hard on that paper, and I know for a fact that Joe was out partying all last week, he still got a better mark than me."
- "I've been running every day this year, but Sarah, who hardly ever trains and I know eats junk food most nights, still came in 20 minutes ahead of me in the marathon – and she's five years older!"

Yes, it's true – life isn't fair (and the only real 'fair' is probably the one with roundabouts), but let's look at what that really means. What I think it means is that there is really no level playing field; no identical starting line from which we can measure our achievements. In some ways this is obvious: living in the western world I'm more likely to have had enough to eat in my childhood, whereas someone born in another part of the world may have been deficient in certain nutrients when they were growing up which will have seriously affected their development. But even within individual societies there are castes or classes; one gender or colour is favoured over another, so that if you're the 'wrong' gender or colour, it is harder to get to the same place in terms of work or status.

And even putting aside social and cultural inequalities for the moment, there are individual differences, even at birth. This seems obvious in cases of learning difficulties or disability, but minor differences in aptitude or temperament at a young age may translate into huge variation by adulthood.

Athletics

I was never particularly athletic at school. It would have been easy to become entirely disillusioned with physical pursuits altogether, but for one innovation that was introduced by our relatively progressive sports teachers. Instead of focusing always on the interpersonally competitive, we were invited to compete with ourselves, to keep records of our times and achievements in running, high jump, long jump, shot or whatever; to pay no heed at all to anyone else's, but simply to try to improve our own against our previous best. And doing this would, of course, also bring more encouragement from the sports teachers.

So we really cannot compare ourselves with another and have it mean anything about how 'well' we've done – only how well we can perform the particular task in relation to another.

However, it is useful to understand something of why we might be doing this comparison, even if it seems unhelpful in your life right now. I think this is another leftover from the prehistoric age, when of course this model of the human being that we are currently running was (more or less) finalised. Imagine you are comparing yourself with a former school classmate who seems to have got on much further than you career-wise. You feel envious, and bring yourself down by comparing your achievements to his. I think that what is sometimes being replayed here is the old caveman drama, wherein he who can slaughter the most gazelles gets the girl(s). In short, this may be a primitive program that has little if any use in 21st century life. But that doesn't mean it should be ignored! Like any other part, it is helpful to acknowledge it and thank it for its contribution.

And I am not saying we shouldn't try to do better at those things we wish to do better in, but please don't make it an indicator of your worth as a whole. This brings us back to the 'newborn baby' question:

Newborn Baby

You are in a public building with a number of other people. There is also a newborn baby in its carry-cot. Nobody seems to know where it came from. What can it achieve, this newborn baby? Not much – it can drink milk, make some noise, fill its nappy. Of course, it may achieve something in the future, but it may not, or it may turn out to be a serial murderer! Nobody knows. Suddenly the fire alarm goes off, and you have to evacuate the building. Do you leave the baby behind? After all, it can't achieve much…

Well, I'm guessing you don't! But if you believe you should take the baby with you, then what that means to me is that you already know that when it comes down to it, to matters of life and death, human worth is not based on achievement. Otherwise you'd leave the baby behind – after all it might slow you down. You already know that human worth is there first.

So while I'm not decrying achievement, it is, in a sense, an optional extra to human existence. We don't have to do anything – except breathe – to claim our full human rights. Like we said before, firemen don't ask for CVs when they're rescuing people from burning buildings. But another question about low self-esteem is where these horrible views of the self come from. We can point to our upbringing, or school or anything else in the past, but we hear the comments in the present, don't we?

This is the story of the self-critic. Sometimes this seems to be a particular voice from the past. When you get down on yourself and start calling yourself names, does it sound like anyone in particular? If it does, a really useful strategy is simply to say, "Hello Dad/Mum/whoever – I don't need your comments right now, but thank you for your contribution." Often, however, it's more a composite entity, put together over years from all the negative comments that ever hurt you and came from people who mattered to you.

McKay and Fanning, in their book *Self-Esteem*, suggest keeping a diary of critical comments to try and find out what their purpose is:

Critical comment	Helps me think, do or avoid

We may find that the self-critic has a protective role – if it puts you off attempting something difficult, you may avoid the risk of failure. But by becoming aware that it is the self-critic speaking, you can decide for yourself whether you wish to take the risk anyway (AIYOBI!).

Another way of working with the self-critic is to use Empty Chair, Voice Dialogue or the Big Mind process. That way you can get it from the horse's mouth, so to speak. Particularly helpful is to explore different stages of the self-critic: the immature self-critic (often vindictive), the mature or wise self-critic (genuinely in the employ of the protector – this critic can give you good reviews as well as bad), or have you suppressed the self-critic and s/he's operating undercover? In which case, speak to the *disowned* self-critic.

On a daily basis, remember that the antidote to an overactive self-critic is compassionate mind, or the perfect nurturer (see Chapter 10). As an experiment, try extending the compassion to the self-critic him- or herself. Because s/he has a job to do as well (as the Buddha saw with Mara – see story on p125)

My self-critic gets me up in the morning early to write this book. ("Out of bed, you lazy bastard!") So if you don't like it, blame him...

But all this theory, as ever, only goes so far. We need to translate it into action (or non-action) in the world. To do this we need to think about which of the little Is need developing. Because the chances are that our self-critical thoughts may be preventing us from having the experiences we would like to be having ('you don't deserve it, you're worthless' etc.).

For the problems around low self-esteem lie between two polarities: at one end, you're actually having a perfectly good life, but your appreciation of it is coloured by your sense of being in one way or another not good enough. At the other end, it may be that *because* you feel not-good-enough in one way or another, you are not getting out there and having the life you want.

One metaphor that has been useful to some is that of the pot-plant: if you are trying to grow a plant and you want it to flourish, what nutrients do you need to put in it? What about your life? Are you feeding in the right nutrients for a balanced life? Think of the activity window, or if you like, let us revisit the department store, this time to check that all the departments we want are activated.

NATURE	SOCIAL
CREATIVE	PHYSICAL

So once again, what are the departments in your life? What are the dreams that you haven't fulfilled yet? Do you still want to? Have you forgotten what they were? Often people who have for a long time been living lives that appear to have been dominated by others' needs or circumstances (like mothers, for example) have lost sight of what it was they wanted to do or be. Think back to what you liked doing when you were little. Did you dance? Paint? Sing? If you're not sure where to start, try the activity window and build from there. Or, like we did in the schema section in Chapter 7, just enumerate the departments of your life, both current and dormant, and see if there are any neglected areas that you need to reawaken for your own sanity. Here is a possible framework:

Department Store

Family (immediate)	Relationship	Work	Health & appearance	Outdoor pursuits (walking, gardening)
Sexuality	Family (extended)	Days out	Financial	Housework & maintenance
Arts (doing): painting, dance, music etc.	Making or fixing things	Spiritual or religious	Academic	Holidays
Social/friends	Arts (visiting galleries, theatre, concerts)	Political involvement	Social action/ volunteering	Sports/ physical exercise

I am not implying that all of these departments should be active at any given time; but are there areas that you care about that you are not doing? It may be that what you need to do at this point is put this book down and go and instigate some of these activities. "Get a life", as they say.

OK, now it's minutes or months later and you've got more of a balanced life, but you're stuck on the other pole of low self-esteem: you're evaluating your worth/contribution etc. as less than it really is. In other words, you're *doing the stuff* (good), but you're not *getting the juice* (bad). Of course, much in this book has already addressed these issues, e.g. sense of being plugged in (Chapter 8), mindfulness (Chapter 9), compassionate mind (Chapter 10), but here is where we need to pick up the idea we mentioned at the beginning of the chapter: the competing memories problem.

COMET

We definitely need to do something about regaining access to those little Is, or the modes that are OK; that do work well and allow us to feel good about ourselves, but somehow we've lost touch with them. One kind of CBT that does this is called Competitive Memory Training or COMET.

Instead of focusing on the negative view of yourself, write some little stories or vignettes about the good experiences you had that show your useful qualities. It's like a positive log, but with more detail. And just as it is important to look at your positive log regularly to remind yourself, so you can set aside some time – daily is good – to focus on these stories.

If you remember, in the section on Compassionate Mind we explored how it is important not just to think about what your perfect nurturer is saying, but also how it feels to be hearing it, and any other sense-memory associations (sight, smell etc.). So it is with this technique: the more channels you can activate, the better chances you will have of finding the right memory and having the effects of that 'stick'. So when you're re-reading these stories to yourself, make sure you sit (or stand) in a posture that feels good: upright; alert; alive. If you like, play some music that reminds you of yourself in positive modes; that has links to times when you really succeeded or felt loved or appreciated.

PUTTING IT ALL TOGETHER

So let's put together the two bits – we can think of them as 'getting a life' and 'appreciating the life you've got' – in an exercise adapted from McKay and Fanning's *Self-Esteem*, called the 'self-concept inventory'. First, take the personalised department store you've just done (or use the version at the back of the book).

Now, in each box, write words or phrases about how you think you are in that department of your life. Look at what you've written! Some, I hope, will be positive; some neutral (under appearance, for example, you might have put your height in inches or centimetres – it's neither good nor bad, just a fact); and if you're reading this chapter, there are probably some negatives; some things you don't like. So if you are not as tall as you'd like to be, you might be calling yourself a 'short-arse'. That's not a fact, that's a negative. Try to make sure you have some of each in each box: at least one positive, one negative and one neutral.

Dealing with negative statements

The next thing to do is to look at the negatives. After all, we all have aspects of ourselves we don't like – that's normal – but we may be seeing these negatives – thanks, perhaps, to an overly-enthusiastic self-critic – in a more extreme way than is useful. So in the next three-column table, re-evaluate the negatives. Use whatever works – go back to the thinking errors and the four kinds of disputing (Chapter 4); try to use objective rather than pejorative or 'self-downing' language and expose the overgeneralising that you're doing by using *negative assertion* ("I may be two or three inches shorter than I'd like to be, but I didn't have any choice in this, and it doesn't make me a runt or a short-arse, or mean that my contribution is any less than those of tall people, or that I'm less lovable") and put in exceptions ("I may not be good at fixing things – you don't have to be good at everything – but those shelves I put up six months ago are more-or-less straight and still holding the books, which for me is quite an achievement"), and also intentions for change that are manageable.

Use the chart on the next page to record some of your own negative statements and how these might be reframed.

Area of life	Negative view	Reframed negative view
Family	I'm a lousy parent	I've been working long hours recently, so I haven't spent as much time with the kids as I'd like. But I'm really there for them at the weekends, and they certainly enjoy being with me. But I do want to work less so I can spend more time with them.

ACCENTUATING THE POSITIVES

Next, we need to go back and look at the positive comments you put in the first 'store'. Are you sure you've put them all in? Think of compliments you've been paid; little successes of whatever kind – which boxes do they go in? *Please don't discount the positive!* Do a survey amongst your friends, and find out what they like about you. I know that in the UK this is very unusual, but you'll be surprised by how much your friends like doing this (after all, they're not having to say anything positive about themselves!). Another way of finding hidden positives is to think – like we did with the unlovability schema in Chapter 7 – about the things you admire in others. This is a good exercise to do with a close friend; you can discuss each other's positive points together. Who are your heroes? They don't have to be real, just inspiring! Almost certainly, if you really admire someone you probably have some of their qualities in yourself – although you may not realise it, and albeit to a lesser extent. But it often takes a friend to see that.

Now use the positive log form, preferably every day for the next year at least, to gather more evidence (from past and present) for the truth of these positives, and/or use the COMET techniques: writing the vignettes, re-accessing those positive times and events in your life and training yourself to bring them to the fore with increasing ease.

Some time later you can redo the department store. Replace the negatives with the reframed negatives; add in the new positives and keep the neutral, factual observations as they are. Now you have a more accurate and helpful description of who you are. You can use this as a corrective when you start to think badly of yourself, or to be more precise, when the self-critic has conned you into thinking that what s/he says is true. It's helpful too as a baseline when doing ABCs to help you with the 'pantomime' disputes (see Chapter 4). But in a way the key insight is the awareness that *these are all parts* of the whole and should not be mistaken for the self – why identify with a particular part as being you? More helpful to see yourself as the one who is aware of all these parts, or even the awareness itself...

New department store
(Draw your own or use the blank one in the back of the book if you need more space.)

Department Store

Family (immediate)	Relationship	Work	Health & appearance	Outdoor pursuits (walking, gardening)
Sexuality	Family (extended)	Days out	Financial	Housework & maintenance
Arts (doing): painting, dance, music etc.	Making or fixing things	Spiritual or religious	Academic	Holidays
Social/friends	Arts (visiting galleries, theatre, concerts)	Political involvement	Social action/ volunteering	Sports/ physical exercise

PERFECTIONISM

This brings us to another aspect of low self-esteem; the curse of perfectionism. Perhaps because we think that fundamentally we're not good enough, we try to compensate through achievement. We can see it as another aspect of our primitive reaction to threat, like dogs peeing on lampposts – we have to make our mark and try to stake our territory!

Some would see that as a futile gesture in the face of impermanence and death. But naturally, a pattern of extreme effort in relation to our study or work performance can yield both fruitful *and* damaging results. To examine how that works in your case, use the cost-benefit analysis that we looked at in Chapter 7.

There is something of a debate among psychologists as to whether there is such a thing as healthy perfectionism. If there were, it would relate to the pursuit of valued goals and the fulfilment of your potential, so that you got what you wanted written on your tombstone. (Hopefully it would not also say *Never had any time for his family, and was so busy he forgot how to have fun*.) But there are people who (mistakenly or not) do feel that they are on a mission. If you are one of those, but you don't want to fall down the pit of perfectionism, then I have some suggestions. Apart from the obvious difficulties (overwork, lack of sleep, worrying, lack of relaxation or downtime), there are three major pitfalls to perfectionism, and they all relate to evaluation:

1. By whom am I being evaluated?
If your perfectionism has a people-pleasing element to it (you are trying to achieve in order to be loved or respected, rather than to prove your worth to yourself), then there is a tendency to hand over the evaluation of your work to others: "It's only good enough if Joe says so." Yet others vary, and while good feedback is obviously nice, the cliché "You can't please all the people all of the time" is relevant here. Also the fable about the man, his son and the donkey (from Aesop, see below). So while feedback from others can often give valuable insights, in the end it has to be your call as to whether a piece of work is good enough or not.

2. How often am I being evaluated?
Perfectionists nearly always spend too much time evaluating. Ironically, this takes time and energy away from whatever you're supposed to be engaged in. Remember the exclamation mark from PACER! (Chapter 1). Decide beforehand how often you are going to evaluate, and if you find yourself thinking about how well or badly it's going during the process, simply recognise it as an evaluation thought (a sort of mental indigestion) and return your attention to the task in hand. Actually, frequent checking of how you're doing is a characteristic of some people's *relapse signature* into depression, so if you notice it happening a lot, and you think you might be vulnerable in this way, take appropriate action (activity scheduling/ window; AIYOBI!; mindfulness practice).

3. Measures: against what am I being evaluated?
How do you know what is good enough? How can 'good enough' be good enough? I suggest a two-level grading here. Of course you don't want to sell yourself short, but you also don't want to blow a gasket. So set yourself a target you would really like to go for as your ideal; as a way of setting your sights and creating a vision that would be the perfect expression of what you seek to achieve. Give *seeking mind* full rein! But have a second mark that is much more easily achievable, probably with one hand tied behind your back if you had to. Now *this* is the one that is the good enough benchmark,

which you will regularly achieve even in the bad times. *Anything above this deserves fulsome credit!*

Going to market (from Aesop's Fables - ca 620 and 560 BCE)

A man was taking his donkey to sell at the market, accompanied by his son. It was a sunny day, and they were walking along quite happily, the boy riding the donkey. Some bystanders, noticing this arrangement, shouted to the boy, "Don't you have any respect? Your poor father, working all these years, having to walk, while you behave like a king riding the donkey". They shrugged their shoulders, and changed places accordingly, the father riding the donkey, while the son walked in front.

A little while later, they came across another group of passers-by, who also shouted out at them,

"What's with this donkey abuse? As if the donkey hasn't worked hard enough all his life, and there you are, a man of considerable weight, squashing him into the ground?"

They became increasingly flustered, trying different permutations as the onlookers dictated; in the end the man had the donkey across his shoulders with the boy on top!

So now you have some principles for dealing with low self-esteem:

1. Don't judge the self as a whole.
2. Don't automatically accept the views of the self-critic – s/he has an agenda!
3. Recognising this, if you want to work on some parts of yourself, then fine!
4. Use COMET/positive log regularly to access positive memories and keep them to the fore.
5. Your worth is not dependent on achievement (human worth is innate), so...
6. Be compassionate to yourself, unconditionally!
7. But if you *are* on a mission, make sure *you* are in charge of evaluation.

The Way

To study the Buddha way is to study the self
To study the self is to forget the self
To forget the self is to be enlightened by all things

Dogen Zenji

Further reading:

Matthew McKay and Patrick Fanning (1996) *Self-Esteem*, New Harbinger Publications
Melanie Fennell (1999) *Overcoming Low Self-Esteem* and (2006) *Overcoming Low Self-Esteem Self-Help Course* (three volumes), Constable Robinson
Windy Dryden (1998) *Developing Self-Acceptance*, Wiley
Tara Brach (2004) *Radical Acceptance*, Bantam Books
Christopher K. Germer (2009) *The Mindful Path to Self-Compassion*, Guilford

CHAPTER 15: BIPOLAR AFFECTIVE DISORDER (AND MOOD SWINGS)

Tackling unhelpful thoughts – The faulty feelometer – Two-list therapy – Rating moods – Acting counter-intuitively – Mindfulness

Bipolar affective disorder – which used to be called 'manic depression' – is a biologically-driven disorder which can cause great distress, both in the depressed phase and also as a consequence of some of the unhelpful things that the person suffering from the condition does during the 'up' phase.

There is also a version of this disorder (bipolar 2) which still has the cyclical element, but lacks the extreme manic 'up' states. If you have been given a diagnosis of bipolar affective disorder, it is unlikely that simply reading a self-help book by itself is going to sort you out! But using this book with the help of a medical or mental health professional may be of some help, and see the specialist self-help material recommended at the end of the chapter.

Naturally people with bipolar aren't different in *type* from the rest of us, and there may be some of you reading this whose moods are more up and down than you would like, but who would not qualify for a diagnosis of bipolar disorder. Hopefully you too will find these strategies helpful. Essentially only dead people have no variation in mood, but it is a matter of *how much* the mood swings as to whether it's a problem.

Whether you suffer from bipolar 1 or 2, or just mood swings, all the advice in Chapter 13 relating to unipolar depression applies to you too when you're in the 'down' part of the cycle, particularly the behavioural stuff (activity scheduling, activity window, Act In Your Own Best Interests (AIYOBI!)).

Of course, if you are in the 'up' phase the strategies need to be different. In that part of the cycle, *rational* mind (or even anxiety) can be your friend, helping you to head off your more extreme plans, ambitions and whims. Here I reproduce a table from Jan Scott's *Overcoming Mood Swings* to give you a flavour of the sort of corrective thinking needed:

The two-column technique for tackling unhelpful thoughts when high

My idea: Give up work and use the money I get on leaving to buy a farm	
Reasons - *for acting on my idea* (benefits to me, constructive aspects, gains)	**Reasons** - *against acting on my idea* (risk of harm to others, destructive aspects, losses)
I've always loved the idea of living in the country	My wife prefers living in cities
	The children would have to leave school in the middle of their studies
	My wife and children would leave all their friends behind
I can learn a whole new set of skills and become a farmer	I don't know the first thing about running a farm
	There may be tensions at home. My wife would also have to learn new skills. If she doesn't want to do this, it will damage our relationship.
	My wife and children might not agree to move to the country
	Farming is actually a very busy job and some tasks have to be done at set times, so I may have less freedom than I think
I'll be able to do what I want, I'll be my own boss and make lots of money for my family	Lots of people are struggling to make money in farming
	The thing I like best about the countryside is visiting it; that doesn't mean I would enjoy working there
Conclusion: I still think I want to live in the country, but I may not actually want to run a farm. Use 48-hour delay and contact Ruth and Mark (third-party advice).	

Of course this is just one example, and all the cognitive and behavioural strategies (see Chapters 2–5) can be brought into play according to the nature of the specific problems you encounter.

In his otherwise excellent TV programme about bipolar disorder a few years ago, the actor and TV presenter Stephen Fry, who to his credit is open about being a bipolar sufferer himself, interviewed many sufferers from the condition that he knew, mostly in the world of the media. These were people who had been able to turn their manic phases to good use as creative expression. The majority of them said that if they could magic the condition away and become 'normal' they still wouldn't do it, because it had been so valuable to them creatively, and also they just loved the 'highs'. I want to say **"Beware!"** Most people I have worked with would give their right arms to be free of this condition, because the highs are unmanageable and transient and get them into all kinds of trouble – overspending and sexual disinhibition, to name but two common problems – and can have disastrous consequences for family and relationships, not to mention health. And only a very small proportion of this group (like any other) actually 'make it' in the creative world.

What seems clear is that for many (if not all) sufferers, the higher the 'up' phase, the deeper the depression that follows it. So the CBT approach attempts to act as a moderating influence: if the peaks are lower, then the troughs are not so deep. But the difficulty with this approach is that it requires you to be *counter-intuitive*, because the way we feel like acting when we are 'up' – partying, staying up all night, going on wild spending sprees – is precisely the route to going even higher and wilder; possibly into psychosis, and then crashing into the pits of depression.

So we need to accept and remind ourselves that the reason we are in treatment for this problem is that our feelometer is out of order – like having a car with the speedometer on backwards – and so we have to use more objective guidelines for how to act, rather than doing as we feel. To carry on the car metaphor, if your speedo isn't working and you still have to drive, then you need to see how fast the trees are going by – some external guide – to get an idea of your actual speed. So you need to come back to AIYOBI! again. Never mind (for the moment) what I feel like doing – what's really going to be helpful?

TWO-LIST THERAPY

To start with, devise two lists of activities: one we can call *grounding* activities (i.e. those activities which, often quite literally, connect you to the earth: cleaning the toilet, weeding, mopping the floor and so on), and another which we could call *inspiring* activities (socialising, partying, listening to inspiring 'up' music, vigorous physical exercise and so on). Normally we tend to do things from the inspiring list when we feel good – i.e. 'up' – and the other grounding stuff perhaps only if we have to. However, given our faulty feelometer, *what we feel like doing at any given moment may be the worst thing for us*! So the strategy is simple if not easy:

1. Notice whether you are in the **up** or the **down** part of the cycle; and
2. Do activities from the *inspiring* list if you're **down**, and activities from the *grounding* list if you're **up**.

What we're trying to do here, boring though that may seem, is to use the midpoint, neither up nor down, as the place we're always trying to get back to. So make your list of inspiring and grounding pastimes in the box below.

Sometimes it will be about doing the same thing in a different way, e.g. exercise: when you are feeling 'up', the temptation will be to go for an all-out, full-on session at the gym. On the other hand, the thought of a long-distance cross-country jog probably doesn't appeal (no 'buzz'), so guess what you need to do? That's right – when you're *up*, do the cross-country; when you're *down*, do the vigorous session at the gym to burn off that depressive lethargy.

Grounding Activities	Inspiring Activities

Rating mood level

As we said, we want always to be veering towards the midpoint, so we need to have a more precise indicator of how we feel. After all, there are different levels of up or down. There are different scales you could use, but I suggest a -5 to +5 rating to emphasise the midpoint at 0. The person who has the best idea of what these different levels all feel like is of course you, but you may not have logged them systematically. It may take a while to build up a profile of these different mood levels, but be patient and log them in. That way you can build up an invaluable template that you can use as a reference to guide you.

Mood Index	Characteristics
+5	(ecstatic, totally uninhibited etc.)
+4	
+3	
+2	
+1	
0	(neutral, neither good nor bad)
-1	
-2	
-3	
-4	
-5	(suicidal, absolutely self-hating)

PUTTING THE TWO TOGETHER

Now go over the activities list. You will find that some activities are not absolutely grounding or absolutely inspiring, but somewhere between the two. You can draw a continuum from one to the other and put the activities somewhere along the line:

  Very Grounding Quite grounding Neutral Quite Inspiring Very Inspiring

Now to put the two together. In the next table, on the opposite page, you will see that we have arranged activities according to mood, so that the higher the mood, the lower or more grounding the activity and vice versa. So a +5 mood would require a very grounding activity, like cleaning the toilet, whereas a +3 mood would only demand a moderately grounding activity, like some gentle yoga, or gardening (but really getting your hands dirty, not making some grand plan for a horticultural makeover of the entire street!). On the other hand, a -3 score really needs you to get out there and talk to some people, while -5 (in theory) requires a really intense level of activity. But actually, anything above +3 or +4 or below -3 or -4 indicates that you should probably call whoever you see to get help, and you're unlikely to be following any advice of the sort given here. But if we can catch the process at an earlier or more moderate stage, hopefully this procedure can help you from becoming too extreme in either direction. As you become more skilled at doing it, you can be more creative by using a *range* of activities, as long as the *balance* comes out as a counterpoint to your score on the mood index. Remember, the focus should always be to get back to the level, even if that doesn't *feel* right at the time!

Mood Index	Appropriate Activity Level
+5	**SEEK HELP!** *Very grounding e.g. clean toilets*
+4	*Seek Help! Stay in touch with people who are solid; do whatever grounds you.*
+3	*Careful! Gentle and mundane things best*
+2	*Try to do ordinary things*
+1	*Most things OK: emphasis on staying in the here-and-now*
0	*Whatever you like within reason*
-1	*Try to tick boxes from the activity window, something creative?*
-2	*Don't hide away, get with some people, do some exercise*
-3	*Phone a friend, listen to inspiring music, dance etc.*
-4	*Seek Help! Vigorous exercise, be with people who cheer you up*
-5	**SEEK HELP!** *Very inspiring! Don't be on your own, keep moving etc.*

Activity	When ok?
Yoga with Sylvia and Fred	Pretty much always
Days out with John, Brigid and their kids	Usually fine, but not if I'm +3 or above - the kids are excitable and get me too wound up
Hip-hop parties at Glen's	Only if I'm +1 or less!
All-nighters with Richard and Pablo	Just don't go there!

What I have put in the boxes in the completed chart above are only suggestions. Another way of approaching the same question, particularly in relation to heading off going high, is to start from the kind of activities you know you do when you're beginning to go 'up', and rate them on an acceptability scale. You're probably aware, deep down, that hanging out with certain people, for example, is just never a good idea, while others can be great company if you're feeling reasonably grounded, but can take you much too far into the stratosphere if you already a bit high (say +2 or above).

Now do yours!

Activity	When ok?

Finally, the dreaded question of medication. Unlike some other emotional or mental problems, bipolar disorder, however it started, has a strong biological component. This means that medication is usually going to be a long-term or permanent feature – it's more like taking insulin for diabetes than taking a course of antibiotics to make you better, after which you stop. But of course, particularly when you're high, you'll think that "There's nothing wrong with me, so I don't need to take these nasty pills any more."

Unfortunately, that doesn't work. It may be that you need to readjust what you are taking from time to time, but *only* in collaboration with your medical practitioner, whether GP or psychiatrist. Generally speaking, if you find yourself wanting to come off your meds, the first thing to do is to check where you are on the mood index – if you're outside the +2 to -2 bracket, take those thoughts *just as symptoms of the problem,* refocus your concern onto doing appropriate activities and keep taking the meds at the prescribed level. If you're inside that bracket and there's a good reason for changing the medication, e.g.

worsening of side effects, go and see your doctor and discuss it with them.

Once the medication is (more-or-less) sorted, and having read this chapter, you have started to get a handle on the idea of bringing your mood back to a level, you may find you could do with some extra techniques to help! It is our old friend *metaperspective* that is needed here: most people get the hang in theory of what they're meant to do, but sometimes the moods shift so fast, or are so absorbing, that they're on a high before they know it and the consequent drop follows like night follows day. The key strategy needed here is *mindfulness*. The more aware you are of what's happening 'in there', the more chance you have of heading it off at the pass.

So once you're stabilised enough to be able to tolerate it (an interview with a mindfulness programme leader should be able to establish if this is the case), then I recommend getting yourself onto an eight-week programme. It probably doesn't matter hugely if it is billed as Mindfulness-Based Cognitive Therapy (MBCT) or Mindfulness-Based Stress Reduction (MBSR) – either will give you the increased detachment from your mind-contents that you need to help you spot what is going on at an early enough stage to help you change direction in time, provided of course that you keep up the practice! See Chapter 9 for more details about mindfulness, and the appendices at the end of the book for details of how to find a programme near you.

I have worked with enough people suffering from this disorder to know that it can be absolute hell in all kinds of ways. I have also known people who have bipolar affective disorder who didn't tell me for years (and I would never have guessed if they hadn't), so well did they manage their condition with a balance of medication and activities. Some are lucky that the medication works well – please keep persevering with your medical practitioner until you find the right, or the best possible, combination for you. And please don't let anything I have said in these pages prevent you from enjoying the genuinely creative aspects that you can access – just keep them in balance!

Ordinary Mind

A monk asked Joshu,
"What is the Way?"
Joshu replied,
"Ordinary mind is the Way"

Further reading:

David J. Miklowitz (2011) *The Bipolar Disorder Survival Guide: What You and Your Family Need To Know,* Guilford Press
Jan Scott (2010) *Overcoming Mood Swings: A Self-help Guide Using Cognitive Behavioural Techniques,* Constable Robinson

CHAPTER 16: PANIC

Theory A and Theory B – Decatastrophising body sensations (what the head thinks the body is doing) – Panic formulation – Panic diary – The panic lizard and his emergency telephone (please answer it)

Lots of people have the odd panic attack; it is hard to know how many because if you just have the one, or very few, spread out over a long time, you might not even bother trying to seek any help for it, so it doesn't get recorded. A much smaller percentage of people have *panic disorder*, where the repeated incidence of panic attacks is distressing and incapacitating. Another group has panic as a secondary symptom of another mental health problem, e.g. depression or generalised anxiety disorder.

What is pretty certain is that *nobody* likes having panic attacks. That's hardly surprising. Your heart starts to race; you might find yourself drenched with sweat; maybe you think you're either going to throw up or wet or soil yourself or both; you feel dizzy and faint and all sorts of horrible ideas come up about what's going to happen to you: is it a heart attack; a stroke; am I going to DIE, for God's sake, or collapse in a heap on the floor with everyone looking at me...?

So quite understandably, people come to therapy with the aim of getting rid of these horrible symptoms, but everything you do to try and get rid of them somehow seems to make them worse. In CBT, the first thing to try and discover is whether the thing you're afraid will happen is *really* likely to happen. One particular common fear in panic is that you're going to have a heart attack and die. Of course the responsible thing to do first is to get yourself checked out medically to ascertain that you don't have a heart condition. Assuming the medics have given you the all clear and you have a reasonably healthy heart, then we have a question to answer: your heart is OK. Yet when you are in certain situations (or at random times), you *feel* like you're going to have a heart attack. On the other hand, you have had many panic attacks, and you're still walking around without ever having had a *real* heart attack. How come?

Well, you might say, the only reason I didn't is because I (............). Now whatever you put in between the brackets is what we call a *safety-seeking behaviour*, or safety behaviour for short. You may remember we looked at them, together with the vicious daisy, in Chapter 1 under *Formulation*. You might want to reread that bit now.

Of course, your particular version of panic might not be about having a heart attack: it might be about passing out, or making a fool of yourself, or losing control (which sometimes means 'going mad'), or dying by some other non-heart attack means, or something else I haven't thought of. Whatever it is, it will seem *catastrophic* to you, which is why you did whatever safety behaviour you did to prevent it happening. In fact the CBT understanding of panic is that it is a *catastrophic misinterpretation of bodily sensation*, although as we will see below, this is not always the whole story. But another way of saying the same thing is to realise or remember that panic is what the head makes of what the body is doing when the organism appears to be under threat.

Like in the heart attack example, the chances are that whatever it is you're afraid will happen hasn't *actually* ever happened to you, or at least not in recent times. But every time you do whatever you do to head it off – like sitting down, holding onto something, breathing in a certain way, seeking reassurance or even reminding yourself repeatedly of what the therapist said in the last session – you make the scary possibility seem more real in your mind, otherwise why would you be doing whatever it is? As the saying goes, actions speak louder than words. This is especially true in panic. Whatever it is you do to prevent the feared event occurring, by doing it you are actually telling yourself at a deeper level – the metamessage – that it is a 'real' probability.

So, how can we look at this in a different way?

The first thing is to get some *horizontal metaperspective*; some 'standbackability'. Is what's going through your mind when you feel panicky true or helpful?

In fact, the development of the CBT panic model by the psychologist David M. Clark is one of the first examples of distinguishing a thought about something from the message it carries. He put it in these terms: in these situations, there are two theories. There is a difference between Theory A ("I'm going to have a heart attack") and Theory B ("*I'm afraid* I'm going to have a heart attack"), which is a fear or worry problem rather than a heart attack problem. Each theory would naturally lead to a different set of behaviours. Sticking with the heart attack example:

Theory A	Theory B
(Thought) "I'm going to have a heart attack and die"	*(Thought)* "I am afraid about having a heart attack and dying"
(Behaviour) Slow down, see a cardiologist, do whatever I need to do to avoid death!	*(Behaviour)* Do whatever I need to do to deal with the *fear* problem (get some CBT!)

So now we have two potential alternatives, and the route through therapy is about testing which theory has the most or best evidence. In this way (to use the jargon) you can *disconfirm the threat belief,* but you have to look and see if what you're doing is confirming Theory A, or at least preventing you from discovering that Theory A isn't true. Because of course, if you were really at risk of a heart attack, then the best course of action *would* be to see a cardiologist, or at least a paramedic. But if you aren't, and it's really a panic problem yet you're still acting as though it were a physical medical problem, then you are confirming the Theory A to yourself by your behaviour, which keeps the whole thing going!

All very well, you say, but *how* do I know whether this is a Theory A or a Theory B problem? Not all the things I'm afraid of can be checked out medically in advance, like a heart condition. What about fears that I might pass out? Or lose control? Or go mad? Or shame myself in public?

Well, a key question will be, does it get worse the more you worry about it? Because if it does, then it's a worry or fear problem. One way you can test this is by simply reading the panic list below; a list of words that remind you of panicky feelings.

Panic Word List

Breathlessness - Suffocate

Chest tight - Heart attack

Numbness - Stroke

Dizziness - Fainting

Palpitations - Dying

Breathlessness - Suffocate

Numbness - Stroke

Palpitations - Dying

Chest tight - Heart attack

Palpitations - Dying

Unreality - Insane

Dizziness - Fainting

Unreality - Insane

Dizziness - Fainting

Breathlessness - Suffocate

Chest tight - Heart attack

Breathlessness - Suffocate

Unreality - Insane

Palpitations - Dying

Dizziness - Fainting

Chest tight - Heart attack

Dizziness - Fainting

Unreality - Insane

Palpitations - Dying

Numbness - Stroke

Chest tight - Heart attack

Dizziness - Fainting

Palpitations - Dying

Breathlessness - Suffocate

Unreality - Insane

Numbness - Stroke

Chest tight - Heart attack

Breathlessness - Suffocate

Dizziness - Fainting

Numbness - Stroke

Numbness - Stroke

Unreality - Insane

Palpitations - Suffocate

Chest tight - Heart attack

Palpitations - Dying

Breathlessness - Suffocate

Unreality - Insane

How did that make you feel? More panicky? Then it's a psychological rather than an in-the-world problem, which is *Theory B* and therefore leads to a different course of action from whatever your safety behaviours were.

Let's look in detail at the different scary ideas you have about what might happen to you:

Heart Attack/Stroke/Die

As this is the example I have mostly used in this section, there is not a lot more to say about the heart attack/stroke bit of this. Assuming you've had the necessary medical checks to establish that you are physically OK, then it's certainly Theory B isn't it?

Of course, the fear of death is entirely normal. Some would argue that people lacking a fear of death are the ones who have something wrong! (See Chapter 20 on health anxiety for a fuller treatment of this issue.) But the idea that I will die right now in the middle of a panic attack; that somehow it will be so intense that my system can't stand it, is the particular fear in this kind of panic. So although it may not seem like it, you are actually in a no-lose situation here. Because if you did die, that would be an end to the panic problem, wouldn't it? OK, bad joke...

But where I am placing my bets is on the idea that if you allow yourself to go into that feeling, then you will *really* discover that this is a *really* unpleasant feeling that does not result in death, or a stroke, or a heart attack. But don't take my word for it...

Pass out

Unless you suffer from blood-injury phobia, which is a specific phobia where you faint at the sight of blood, you cannot *truly* faint in a panic attack. Why is this? Because in order to faint, your blood pressure has to *drop*. When you panic, you *feel* dizzy and faint because the blood is going from your head (where it is not needed – you don't need to think if you're about to be eaten or attacked, you need to run or fight!) to your arms and legs to give you extra power. And your blood pressure is actually going *up* when you panic. So if you are worried about fainting deliberately try getting more anxious, then you won't faint!

Lose control or go mad

This is a really interesting one. On the one hand, it's *all-or-nothing* (also known as *black-and-white*) thinking. Are you *supposed* to be consciously in control of every aspect of this organism's functioning? Of course not. And there are some activities (e.g. sex) where losing control is actually necessary for it to be any good (*pace* tantrics). But when *is* it necessary to be extra vigilant and more in control? That's right – when you're under threat. So the feeling of wanting to be more in control turns out actually to be a *symptom* of anxiety rather than its cause. Of course, when I'm under attack I want all the troops back from leave and ready to fight...

On the other hand, have you ever really been totally out of control? What does that look like? Even if you gibber, drool and act as weird as you can possibly manage, aren't you really doing that deliberately? However, if this is your fear you're probably trying to 'act normal', or even 'super-normal'. Now that *will* make you feel like you're going bonkers, otherwise why would you be trying to act normal? Take yourself out of the mental straitjacket and experiment with being a bit eccentric! Discover that life is more fun like that – of course, this links into the next one...

Embarrass myself and have everyone looking at me
Particularly if we have very firm rules about having to be strong, together and competent always and everywhere, we may see any kind of mental health difficulty as a weakness and a threat in itself. We don't want to be seen as weak in the boardroom, on the football pitch, or in any other gladiatorial arena, do we? The orange juice story is relevant here (see Chapter 21) – we are not defined by what others think of us. *But we were, or at least thought we were, as children.* What other people said about us and to us was how we learned what sort of a person we were. It may be that there were embarrassing events in our childhood, in response to which we made a decision to never, ever let that happen again.

Whenever the Protector gets a whiff of a potentially shameful situation, it thinks it's time to get the guard up and fight or flight. We will discuss this more under *Social anxiety* in Chapter 21, but there are two main things to be aware of here, in addition, perhaps, to recognising that a powerful program from the past has been triggered. These things are:

1. Anything you think you know about what others are thinking is subject to the thinking error of *mindreading* and therefore not to be trusted.

2. If your attention is based in how you think others are perceiving you, it's in the *wrong place*! Your attention belongs *in you*, looking out, not *outside* (in others) *looking in*. So refocus, either by using mindfulness to relocate in the body and then

looking out, or focus externally by deliberately concentrating on what others are saying, doing, wearing etc.

Of course to test this out, you need to enter the situation, and maybe even try that old technique of *shame-attacking*. At whatever level seems possible for you (wearing odd socks or unfashionable clothes from a charity shop; pretending to be stupid or drunk), deliberately act out some version of the scary fantasy and see what happens; even, if you're up for taking the risk, combining this with the 'pass out' idea, by pretending to faint in a public place and seeing what others' reactions are.

Sometimes it's good to do that one with a friend or therapist so they can tell you what's happening (it's hard to see when you're pretending to be unconscious).

So let's put your version of this into some kind of formulation:

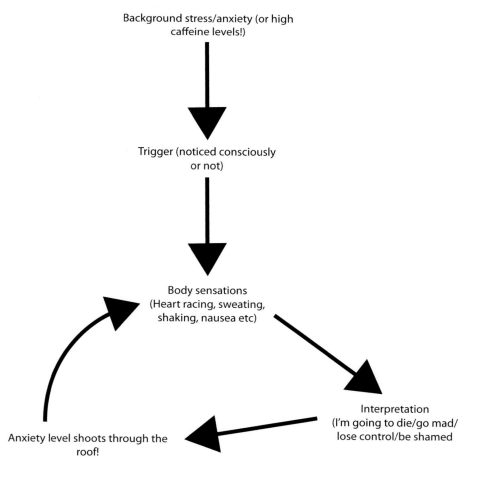

And when the anxiety shoots through the roof, of course the body sensations are correspondingly amplified, which seems to confirm the interpretation.

So what do we need to do? Well, actually the first thing we need to do is to notice *what we are already doing that is* **preventing** *us from discovering whether or not what we fear is actually going to happen!* So when the anxiety goes through the roof in response to your idea about what these sensations mean, what do you do to make yourself safe?

Some possibilities:

Interpretation	Safety behaviour
I'm going to have a heart attack	Sit down, reduce activity
I'm going to lose control/ go mad	Try to 'act normal', control my thoughts
I'm going to pass out	Sit down, put my head between my knees
I'll make a fool of myself	Try to appear normal, becoming self-focused

Of course there are many variations. But the point is that each of these safety behaviours[14] either prevents you from discovering whether what you fear is true or not, or actually seems to confirm the scary hypothesis, e.g., why would I be trying to 'act normally' if I wasn't at risk of completely losing the plot? So, if you haven't already done so, do your own formulation using the DIY Panic Formulation chart on the next page.

Safety Behaviours/Avoidances

How do you make the anxiety go down? Or 'make it better'? Or stop the feared consequences occurring?

Interpretation	Safety behaviour

---

14   This may seem to contradict what we were saying in the behaviour section above. But the key point is what the effect of the safety behaviour is. If it prevents you from discovering whether what you fear is real or not, you need to drop it. If it acts as a helping hand to get you into a situation you'd otherwise be too afraid to enter, you may need to adopt it temporarily.

DIY Panic Formulation

Background stress/anxiety (or high
caffeine levels!)
What are yours?

↓

Trigger (noticed consciously or not)
Did you notice one?

↓

Body sensations
(E.g. pains in chest,
sweating, shaking, nausea etc)

Where do you feel that in your body?

*What goes through your mind when
you feel that? What does it mean to you?*

Mood/Emotion
(E.g. anxious - any others?)

Interpretation
(I'm going to have a heart attack/
lose control/pass out/be shamed...)

How does that make you feel?

So here's the *really* scary bit. Now that you've worked out what it is that you fear, and what that means, you have to find out whether it's true or not. So if you think feeling breathless and lightheaded in the supermarket means you're going to go mad if you stay there, *and* you can see that this is not rational or likely, then what have you got to do?

That's right – do the behavioural experiment and take yourself into the supermarket to find out what happens if you *do* stay there and feel the feelings and not do any safety-behaviours. Of course, this is putting yourself through a rather uncomfortable process, and in that is the key to working with most if not all of the anxiety disorders: learning how to become *comfortable* (or at least tolerant) with *discomfort*. That doesn't mean you should be hard on yourself, or self-critical, if that is too hard a step at the moment. As with all these experiments and techniques, we have to start from a place of self-compassion. Give yourself credit for what you can do, and don't beat yourself up for what you can't – you'll see why in a minute.

One of the reasons that it sometimes seems difficult to do these experiments is that it feels like there's a split between what I understand rationally (I *know* I'm not really going to have a heart attack/go mad/ pass out etc.) and how it feels at the time (it *really feels* like I'm going to have a heart attack/go mad/pass out etc.)! Here it's useful to treat different parts separately, as though they were different minds – like in the Big Mind process (Chapter 10)[15]. One of my clients talked about his 'mind-mind' and his 'body-mind'. So here 'mind-mind' may know that you won't experience whatever the catastrophe is that you fear, but 'body-mind' or 'animal-consciousness' still hasn't got the message. So we have to take 'body-mind' into the situation (leading it by the hand, as it were), gently, to help it discover what is actually the case. If it feels too scared, don't force it – just *work the edge*, like how you do the yoga or chi gong in the mindfulness programme. Stay with the discomfort (keep holding body-mind's hand!), noticing mindfully what is going on. Try to allow discomfort, without pushing it into abject terror. Let the watchword be 'challenging, but not overwhelming', and when body-mind has had enough, listen. You can always come back next time, but if you freak him or her out – like the frightened animal s/he is – it will be that much harder. In fact, treating your anxious part like a frightened animal you are trying to retrain will give you a good idea about how to pace your experiments. It's a balance between being compassionate while still letting body-mind have sufficient experience of anxiety to see that the anxiety is misplaced!

So now you're in a position to do most if not all of the panic diary (see below). Try filling one in and see how you get on. You'll need to set up one or more behavioural experiments to test out body-mind's hypothesis versus mind-mind's!

If it feels really tough, and body-mind just isn't letting you go there, you may need to take a more graded approach, as in exposure and response prevention (outlined in Chapter 5). Patiently, work out what's manageable right now, and work up from there. As Lao Tze said, the

---

15 OK, there seems like a contradiction here: on the one hand, panic is 'what the head thinks the body is doing', on the other, 'mind-mind' knows rationally that it's not going to happen. To be more precise: somehow the old brain/mind senses threat, and this triggers body sensations. *Automatic* thinking kicks in with the die/go mad etc. interpretations. *Rational* mind can tell you it's not the case, but it takes *deliberate and compassionate mind* to stand back from the content sufficiently to engage sympathetically with the process: "It's OK – your alarm's gone off."

journey of a thousand miles starts with a single step. We go from where we are, and *work the edge*.

PANIC DIARY

Situation or trigger (Where, when, what was going through your mind, what were you focusing on?)	Anxiety Rate % intensity Time duration	Safety behaviours and avoidances What are you doing that prevents you finding out how it really is?	Is there a different (rational or 'mind-mind') interpretation (Theory B)?	New behaviour? Design experiment
Physical symptoms (What is 'body-mind' saying?) Heart racing Sweating Nausea Feeling faint/dizzy Shaking Choking Hot/cold Pain (where?) Feeling unreal Other: state what	Interpretation What does body-mind think these sensations mean (Theory A)?	Effect of safety behaviours/ avoidances Do they confirm Theory A?	What is body sensation *really* about – what is the actual threat in my life (if anything)?	Re-rate anxiety % intensity Time duration

What we are trying to do here is learn to reset our alarm system (which body-mind has been in control of). Once we discover that the panic alarm system has somehow got to a hair-trigger setting, a bit like a burglar alarm that goes off when a mouse runs across the patio, and by learning that this is what has happened and not acting like the mouse is Burglar Bill, we can recalibrate the alarm and all will return to normal.

OK, I know I'm not going to die or go mad, but I'm still having panic attacks

But sometimes you may have already learned, perhaps through CBT, that the scary possibility that you first thought would happen is not going to happen. You remember these are usually:

- I'm going to die (through heart attack, stroke or similar).
- I'm going to lose control, which probably turns out to mean that I'll go mad.
- I'm going to pass out or faint and either seriously embarrass myself (everyone looking at me) or be ignored and abandoned.

But although you know none of these are really true, you still have panic attacks. Probably you're not as frightened of them as you were, but they're still really unpleasant.

To understand in more depth what is happening here and how to treat it, we need to go back to evolution, with more than half a nod to a brain scientist called LeDoux and his (e.g. 1998) work. Essentially, the panic system is very primitive. It resides in the older part of the brain, and we can say that it hasn't changed much since we were lizards. Lizards have many fine qualities, but they aren't very sophisticated, intellectually speaking. On the other hand, our lives as 21st century humans are extremely complex. There is a big difference between various situations in which one might feel anxious: humiliation in a bar; not having done one's tax return in time; possibility of serious illness etc. But to our lizard, they just mean one thing: THREAT!!! Like something's going to eat me, NOW. So the lizard presses its red emergency telephone button (as it were), to warn us.

Now this telephone, once pressed, sets off a hell of a racket. It has to, or we might not take any notice. After all, if the alarm system went "tweet, tweet", it wouldn't be very effective. And from the lizard's point of view – bear in mind, if we get eaten, it gets eaten too – we need to be in fight-or-flight mode, so the alarm has to jangle us out of whatever we're doing.

Yet, from the perspective of our conscious mind, all that's happened is that for some unknown reason, we're getting all these weird, unpleasant symptoms, yet there's not a sabre-toothed tiger in sight. It's understandable, then, that you do all kinds of stuff to suppress the symptoms, like taking a valium or something. Of course this makes the lizard go to sleep, but when it wakes up again, it's even worse! "Damn, fell asleep on the job again – sound the alarm, something might have happened!"

There are two other problems: One, this old-brain lizard *is* rather old. So just because there's a panic, it doesn't necessarily mean there's anything to panic about. Two, when people get upset *about* having anxiety, and tell themselves "But I shouldn't feel anxious here" then the lizard takes it personally. In fact it's a serious threat: "They're ignoring my alarm; I'll have to ring it louder to make them take notice." So what does he do? Presses the emergency button again and makes it worse. Actually, *any self-critical thinking* is experienced as threat, and remember, the lizard just can't tell the difference between externally and internally-generated threats. Something pokes him, and he presses the button.

So how does this natural history lesson help you to deal with panic? Well, firstly, by helping you not to run away from the panic symptoms. Would you run away from the telephone because you didn't like the sound of the bell? Remember that the symptoms *have* to be jangly, to put us on alert. So what do you need to do if the phone rings? Answer it, of course. How do you answer it? *By breathing into or focusing on the area of the body where the symptoms are strongest.*

Now this is odd, because it seems like we're just going back into 'body-mind'. But here we need to make a fine and subtle distinction between two kinds of 'minds-in-the-body'. One is actually the *primitive* voice; the voice of the panic lizard if you like. That's the one that automatic thinking/the self-critic gets hold of and makes stuff worse. ("Oh my God, if I'm still having panic attacks after all this treatment I must be a complete idiot.")

The other is the voice of body-awareness: patiently, kindly, compassionately investigating what has got trapped in here by breathing into the part – usually the belly or chest – where the panic sensations are strongest; gradually allowing the closed fist inside to unfurl and reveal what is hidden.

Often, it's really obvious what's up – usually something that is troubling you in your life, but is not an immediate physical threat, so you hadn't recognised it as a cause for panic. Sometimes, even with the mindful, compassionate investigation you can't access what it is, or at least not yet. This may mean the lizard tripped over his feet again and pressed the button by mistake. Don't be cross with him, or he'll press it again (it's all he can do). But if it's happening repeatedly, then either it's a simple 'neural habit' or, more likely, there is something happening that the lizard perceives as a threat. This may be an association from the past (lizards don't understand time); but it may be that 'it' is reluctant to emerge.

I have noticed sometimes that clients, when they try to breathe into the centre of the panic, encounter what they describe as a 'knot' or a 'closed fist'. This may be something they/you have suppressed repeatedly, maybe since early childhood. In that case we need to treat it a bit like a shy child that has been ignored for too long. We may have to sit with it awhile, to let it open up in its own time. This is compassionate mind (Gilbert 2005) in operation. As it unfurls, we can do whatever we need to do with what comes up. If you are working with a therapist you might want to do some imagery rescripting (see Chapter 10) with the emerging content.

One difference that occurs when this approach is taken concerns what happens with the panic symptoms. Using this 'answering the telephone' technique seems sometimes to get rid of the panicky sensations more quickly! Instead of the symptoms subsiding gradually (which is, after all, much better than staying at a high level), when you hit on *the material driving the panic*, they just evaporate instantly. I can give a couple of examples of this:

a) A person is in a therapy group, actually having a panic attack. On being requested to breathe into it, he suddenly gets an image of his mother, and becomes upset as their relationship has problems. I ask, "Where are the panic symptoms now?" "Oh, they've gone," he says.

b) As above, in a group situation. The client has done the basic CBT work and knows that if she panics she is not going to have a heart attack, go mad, etc. Nonetheless she is very hard and analytical towards herself about her work situation. I ask her what is going on inside as she panics; what she is aware of. She then describes 'getting a message': literally, "Listen with your heart," it said. At that moment, the panic symptoms disappeared instantly.

A third client, who suffered not panic but longstanding anxiety and depression, had difficulties with a parent. The anxiety was experienced as a heavy lump in the centre of the chest. Through Gestalt-style empty chair work, this was explored, and lessened with repeated interventions, including the mindfulness programme, during which it gradually disappeared. Again, compassionate 'body-mind' investigation into bodily-felt tension revealed and provided a route through psychological difficulties.

It will be obvious (at least to those who have read the earlier part of the book) that we are using mindfulness techniques to help us answer the anxiety telephone. It is preferable that this is done in the context of a regular, developing mindfulness practice. Unfortunately, some people have used mindfulness techniques as safety behaviours, just to try and make the panicky symptoms go away. Please don't use them this way, because it won't work, and will make you think that mindfulness isn't effective. It is extremely effective, but use it as a way of *staying with* whatever is going on, not trying to suppress it!

How can we sum all this up?

First, *panic is your friend*, even if it doesn't feel like it. It is, if you like, an arm of the Protector – albeit a very old arm that has a lot in common with a lizard.

Second, when the alarm goes off, don't fight it! It's just an alarm. It's a communication from one part of the self to another, trying to let you know that (it thinks) something's dangerous.

Third, it makes sense, therefore, to look around if you feel panicky, just to honour the lizard and check you are not under immediate threat. ("Oh, perhaps I shouldn't be walking on this motorway!")

Fourth, assuming you aren't really under threat to life and limb, take a Theory B position ("OK, I *feel like* I'm about to be eaten by a sabre-toothed tiger, but that's just because my primitive alarm's gone off. Thank you, lizard, for trying to keep me safe"), but don't act like it's a Theory A situation. Stay in it and let the lizard calm down by itself.

Fifth, if it's happening a lot, try to access the panicky feelings deliberately and breathe into them to see if anything is revealed (you may or may not want to do this in the supermarket). Is there a current threat in your life which you are not acknowledging (job, relationship, finances), or is it that something you do or somewhere you go triggers scary reminders from the past? Either way, try to deal with it (explore, not suppress), and get help if you need to.

The main thing, above all, is not to be afraid of these panicky body sensations, but rather to treat them, at least potentially, as a messenger bearing possibly vital, but probably not immediate, information from another part of the self. So although they may be unpleasant, they are to be welcomed. This 'approach rather than avoidance' attitude towards your own internal world is of course to be encouraged as being good for your mental health generally.

Further reading

Clark, D. M. (1988) *A Cognitive Model of Panic* in *Panic; psychological perspectives* (ed. S. J. Rachman and J. Maser), Erlbaum
Gendlin, E. T. (2003) *Focusing*, Rider Books
Gilbert, P. (2009) *The Compassionate Mind*, Constable Robinson
LeDoux, J. (1998) *The Emotional Brain*, Phoenix/Orion Books

CHAPTER 17: SIMPLE OR SPECIFIC PHOBIAS

Explanation – Different types – Origins– Blood injury phobia – Situational and environment phobias – Specific phobia of vomiting

There are a number of areas of life that many people find problematic, even though the rest of their lives seem broadly OK. It is just that a particular kind of something-or-other produces a level of fear or extreme reaction that makes being with whatever-it-is virtually impossible.

This is a category that has already been almost completely covered in the preceding chapter. Essentially, in most cases, the protocol is the same as for other anxiety disorders, especially panic.

As always, we begin with some kind of formulation (see Chapter 1): this helps us both to understand and accept the condition. Probably the vicious daisy is the simplest and most effective method; as it is a simple phobia, i.e. you know what it is you are afraid of, it should be fairly simple to state what the threat belief is at the centre of the daisy. What is also useful about this exercise is that it helps tease out what it is about the particular thing that scares you: the scuttling of the spider, the (perceived) coldness of the snake, the fear of choking in vomiting and so on. This is where CBT is more targeted than behaviour therapy, so we don't just throw you in with the lions!

Having identified what it is that is scary about the thing you are afraid of, and your safety behaviours that seem to confirm the 'truth' of your belief, we then set out a series of behavioural experiments for you to discover whether what you *expect* to happen actually happens or not. You may need to precede these with some further cognitive work (e.g. an ABC) or put it in some kind of historical context: "When I was three I was tormented by a Basset Hound and have been scared of dogs ever since."

It will probably be helpful to use a hierarchy and firm up the results of your behavioural experiments with some exposure and response prevention to retrain the scared animal in you, as well. Discovering that nothing terrible happens if you are in the same room as a spider (behavioural experiment) is not the same as being in the same room as a spider *without anxiety*, which is what can happen after repeated exposure.

As always, compassionate mind is helpful. Remember, if you get down on yourself for having the phobia, then your 'panic lizard' in the amygdala experiences it as another level of threat. This becomes associated with the phobia and reinforces the anxiety – which is just what you don't want. So *be nice* to yourself about it.

I am curious about the fact that some phobias are more common than others: why are more people afraid of snakes than lizards, for example? Or spiders than flies, especially as flies are probably more dangerous to us? I suspect that some of these threats may be encoded in some kind of genetic memory: after all, in some parts of the world, snakes and spiders are (or were) dangerous. So when you're being compassionate to yourself for having shot up a tree on seeing a harmless grass snake, say, "There, there, it's only your inner caveman (or woman) getting upset – we had some scary times with snakes back in the Paleolithic!" and go back to working on your hierarchy.

But although we can use the panic model to deal with specific phobias – as they generate symptoms of panic when activated – nonetheless there are some particular points to be noted and some individual characteristics of certain kinds of phobia.

Amongst professionals, there has been a tendency to divide up phobias into five types, for example as in the US Diagnostic and Statistical manual (DSM-IV):

1. B-I-I or Blood-Injection-Injury phobia (fear of needles, blood etc.).
2. Animal phobia, e.g. fear of spiders, snakes etc.
3. Natural environment phobia: e.g. fear of heights or the dark.
4. Situational phobias: fear of flying, going over bridges, driving etc.
5. Other types, including for example fear of vomiting (known as emetophobia or Specific Phobia of Vomiting (SPOV).

We also need to mention agoraphobia: not, as some people think, fear of open spaces, but actually "fear of the marketplace" (from the Greek *agora*). Most instances of agoraphobia are the result of having had panic attacks and being so frightened of them that the person refuses to go out again and just stays indoors. A graded exposure programme using the panic model will probably be the best course here.

In a moment we will take the five types in order, but first a little on the history of treating these problems. Once the psychoanalytic approach to these issues had been more-or-less discredited, the behaviourists' approach gained favour. This often relied on 'flooding', wherein the person was flooded with stimuli relating to their phobia and eventually emerged – with any luck – no longer afraid. (Or completely traumatised...)

Bringing in a cognitive approach has meant that we can try to work out *what it is about the particular scary thing* that upsets the patient, and then target the experiment accordingly. So, for example, someone afraid of spiders may fear that they will get bitten and be poisoned; someone else may fear the 'scuttling' that spiders seem to do. Holding a tarantula might be terrifying for the first type but not the second (tarantulas don't scuttle).

If we then bring in the graded approach of Exposure and Response Prevention, we can both target treatment accurately, and not frighten the animal we're trying to retrain, because it is usually pretty clear to the patient that this fear is not rational. That makes it even more obvious that it is the animal we're retraining, and the exposures have to be graded accordingly. It might even involve allowing the person to use some particular safety behaviours but only if that helps him or her (you!) to gain some useful information.

Many phobias can be seen as having had a function in Stone Age or earlier times. We will discuss these as we go through the different types.

1. Blood-Injection-Injury aka Blood Injury Phobia

This is different from other kinds of anxiety in that the arousal goes up initially, but then drops, with the result that the person is very likely to faint. This can be inconvenient in any number of situations! It also overlaps needle phobia. As the arousal pattern is different, so the treatment is different too.

Once you have a formulation, so that you know the situations that you are likely to go woozy (or worse) in, then we need to do two things:

1. De-catastrophise the business of fainting. Of course it's not pleasant, but it's only dangerous under particular conditions (if you're a neurosurgeon in the middle of an operation, or a tightrope walker, for example). If necessary, particularly at the beginning of treatment, warn anyone who needs to be warned that you are likely to pass out when you have your pre-holiday injection for whatever it is. They will usually be much happier that you told them so they can be prepared. As always, take reasonable care of yourself.

2. Unlike every other instruction in this book, when you feel you may pass out, DON'T RELAX! In fact, deliberately tense up. You can try pushing your forearm sideways into your belly to increase the sensation. And/or clench your larger muscles (like thighs and buttocks). This is a behavioural experiment to see if you can reduce the fainty-type symptoms by artificially keeping your blood-pressure up. As with other kinds of anxiety, it's worth using a hierarchy (see forms appendix...), and starting with situations that you just feel a bit dizzy or woozy in, and building up to those in which you are more likely to completely pass out.[16]

While this is only conjecture, one reasonable and possible explanation of why some people have blood-injury phobia is that it was a potentially life-saving reaction in the face of battle: if you collapse and pass out, the (victorious) enemy will think you're dead and leave you alone...

2. Animal Phobia

Various kinds of animals frighten different people. As I hinted in the introduction to this section, there is probably an evolutionary origin to some irrational fears of particular animals, while others may come from particular personal difficult experiences. I suggest three stages to treatment:

1. Formulation: Identify what it is about the animal that is frightening. The 'awfulness' if you like. Identify the probability of it happening to you (being eaten by a shark is undoubtedly unpleasant, but they're not often found in the municipal swimming baths...)

2. Use the cognitive techniques already described (ABCs etc.) to get some perspective on the likelihood of whatever you fear happening to you.

---

16 It's important that you have this condition diagnosed by a professional. If you haven't got blood-injury phobia, but panic with a fear of passing out, the second part of this treatment would just become a safety-behaviour

3. Do the behavioural work: set up particular behavioural experiments to see what you can discover about e.g. being close to snakes or spiders. Do they actually do what you fear they will do? Once you are clear about what is rational,(but) if you still feel frightened, gradually work up a hierarchy so you can re-train your own animal.

3&4. Situational and Environment Phobias (Heights, Planes, Bridges, the Dark etc.)

I am taking situational and natural environment phobias together as the treatment is very similar, as it is indeed to animal phobias above. Initially our formulation is largely concerned with what it is about the thing you fear that you find particularly frightening. Are there associated images? Where do they come from (if you know)? Do they relate to fear of death (this is dealt with in some depth under health anxiety (Chapter 20))?

Once you have worked out what it is you are afraid of in particular, then use cognitive techniques to discover whether your fear is justified or useful. But bear in mind that primitive part may also be having an input here: for example, I have worked with many people who have a fear of flying, which is often worse if they are already anxious about something else. I usually end up saying something like:

"Of course you're scared of flying, you'd be mad not to be. Sitting up there at 30,000 feet in a tin box? Obviously crazy!"

Because to our primitive side, it is clearly madness. Of course, I'm not suggesting people really don't fly. But I am suggesting that people allow themselves – their panic lizards, if you like – to feel anxious when they're taking off or whatever. Because it is often, I think, that the person is telling themselves that they *shouldn't* feel anxious in this situation that is causing the problem. So you soothe the lizard,

"I know you're feeling anxious, and I don't blame you, I don't really understand how these things stay up in the sky either. But in fact nearly everyone gets where they're going and there's no reason why we shouldn't...just see, we'll be all right"

When you're satisfied that you can see that your fear is at least excessive if not entirely misplaced, then it's time to start working out a combination of behavioural experiments and, if necessary, an exposure hierarchy. List all related situations, start with the easiest, and work your way up. Remember, one tick means you're working on it (but it's still making you anxious), two means it's no longer making you anxious. Don't try to do it all at once.

5. Other types: Specific Phobia Of Vomiting

The most common of the other types is specific fear of vomiting; this can partly be dealt with in the way that we have dealt with most of the others. Except that, as in Blood Injury Phobia, what is feared may actually occur, simply through the anxiety, of which nausea, including sometimes actually vomiting, is a recognised symptom. If this is your problem, you may also wish to look at the chapters on Obsessive Compulsive Disorder (OCD) (19) and Health Anxiety (20) with which it often co-habits.

The first question to ask, is, are you afraid of being sick yourself (and what is it about that that you fear?) or is it seeing others vomiting that distresses you? Strangers or those in your family? If it is about contamination or responsibility it may well really be OCD. If you think that vomiting is a sign that you have something wrong with you (despite medical reassurance) it may well be Health Anxiety.

Assuming that it is none of these, and that it is just you being sick that bothers you, what is it about this that is so frightening? Some people particularly fear choking for example, having heard of some rock star choking to death on his own vomit having consumed a whole bottle of spirits (that being the point!). For others it is just the smell or the noise. I suggest that there may somewhere in the mists of antiquity be an evolutionary benefit to being repulsed by sickness (avoiding contagion, perhaps, in the days before antibiotics?).

Whatever the cause, the fear is not rational, so therefore targeted exposure is likely to be your best bet. Initially talking about it is one place to start, old Billy Connolly clips of 'Ralph and Huey' can provide a stimulus. This will help to decatastrophise sickness. From there you can move on to viewing people vomiting (YouTube has some delightful exemplars, and there always seems to be someone laughing in the background). You can then progress by making simulated vomit from perfectly harmless food materials (porridge, vegetable soup and parmesan make a good combination) which you can ingest and pretend to vomit up again.
Of course it's up to you whether you actually want to progress to making yourself sick in the end; I suggest discussion with a therapist is a good idea at this point. But there's no harm in occasional vomiting itself, it's a natural reaction to expel material the body doesn't want inside.

It's also worth doing a vicious daisy to identify any subtle or not so subtle safety behaviours that are accompanying this phobia. Are you restricting your food intake/ avoiding alcohol/ not eating in public etc.? These also need to be worked through, or you will unwittingly keep the condition going.

There is also another level to working with SPOV, and that is where we go back to the 'breathing into'-type technique that we looked at under panic. If you are feeling sick, what happens if you breathe into the source of the discomfort? Does anything else emerge? Sometimes, fear of sickness seems to be linked to fear of disclosure (not wanting to tell the spouse about an affair/ overdraft, perhaps). Or is there something in your life you *really can't stomach*? But you don't want to admit it, not even to yourself?

SUMMARY

Naturally there are various different phobias that have not been covered here, but we have identified some principles for dealing with phobias in general:

1. Formulate your problem: what is it about the thing you fear that disturbs you the most?
2. What safety behaviours are you carrying out that prevent you from discovering whether your fear is true? (including avoidance!)
3. Use ABCs or other cognitive techniques to challenge the basis of the fear.
4. Carry out behavioural experiments to test your new version. If it's a primitive fear, then use exposure to re-train the animal.
5. Does your body have something else to tell you (e.g. in SPOV)?

And as with all the other treatments in this book, don't forget to be compassionate to yourself: cut yourself some slack!

Further Reading

Michelle G. Craske, Martin M. Antony and David H. Barlow (2004) *Mastery of Your Specific Phobia*, Oxford University Press

CHAPTER 18: WORRY

*Worry and worrying – Understanding worry – Type 1 and Type 2 worry
– Coming to a formulation – General strategies: cognitive, behavioural
and mindfulness – Specific worries - Summary*

THE PROBLEM OF WORRY

Worry is a tendency that we all have to some extent, at least at times of crisis. In essence, we are trying to fix something in our heads before it really happens, so that we don't need to feel anxious about it. But if we spend a lot of time in worry mode, we *actually feel more anxious*.

In fact, what I was just talking about wasn't *worry* but *worrying*. Whether you like to use a hot cross bun or an ABC to formulate it, it works best if you put *worrying* in the area marked *behaviour*, rather than *thought*. **Because although we all have different kinds of *worries*, worry*ing* is something you *do*, even if it feels automatic.**

Automatic Behaviour

In common with many others I used to enjoy a cigarette with a pint of beer after work in the pub. And one pint would often turn into two or three. Often, in the middle of a conversation with my fellow drinkers, I would notice a half-smoked cigarette in my hand. I had no memory of it having got there. But as I smoked roll-ups, that meant I had got out the papers and the tobacco, spread the tobacco in the paper, rolled it up, inserted a filter of some sort, licked it, and smoked the first half *before I became aware of what I was doing*. Of course alcohol helps you to operate like this! But **nobody else** did it to me! So smoking was therefore something I could choose to stop doing. Likewise with worrying – although (see below) there may be *some* situations where it is called for.

However, although we put worrying in the behaviour category, it is undeniable that we are talking about thinking here. Previously we talked about deliberate versus automatic thoughts. Actually, worrying often starts with an automatic thought, but the worrying itself is our response to that thought – we treat it as though it were a real event or thing. We will come back to this in a minute.

Worrying has some similarities to rumination, but while rumination is usually about something you did in the past, or comparing yourself to some kind of 'ideal you' and deciding that you fall distinctly short, worrying is nearly always about the future, or about the effects of some past action on what happens in the future. What they have in common is that they are both an attempt to fix stuff in your head, but they are second-rate problem-solving strategies.

Born or made?
Some people describe themselves as 'born worriers'. While it would be foolish to rule out some degree of genetic predisposition to worrying completely, it is almost certain that there was a great degree of learning involved! It would probably be more accurate to say "I've got a master's degree in worrying." Who taught you? Or did you learn it in response to trying to avoid threat (of being told off, beaten, humiliated etc.)? Can you put it in a historical formulation? What unpleasant thing did you decide you were never going to put yourself through again? How old were you? Who was there?

Poking the lizard
However, here we find ourselves in a tricky spot. When we start worrying in order to head off the nasties, we are automatically reminding ourselves that *this is why* we are doing it. The neural connection is established, and before we know it, the panic lizard has stirred from his sleep and is making us feel *more*, rather than less, anxious. As one of my clients who suffered from both panic and worrying remarked, "I've got to stop poking the lizard!"

Origins of worrying
So why do we do this? Different psychologists have focused on different aspects of the problem. One important factor, highlighted by Kevin Meares and Mark Freeston, is 'intolerance of uncertainty'. It seems that some people can't stand not knowing what is going to happen. They think that if they can predict accurately enough, it will all be plain sailing, as they can head off any disasters in advance. Unfortunately this has certain disadvantages:

1. While you're busy predicting, you don't get to enjoy what is happening now, so you don't get the 'juice' that you've worked so hard to procure; and

2. Keeping yourself permanently problem- and future-focused is ***telling yourself that you must be under threat***, and so increases the *general* sense of anxiety. In fact the diagnosis often given to worriers is generalised anxiety disorder (GAD).

It would be wrong to pretend that making predictions is always unhelpful, however. Many of those who suffer from GAD are those who have trained themselves to worry professionally – they have employment that requires them to see problems in advance and head them off, or their jobs actually involve crisis management, or they're parents – so not surprisingly they try to see what crises are round the next corner!

Sometimes the training happened earlier – as I suggested above, you may have initially learned to worry as a child in order to head off criticism, beatings or worse, but then, having got good at it, that predictive ability has been pressed into service in the office, and thereby been reinforced.

So, as is usually the case in CBT, a good place to start is *compassionate conceptualisation*. Which sounds something like: "It's not surprising I've got a tendency to worry – when I was little I had to worry to keep myself safe/from being humiliated/hurt/abused etc., and for the last x years I've been working as a (........) and/or rearing children." Worrying is an occupational hazard of parenting.

What does *your* worry sentence look like? Write it here:

My Worry Sentence
"It's not surprising I worry because --- -- --"

At this point you may want to look back over the chapter on schemas (Chapter 7). How does worrying tie in with your core beliefs and assumptions or rules that protect? Perhaps you have a rule about worrying, which makes it the default option? "I have to worry unless I'm absolutely certain it's safe not to", for example. The worrying program would certainly get frequently activated if you had one like that...

TYPE 1 AND TYPE 2 WORRYING

So now that you have some idea of where your tendency to worry came from historically, what is the process that makes you take up this strategy in the present? The psychologist Adrian Wells has shed light on how this works. This is my understanding of it in a diagram:

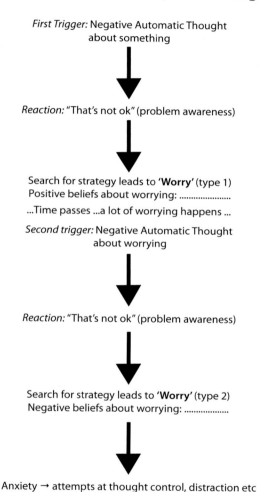

First Trigger: Negative Automatic Thought about something

Reaction: "That's not ok" (problem awareness)

Search for strategy leads to **'Worry'** (type 1)
Positive beliefs about worrying: ....
...Time passes ...a lot of worrying happens ...

Second trigger: Negative Automatic Thought about worrying

Reaction: "That's not ok" (problem awareness)

Search for strategy leads to **'Worry'** (type 2)
Negative beliefs about worrying: ....

Anxiety → attempts at thought control, distraction etc

So from this we can see there are two types of worrying: Type 1, which is worrying about *something*, and Type 2, which is worrying about *worry*. The first is driven by *positive* beliefs about worry, e.g. that it is a useful, necessary and helpful thing to do, or even that if I don't do it I'm being irresponsible (see the next chapter on Obsessive Compulsive Disorder), while the second is driven by *negative* beliefs about worry, e.g. that it will make me ill or drive me mad, or that it is 'uncontrollable'.

Write your positive beliefs about worry – why you think it is a good or, at least, a necessary thing – here

```
╔══════════════════════════════════════════════════════════════╗
║                                                                ║
║                 My Positive Beliefs About Worry                ║
║             E.g. If I didn't worry, I'd be irresponsible       ║
║  ------------------------------------------------------------  ║
║  ------------------------------------------------------------  ║
║  ------------------------------------------------------------  ║
║                                                                ║
╚══════════════════════════════════════════════════════════════╝
```

Now what are the ways in which you think worrying can harm or hurt you, or in some other way is negative?

```
╔══════════════════════════════════════════════════════════════╗
║                                                                ║
║                 My Negative Beliefs About Worry                ║
║                   E.g. I can't control worrying                ║
║  ------------------------------------------------------------  ║
║  ------------------------------------------------------------  ║
║  ------------------------------------------------------------  ║
║                                                                ║
╚══════════════════════════════════════════════════════════════╝
```

As with most other written CBT techniques, you can probably already see, now you've written these beliefs down, that they may not be a totally accurate or helpful way of looking at things in all situations.

Deliberate and automatic thinking
Working at a more analytical level, if we examine this whole process carefully we can see that our problems here are based on a confusion between automatic and deliberate thinking. Because something has appeared in our minds, we think it is a real problem – we have confused a random *automatic thought* with something *real*. If we have a real problem to deal with, we should prepare a *deliberate* strategy.

Productive and unproductive worry
Sometimes, of course, something pops into our heads that is useful and can be dealt with. In his self-help book on the subject (*The Worry Cure*), Robert Leahy distinguishes between *productive* and *unproductive* worry: productive worry is that kind – whatever it is pops into our heads, we see more-or-less immediately what needs to be done, and we either take action or schedule a course of action, and then it quite naturally disappears from our minds.

Real versus hypothetical event worry and probability
Another pair of categories, not quite the same, but overlapping, is that proposed by Meares and Freeston: *real event* worry versus *hypothetical event* worry. But although we could imagine having productive worry about a real event, it is less likely that we could worry productively about

a hypothetical event – although I suppose if we are on the verge of some cataclysmic happening (earthquake; invasion; plague) it might be possible. The distinction is a useful one, though, because it reminds us to question our mind-contents: is the thought that came into my head related to any real possibility? In philosophical terms, does the thought have a *referent*? Or to be less black-and-white about it, how *likely* is it that the feared event will happen?

Whatever words we use to describe them, it seems that there are some situations in which it is helpful to take notice of our automatic thinking. OK, whatever it was just popped into our heads, but it has served as a reminder to do something or take care of something that we want or need to do or take care of. So for worry to be productive, we need to decide what it takes for it to be useful. I suggest the following criteria:

1. The concern in the automatic thought refers to something real or likely.

2. It's my responsibility.

3. I can do something about it (it's in my power)

4. When I've done or planned whatever it is, I can let it go.

So you can see that this will work for paying bills, buying anniversary presents, doing tax returns and so on. These are real things we all have to deal with and sometimes forget about.

Summary of the problem

We all have worries. Some of them are more likely than others; some are more in our control than others. The less tolerant of uncertainty we are, the more likely we are to worry excessively. Having worries is not the same as worry*ing*, which is the repeated focusing of our thinking on things we fear may happen in the future, in order to head off unpleasant events and reduce our anxiety. Unfortunately, a by-product of worrying is that it *increases* generalised anxiety.

We may believe that it is necessary to worry because of what happened to us in the past. In that case we are likely to have some positive beliefs about worry, and it would make us feel more anxious not to worry.

If we have been worrying a lot, we may have begun to notice that the quality of our lives has deteriorated, and we may have begun to worry about the effects of all this worrying (Type 2 worry)! The next part offers some suggestions about what to do (or not to do) about worry.

WHAT TO DO: STRATEGIES FOR WORKING WITH WORRYING

First, as always with CBT, we need to formulate the problem. So if you haven't already done so, write down your historical formulation of worry. Against what did it first emerge as a defence? Disapproval? Physical harm? What did you decide you were going to make damn sure you never had to deal with again?

Again, if you haven't already done so, write down your positive and negative beliefs about worry. Then you can put it all together in a form like this:

Worry Formulation

Early frightening experience(s)	
Made you think you were (core belief):	*Weak? Vulnerable? Unlovable? Bad? Worthless?*
Rules about worrying	*If I worry, then. . .*
Other positive beliefs about worrying	*I can head off crises before they happen*
Negative beliefs about worrying	*It's out of control* *It's making me ill*
Critical Incident: what brought all this to a head? Any similarities to early experiences?	*Laid off work due to stress*
Symptoms:	*Thoughts:* *Body sensations:* *Behaviours:* *Emotions:*

A larger blank version of the worry formulation is available in Appendix 2.

Now you have an overall template of how your worry problem looks, there are a number of different things you can do:

1. If you haven't already done so, do your worry sentence – the 'it's not surprising' statement. "It's not surprising that I have a tendency to worry, given what happened to me/nearly happened to me/what was going on when I was (age), and my occupation as a troubleshooter in the banana industry." As always, be compassionate to yourself – perhaps revisit the perfect nurturer from Chapter 10.

2. Can you change unproductive into productive worry? By this I mean using TIC-TOC: change the Task Interfering Cognition into a Task Oriented Cognition. For example, instead of worrying how long I am going to take writing this chapter, check that I have everything I need to continue – and then continue!

3. Look again at the chapter on schemas. Is the child's interpretation of what happened the most helpful one? If not, maybe you don't have to spend your life figuring out ways to prove you're not (worthless/unlovable/weak/bad)?

4. Test out the positive and negative beliefs about worry. I suggest doing the negative ones first:

   a) Negative beliefs about worry:
   Worrying will make me ill/drive me mad.
   Worrying is uncontrollable.

Worry time

Adrian Wells suggests the strategy of 'worry time' for dealing with these. Instead of trying not to worry, or somehow trying to control your thoughts, allocate half an hour each day to worry. During this time, *worry as hard as you can!* See if it *actually* drives you mad or makes you ill. Of course you will catch yourself worrying at other times of the day, but when you do, just tell yourself "Not now, I'll catch you later" and redirect your attention back to whatever you were doing. My guess is that you will find that you can get a measure of control, even if not perfectly. But even a measure of control means that it is not completely uncontrollable, and nobody that I have worked with (or heard of) has yet driven themselves mad by worrying for half an hour, however intensely. But try it – you could be the first!

It is important to keep your deal with yourself. Please set aside a particular time and do worry during this time. Naturally, when it is not worry time, you will sometimes wonder if worry is still there. And when you look to see if it is, guess what you will find? Yes, it is there. If it helps, you can view it as the Worry Channel. Worry is always playing on the Worry Channel, but that doesn't mean *you've* got to be there all the time. So, in non-worry time, just retune back to the here-and-now. Mindfulness is an invaluable adjunct to this technique.

> b) Positive beliefs about worry:
>   *I need to worry to keep safe.*
>   *If I don't go over all the possibilities, something bad will happen.*
>   *It would be irresponsible not to worry.*

It's not that attempting to predict (and therefore stave off) disaster is always bad. Being good at it has made some people very rich! But looking at it in terms of your psychological health, we need to establish *how much* time it is useful to do it for, and for what kinds of problems, because encouraging anxious prediction triggers the threat mechanism and makes you feel worse. So we need to *test out* these strategies. For example, if you're the sort who always worries about their teenagers when they go out in the evening, try worrying one Friday night, and not the next. Is what happens to them any different? If it is, was it *caused* by your worrying or not worrying? If you *had* worried, would it have made any difference? Now, is there any point in worrying about stuff that is *not in your control?*

> 5. Learn to develop greater tolerance of uncertainty. Of course we survived as a species with the help of our self-protective threat mechanism, which operates on a 'better safe than sorry' principle. But that doesn't mean we should always let it rule the roost. The Protector is not the only guide in town worth listening to, but if you've been very addicted to (the illusion of) certainty (Meares and Freeston quote Pliny the Elder from 79AD: "The only certainty is that there is nothing certain"), then it may be difficult to dive into what seems like the anarchy of uncertainty all at once. So do a hierarchy, just as you would with any other difficult area that you needed to expose yourself to in a graded fashion.

Worry	Behaviour to be resisted	How scary (*not* to act on it) 0–100	One tick/two ticks
Worrying about whether my fourteen-year-old has got to school (despite there having been no problems in the previous nine years of schooling).	*Calling the school to check they got there OK.*	85	
Worrying that I can't eat the food on the day before its use-by date (even though it looks and smells fine).	*Throwing it away.*	60	
Put yours here:			

As you recall, one tick means you're working on it, but still struggling; two ticks means it no longer causes you significant anxiety. So write down all the things that you are afraid might happen and the things you would do to try to head off the uncertainty, rate for the degree of anxiety it would cause you not to do that particular safety behaviour (be that physical or in your head) and tick them off as you work through your hierarchy.

WORRYING AND THE BIG MIND PROCESS

In Big Mind process terms, the intolerance of uncertainty points to an overactive Controller, so it's a good idea to speak to him/her to find out why they're so hypervigilant. This may relate back to early experience and the formation of schemas. You can bet that at some point there was a time when it seemed that you didn't have enough control, and that meant you weren't safe, or got humiliated or something else unpleasant like that. Your Controller felt s/he had slipped up on the job, and is determined to make sure that it doesn't happen again. The Self-Critic probably gets in on the act too. The trick here is to validate what the Controller decided in response to that crisis or trauma, validate it for *then*, and maybe do a little informal cost-benefit with the Controller or Controller/Protector for how that super-controlling strategy is working *now*. Then maybe s/he will be OK with a lighter touch that doesn't have to predict and head off everything.

What to do with my mind

OK, so you've decided not to worry. You're doing worry time, and though imperfectly, you're able to give your mind a bit more of a rest from worrying. "But what else am I supposed to do with it?" I hear you cry. Understandably, your mind has got used to worrying, and it's a powerful neural habit. You're doing a hierarchy, and resisting the urge to try to tie up all the loose ends, thereby allowing a greater degree of uncertainty in your life. But at least in the short term, this may actually be increasing your anxiety, as you don't know what to do with it. 'Worry mind' is sitting there fidgeting like an unscratched itch.

Mindfulness

So here is where mindfulness really comes into its own. Actually, the itch metaphor is a very good one. When you first start sitting meditation, from time to time you get an itch. You interrupt your practice to scratch it. Surprisingly, quite quickly it can come back again in the same or a different place. You scratch it again. Sometimes you don't know whether you're doing an itching and scratching practice interspersed by periods of meditation, or the other way round, so eventually you decide to try to ignore it. You resist it for a while, and then scratch it. After some days (or months, or years!) you manage not to scratch it. To your surprise it goes away. Without you having scratched it. By itself.

The itch is a perfect metaphor for mind-contents, of which worries may be a significant part (!), in meditation. With sustained practice, such as you may develop in the eight-week mindfulness programme, you begin to notice that stuff, including worries, comes and goes. As you develop increasing fridge/sky consciousness, you can allow this stuff to pass by or through, arise and fall all by itself, and you don't have to do anything.

> Sitting quietly
> Doing nothing,
> Spring comes and
> The grass grows by itself.
>
> *Basho*

Thoughts and things

Talking about mindfulness brings us back to what may, in terms of metaperspective, be the most important insight about worries and worrying. That is, to notice that *a thought is not a thing.*

When we react to the presence of a thought as though it were something real, and try to apply deliberate thinking to it, we are already lost in the world of illusion. Because it's just neurons firing! Robert Leahy, in his excellent self-help book *The Worry Cure*, puts it like this:

Your worries involve what you think *reality is. What does this mean? Your thoughts are internal experiences that change every second and are different from someone else's thoughts. For example, your thought "I might end up alone forever" is not reality, is it? You don't really know what is going to happen. It's simply a thought.*

Another thought could be "This is a dog." Maybe this animal is a dog, but the thought is not the dog. I need to observe, to see, to check it out. I need to be aware – right now. A dog is a dog; a thought is not a dog. I can't pet a thought, and thoughts don't bark. Thoughts are not reality. (p98)

Of course it's understandable that we make this mistake. Attaching significance to images goes all the way back to us holding an image of our mother in our baby minds so that we can tolerate her temporary absence without thinking we're going to die if she goes away (because we don't know we're separate from her yet). So our representations of the world, primarily through language (once we've learned it), get confused with the real thing. This is the main drift of Acceptance and Commitment Therapy (ACT). So we need to practise *cognitive defusion.* Talking about Depression FM or the Worry Channel is doing just this – bringing our attention to the difference between (particular kinds of) thoughts and reality.

There is another advantage to a more mindful approach, in addition to being able to discern reality. Once you recognise that a thought about an event is not the event, then you realise that this particular moment is brand new, even if in the 'thoughtosphere' it seems to belong to a category of events you've already experienced. The raisin experiment in the mindfulness programme shows us this – we have never tasted *this* raisin before. And the experience of tasting this very moment is *inestimably richer* than your thoughts about it. It is, as we have said, the difference between reading the menu and eating the meal. In fact, just 'being in your head' or living through your thoughts is like eating the menu – very dry and cardboardy!

This is why the famous Korean Zen Master Seung Sahn used to encourage his students to embrace 'Don't know mind': "Only don't know!"

If you think you know something, you run the risk of simply relating to the concept. Does this experience fit my picture of how it's supposed to be? If you *don't* know, and you *know* you don't know, and you're *not trying* to know, you can really, as the beats used to say, *dig it.*

DEALING WITH DIFFERENT KINDS OF 'REAL' WORRIES

Many of the suggestions about the different kinds of worries here will simply be redirection to other parts of the book or other books, because the extreme version of a particular kind of worry is sometimes a particular diagnosis!

Mostly it will be more helpful to focus, as we have been doing, on the process of worrying rather than the content. After all, as Shantideva (8th century Buddhist scholar) pointed out, "If you *can* solve your problem, then what is the *need* of worrying? If you *cannot* solve it, then what is the *use* of worrying?"

Nonetheless, there may be some snippets of advice for specific worries that could be of use:

People worries
This comprises three different issues:

1. Worrying too much about what people think of me (social anxiety/self-esteem).
2. Worrying that people are out to get me (paranoia).
3. Relationship issues.

Obviously in the first case, look at the chapters on low self-esteem and social anxiety. But one of the most important things to remember is *not to get these two confused* – what people think of me is not the same as what I am, and what I am is, as we know, a composite (Big I, Little I). Please refer to the orange juice story in chapter 21. Actually, this story addresses both the worrying about what other people think of me and the relationship aspect. In short, what the other person thinks of me is up to them. If they prefer pineapple juice, let them go and find some, but as you can't be anybody other than who you are, just be good orange juice!

Paranoia

Worrying that people are 'out to get me' is obviously a distressing state to be in. I suggest, if it is strong, that you go and see your medical practitioner and get some medication and some specialist professional help. If it is unpleasant but not substantially restricting, then use the cognitive and behavioural techniques in the first part of the book. Yes, you are feeling threatened, and you are *attributing* this to other people. Where is the evidence? Try doing ABCs on particular situations, and test out your different hypotheses. How much mindreading is going on?

Relationships

In addition to the orange juice story, if the issue is about your partner or other significant relationship, I would like you to consider two things:

1. What are the *demands* (thinking error alert!) that exist in this relationship? Do we both agree on them? (See the Gestalt prayer, Chapter 27.) Are they manageable? Talk to each other!

2. Which parts (little Is) are uppermost in your interactions with each other? Are they the parts that you both want to be presenting to each other? Do those parts complement or conflict with each other?

If you want to explore this further, see Chapter 27.

Appearance worries

If you worry a lot about your appearance, you may qualify for a diagnosis of body dysmorphic disorder (BDD). If you think this may be the case, and if what's going through your mind right now is, "No, I'm just ugly/disgusting" (and you're over 18[17], then it probably is!), then go

---

[17] I say 'over 18' because in late adolescence and the early stages of adulthood, we are biologically programmed to be in 'mate-attracting' mode – which involves a lot of focus on our appearance until we're (more or less) comfortable with how we look. So I'm distinguishing between the concern and experimentation which is natural as a teenager, and *ongoing excessive* concern as a mature adult.

to chapter 22 below *and* get some help from a CBT practitioner who has experience of working with BDD – they do exist!

In essence, we can break the problem down into different aspects:

a) My worth is defined by how I look.
b) My lovability/likeability is defined by how I look.
c) I feel disgusting in myself, and this shows in my appearance.
d) My appearance will lead to further humiliation.

Or more than one of the above! If they strike a chord or two, then go to Chapter 22. But if you look at those statements and think, "No, I'm just careful about how I look" then maybe all you need to do is to decide how much time and energy you want to put into your appearance. Naturally, if you are a performer or model, you are going to spend more time on it - but beware the impact of your work on your personal life. If you train your brain in certain ways for eight hours a day, guess what? It will likely operate in these ways even in your time off! So try deliberately looking scruffy when you you're not professionally on show, just as a counterweight...

Health worries (including weight, fitness etc.)
I'm always happy when someone turns up for help with anxiety about death. I know they have at least got to the root of the problem, and often it *is* mortality that is at the root of health worries. And if it is this sort of thing that bothers you, then you are in good company. The things that drove the young Gautama from being a trainee prince living the life of luxury to a life of meditation culminating in Buddhahood were an awareness of sickness, old age and death. Again, we will discuss this more in Chapter 20, but if this is more a concern than an obsession, then I would ask you to reflect on the following:

Remember what we talked about under *Cognitions* in Chapter 3. If I can be aware of something, then I am the one who is aware of whatever-it-is, and whatever-it-is is the thing that I am aware of. We mentioned thoughts as a key example – so I am not my thoughts; I am the one who is aware of these thoughts.

Ken Wilber said, as we mentioned, "Suffering is the misidentification of 'I-amness' with an object", thoughts being the object.

But of course, they are not the only kind of object. So can you be aware of your body? Yes? Then in that case, *are you your body or the one who is aware of it?* Or, we could say, the one who is living in it? That makes the body not *you*, but the vehicle you are, if you like, travelling in.

If you are OK with this way of looking at it, then you have already solved all these problems in one fell swoop. Let's draw out the implications. What is it that gets sick and dies? The body; the vehicle you are travelling in. If you have done the Big Mind process, you may be able to answer experientially the question about whether awareness (= I-amness = Big Mind) ever dies. But assuming you haven't, what is the only really truthful answer to what happens to awareness after death? You don't know! But that is not the same as being *sure* that awareness/consciousness is definitely obliterated on death. I am not trying to engender false hope here, only trying to keep within what is our commonly held experience (rather than belief) about life and death.

If 'you' (I-amness) are not that which gets sick and dies, does that mean you shouldn't care about the body? No – in the same way that your car will work better if you take care of it, put petrol in, keep the right bits lubricated and so on. If it gets a dent, you might be upset temporarily (although certainly there are people who are unhealthily identified with their cars), but most people don't feel overly distressed by it. If the fuel is too rich, you adjust the setting on the carburettor, or perhaps change the kind of fuel. It's just a matter-of-fact kind of operation; you don't take it personally. Reduce the fats and increase the exercise, based solely on what improves performance (AIYOBI! again). If you're running an old car, you notice it needs to go to the garage more often, and it doesn't quite have the top speed it used to. But it has a certain charm – 'classic cars' – and if you take good care of it, it will probably run for a few years yet, albeit with a higher level of pollution! And when the time comes for it to go to the scrap-yard, you might look back wistfully on all the great drives you had in it, but you just accept that the end has come. Doesn't that sound like a better attitude to sickness and death?

Money worries
Many years ago, a study of children from economically deprived backgrounds established that they perceived coins as being larger than they actually are. Children who had enough, on the other hand, saw them accurately. If your background is one of deprivation, it makes sense that money will be more important to you than if you were reasonably comfortable growing up. It's a potential threat. Or if at some point you went from being OK financially to destitution or relative poverty, then you are going to be more careful about money matters than if you've always been OK. It is as though the Protector made a decision, saying something like, "We nearly came seriously unstuck before – I must have taken my eye off the ball, and that's never, ever going to happen again." So while others sail much too close to the edge for your liking, you always have to have a healthy surplus in your account, even if

that prevents you from taking advantage of what might be interesting opportunities. The first thing I would say about that is: this is just how it is for you, and it's *not surprising*. If you'd like to change, then it's still important to validate the Protector's decision as a helpful response for then!

At the time of writing, we're just (maybe, hopefully) coming out of what started out being called a 'credit crunch' and then, more sombrely, a recession, so those who had a bit more caution are currently being applauded. So you need to analyse your strategies to see whether your level of caution has served you well or needs adjusting.

All the above is pretty much common sense. Where rationality has often disappeared is where money has more symbolic value for you – if you have made your salary a marker of your personal worth or value. Just as I would say that your worth (lovability, strength, intelligence) is not dependent on or defined by what you do for a living, neither is it indicated by your salary or level of savings. Robert S. De Ropp, in his 1968 book *The Master Game*, described two life-games that we humans often get caught up in: 'Pig in Trough' or 'Cock on Dungheap' – money and status respectively. (He was instead advocating a path of personal development which he called the 'master game' as a more satisfying alternative.)

I want to ask a question if this is an issue for you. What *is* the optimum time to spend in money-seeking mind? Not that it's bad, but if you spend all your time and energy in pursuit of wealth, how much fun do you have? "Oh, it's for my family," you say. Maybe, but how much time do you spend with them? If they'd rather have all that money than spend time with you, then you've really got a problem. And what about the time you get to spend with them? Is it enough?

"But if I didn't work all those extra hours I'd lose my house/apartment!" I have worked with so many people who do a job they hate, for long hours, to earn enough to keep their pile of bricks in which they hardly ever spend any time. Maybe it has a big drive, and fences to keep the neighbours out, so you don't have to talk to anyone! So you get to pay extra for loneliness!

Do you really want to go on living like this? What about a lower-key, local job, that pays less but is more fun and gives you time with your family/partner/friends?

Achievement/overload worries

This leads us right into one of the most common pitfalls for a certain class of people in modern western society (and increasingly, some eastern ones too): Falling headlong into the belief that your worth is dependent on what you do for a living, or how well you perform in your job, you drive yourself nuts by forever trying to raise the bar of what you can achieve. Here comes the coronary!

Remember the newborn baby story? OK, here it is again:

Newborn Baby

You are in a public building with a number of other people. There is also a newborn baby in its carry-cot. Nobody seems to know where it came from. What can it achieve, this newborn baby? Not much – it can drink milk, make some noise, fill its nappy. Of course, it may achieve something in the future, but it may not, or it may turn out to be a serial murderer! Nobody knows. Suddenly the fire alarm goes off, and you have to evacuate the building. Do you leave the baby behind? After all, it can't achieve much...

Well, I'm guessing you don't! But if you believe you should take the baby with you, then what that means to me is that you already know that when it comes down to it, to matters of life and death, human worth is not based on achievement. Otherwise you'd leave the baby behind – after all it might slow you down. You already know that human worth is there first.

We might add that firemen don't ask for people's CVs when they go into a burning building. Fortunately for us, they save everybody they can, even a dog if possible.

So given that human worth isn't a function of achievement but is there first, why are you busting a gut? It may be that you are involved in something that is a good and beneficial thing for humanity generally. Great! Do you enjoy doing it? Is it in accord with who you are – the *ecology* question from Neuro-Linguistic Programming's PACER! model (see *Problems and Goals*, Chapter 1)? If you enjoy it, and it is a contribution you are happy to be making with your working life, wonderful. Does the quality of what you do increase the more you do it? After a certain point, the answer is bound to be no, so I want to suggest that sometimes less is more; that you may be more effective in achieving what you want to do if you give yourself some downtime. Think 'activity window' for a more balanced life (see Chapters 5 and 13).

The other thing is that if you are worrying about it, that time you spend worrying is taking energy away from your performance – you cannot

257

be worrying *and* performing wholeheartedly at the same time. So, again referring back to the PACER! model from NLP, decide when/how often it is *useful* to evaluate how you're doing, and stick to it. If you find yourself worrying about it at other times, treat it in the same way as if you're doing the worry time experiment, that is to say to worrying mind, "OK, I hear you and I'll catch you later at the time we agreed."

Now what about if you don't enjoy what you're doing, and are doing it solely for the sake of others' approval; to make money; to prove you're not worthless; to pay the mortgage on a big pile of bricks...I don't think I really need to say any more, do I?

There is only one reason that I can think of for doing something for a living that you really don't like, and that is that (for the moment) you can't get anything else, and the rent has to be paid. But if that's the case, then for heaven's sake don't do any overtime! And I would also ask you to at least consider Kahlil Gibran's view that if you can't work with love, it is better to sit by the temple and beg alms...but I know that's culturally unpopular right now!

And although we do of course need to be responsible for what is happening in our communities, sometimes we may cause less trouble following the old Taoist rascal Chuang Tzu's example:

Chuang Tzu's Turtle Story

Chuang Tzu, the legendary Taoist sage, was living in the countryside. Affairs of state were in disarray, and some courtiers came to see him to ask if he would come and get involved in national politics. They found him sitting by a river. Chuang Tzu replied something like this:

"There is a ceremonial turtle in the court. It has been dead for hundreds of years, but it appears brilliant, because of all the jewels with which its shell is encrusted. But of course there is only the shell. If you were a turtle, would you rather be like that, or like these happy fellows you see around you, flapping their tails in the mud?"
"Like one of these live turtles, of course."
"Good. Then leave me here to flap my tail in the mud!"

So, to summarise, our worth is not dependent on what we do. In which case, if you're just working to make ends meet, then of course it is more satisfying to do a good job, which means taking care of what you do, but making sure you don't overdo it – lead a balanced life.

But, like the Blues Brothers, we may be on a mission. Then it becomes a question of whether worrying helps us on our quest, which brings us back to productive and unproductive worry: does it lead, more or less immediately, to taking a course of action? If not, it's probably unproductive. On your mission, what is the *optimum* frequency of evaluating? If you find yourself worrying about your performance, just redirect your attention to doing whatever it is until you reach the agreed evaluation point. And when you're not actually engaged in your mission, enjoy flapping your tail in the mud!

'Something bad will happen' (SBWH) worries

Sometimes we worry only with a vague sense that 'something bad will happen' if we don't. The obvious experiment for this is to try worrying and not worrying to see whether more bad things happen when you do or don't worry. The problem of course is that old chestnut which the philosophers refer to by its Latin term: *post hoc ergo propter hoc*, literally *after it, therefore through [because of] it*. Just because something happens following worrying (or not worrying), doesn't mean that worrying or not worrying was the cause of it, though worrying may affect how you react in a given situation – your mind being somewhere else, you are unlikely to be very effective.

If this 'something bad will happen' sense is very strong, to the point where you are trying to do something about it mentally or physically, then the chapters immediately following this on obsessive compulsive disorder and/or anxiety about health will probably be relevant.

Recovery worries: "I'll never get better"

Often people who have been in treatment for some time, or who have had a relapse, say this sort of thing. Of course it is a reasonable worry, especially if you are an inpatient somewhere or you have had substantial time off work. There are two elements here:

1. *Behaviour*
What do I need to do, realistically (given my condition), to take the next steps towards getting discharged/going back to work/ moving back in with my partner? (Remember the PACER! or SMART models if you're setting goals.)

2. *Mind-contents*
What do I need to do to stop being identified with my mind-contents, or using the presence of certain thoughts or feelings as evidence that I am 'not better'? (When clients ask me, "When am I going to get better?" in this sense, I usually say, "I don't know; I'm not better yet.")

The very notion of 'better' in terms of what's going through your mind is antipathy to the kind of attitude that I am trying to encourage in this book. The point is to do whatever you need to do to get back to functioning, while turning towards whatever part of yourself needs working on, secure in the knowledge that you are not your mind-contents! Remember that there will always be worries on the Worry Channel, but you don't have to live on that frequency.

SUMMARY

We all have worries – but it's what we do with those worries that determines whether we get unduly anxious or not. Checking out whether they're real or productive worries to start with will help: is this a situation that is actually happening (not a thought in my head), and that it is reasonable for me to want to do something about? If so, do it, or plan it, and then forget about it for the time being. If it isn't real or productive, but just a product of my difficulty in accepting uncertainty, then watch it, don't do anything, let it go if you can. Try worry time as a way of limiting worrying, as well as discovering that in short bursts it's neither harmful nor dangerous.

Further Reading

Meares, Kevin & Freeston, Mark (2008) 'Overcoming Worry' Constable Robinson: London
Leahy, Robert L. (2005) 'The Worry Cure' Piatkus: London

CHAPTER 19: OBSESSIVE COMPULSIVE DISORDER

A formulation – Experiment and exposure – It's not me, it's my OCD – Suppressing thoughts – Radio OCD and mindfulness – Big Mind and OCD – Exposure and response prevention (again, and again) – Hierarchy – Relapse prevention

David Veale and Rob Willson, in their excellent *Overcoming Obsessive Compulsive Disorder*, reckon that about one in a hundred people suffer from OCD to some degree. I would suggest that at a sub-clinical level, it is much higher than that. Lots of us check our front doors when leaving the house, but you just shut it and heard it click, so why would you need to push against it again? Or you've just cleaned up something unsavoury, and because you're reasonably dextrous you didn't get any of it on your hands, yet you still go and wash your hands with antibacterial soap...in short, you have had a particular kind of thought – an *obsession* – and that means, for you, that you have to do something about it – the *compulsion*.

But for many people, obsession is considerably more trouble than just being a bit over-cautious when leaving the house, or being a bit over-conscientious about hygiene. Somehow you have got to a point where your life is filled with 'meaningless' ritual (although as we shall see, there is often meaning in it), or you keep going round in loops of repetition, or there's a continual battle in your head as you try to neutralise bad thoughts, or some or all of the above.

As with everything that we work with in CBT, the first step is to try to get some kind of formulation. The vicious daisy (see Chapter 1) is very useful here, but to begin with let's start with an even simpler version:

OCD Formulation

Trigger event (internal or external)

Intrusive thought, image or urge
+
Misinterpretation (metacognitive/strategic)

CONFIRMS

Anxiety reduces - phew!

Anxiety increases! Help!
Other (negative) emotion?

Do ritual, neutralising or
escape/avoidance

Let us go through this diagram. The first bit, the trigger event, may be absent – sometimes a random intrusive thought *is* the trigger event. But sometimes there is something that happens – somebody brushes into you, or you have an innocent automatic thought – but then there is an intrusive thought, image or urge. "Suppose he's got AIDS," you think. For most of us who don't suffer from OCD, it would stop there, or at the most you might think "That was a barmy thought; so what if he does?" or something like that. But as some of you will know, for OCD sufferers, there may well be another layer. This is what I have called 'misinterpretation'. It can be of two kinds:

1. Metacognitive. This means it is a reflection on the *meaning of the presence of* the thought itself: "If I had this thought, that must mean it is real."

2. Strategic. This means I have to do something about it. This is usually about **responsibility**, which is a key theme in OCD: "If he's got AIDS and I don't purify myself, then my family might get ill *and it'll be my fault.*" Of course this second one builds on the first – if having the thought

didn't mean it was 'real' then I wouldn't need to do
something about it.

So something has happened, at least in your mind, with imagined terrible
consequences; you therefore feel very anxious. There may be other
negative emotions about as well. As you think it's your responsibility to
head off this impending catastrophe, you have to find a way of doing
something about it. Whatever it is that you do – the ritual or neutralising
– somehow seems to make you feel better, or at least (in your view)
prevents you from feeling any worse. So the anxiety goes down, but in
that very reduction apparently confirms the misinterpretation that you
made in the first place. Let's take an example:

OCD Formulation - example

Trigger event (internal or external)
*Brushing against a scruffy-looking
street person*

Intrusive thought, image or urge
'He might have AIDS'
+
Misinterpretation (metacognitive/strategic)
'If I thought that, it might be true'
'If I don't do something about it, I'd be irresponsible'

CONFIRMS

Anxiety reduces - phew!
Also guilt disappears

Anxiety increases! Help!
*Also guilt (felt at the prospect
of not doing something)*

Do ritual, neutralising or
escape/avoidance
Go home immediately and wash with antibacterial soap repeatedly

Of course, even if the unfortunate street person did have AIDS, you
wouldn't catch it by brushing against him. But because the anxiety has
gone down, and the guilt disappeared, your washing action seems to
have been effective – it has been reinforced. So you have conditioned
yourself, and the next time something similar happens, you take the
same course of action.

As we have said, OCD can take many forms, not just washing or contamination issues – people may feel they need to check repeatedly, or repeat certain actions because they are worried they haven't done whatever it is properly. Sometimes people hoard things because they fear the consequences of getting rid of them. Perhaps the most subtle is the need to neutralise 'bad' thoughts – there is no externally visible ritual, but the person is working away in their head to somehow change the feared outcome of having a particular kind of thought. There are also combinations of these different styles of OCD.

The traditional treatment for OCD was called Exposure and Response Prevention, and it still forms an important part of how we work with the condition, but in the old version, the person was 'dumped' in the situation they feared and not allowed to do anything about it, with the hope that the anxiety would fade through habituation – they would get used to it. In its crudest form this was abusive! Fortunately, CBT has moved on from this. Particularly through the work of Paul Salkovskis and his team, we now pay much more attention to the *meaning* the obsession has for the person. So instead of the person having to expose themselves to whatever they feel is the threatening situation without knowing why, we explore what precisely it is about the situation that frightens them and see if we can find a way of testing out that belief. In short, we have moved from *exposure* to *behavioural experiment.*

One technique that we use to look at the meaning is the same as used in cases of panic: Theory A and Theory B. Is the problem (in the example situation above) that you and your family *will* all get AIDS and die and it'll be your fault (Theory A), or that *you are worried that* you and your family will all get AIDS and die (Theory B)?

Fortunately, most people who suffer with OCD recognise that their fears are largely irrational. You're not stupid; you know that AIDS is not transmitted by casual touch. But (and here's the sting in the tail) "What if...?" you say. "What if somehow...?"

Another of Paul Salkovskis' contributions in this area has been the formula for anxiety: the level of anxiety is determined by the *probability* of the feared event's happening multiplied by the *awfulness* of it, all divided by the person's *coping* and *rescue* factors.

$$\text{Anxiety} = \frac{\text{probability} \times \text{awfulness}}{\text{coping} + \text{rescue}}$$

So the rational part knows that the probability is very low, even if the awfulness is very high. Unfortunately, because in a probabilistic universe we can never be absolutely certain about anything at all, that seems to leave the gate open for the awful thing to happen! And in common with serious worriers (of whom OCDers can be seen as a particular type) persons with OCD tend to have a very low tolerance of uncertainty, and the more we ruminate, or even check (!), the less certain we become.

"Can I be **absolutely sure** that x won't happen?" I often hear.
"No," I say truthfully (and watch the panic rise).

One way that people look for confirmation that they have certainty is to try to get a sense of *feeling comfortable* about whatever it is. When they don't, this can be described as having 'not just right' experiences. It's surprising how hard it is to deliberately feel comfortable if you're looking for it. Why is this? Because seeking for 100% certainty, or a 'just right' experience, is just another version of 'seeking mind', which as we know is never satisfied. And as with the other anxiety disorders, we have to learn to become comfortable with (or at least able to tolerate) discomfort.

So how *can* we deal with this uncertainty? We have to go to the people who know best; who even make a living from uncertainty: the bookies! How do they determine whether something is likely to happen or not? They work out the odds. Now before you rush down to your local turf accountant to see what they'll give you on whatever your feared catastrophe is, I just want to say that we can do this in a relatively simple manner by asking ourselves the question, "Where will you put your tenner?" Will you put it on the feared event happening, or against the feared event happening? Remember, you'll lose it if you get it wrong!

To give this extra juice, if you see rationally that x is *unlikely* to happen, but you act as though it *is likely* to happen (by doing a ritual or neutralising or avoidance), then I suggest you donate the tenner to a cause you really *disagree* with. You probably won't do it very often! This brings us back to the vicious daisy – remember, *we keep beliefs strong by acting as though they are true.*

Often the belief at the centre of the daisy in OCD is a rather vague 'something bad will happen' (SBWH) if you don't do whatever the ritual is, so quite naturally you tend to do whatever it is in order to fend off this SBWH. But in doing this, you are playing the *Asterix* game – by *acting as though* the sky will fall on your head, you seem to confirm its likelihood; its probability. Fortunately, this tactic works both ways – if you act as though the sky will *not* fall on your head, you reduce the likelihood in your own mind. Especially if you notice that whatever it is *doesn't* happen, or that eventually the anxiety reduces of its own accord.

Fill yours in here:

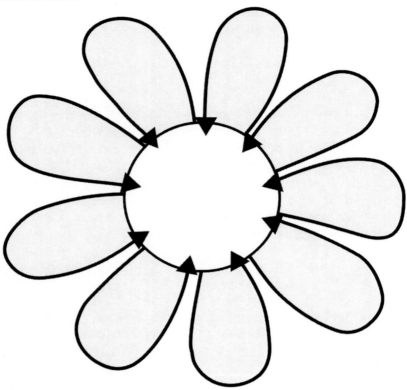

Historical origins

Often when we examine the nature of the ritual, there is a clue as to the sort of belief, or perhaps a particular incident, that lies at the heart of it.

For example, amongst people who are particularly concerned about contamination there has sometimes developed a belief that they are disgusting and in need of purification, as a reaction to an incident or series of incidents from their childhoods. (I stress this is not always the case.) Or someone who is concerned that something bad will happen to others as a result of their action or non-action may have been brought up with a particularly strong belief in original sin, or a strong sense of moral responsibility.

We cannot always find sense in the particular ritual, but that doesn't mean there isn't some kind of logic in it. Fortunately it's not essential to know where it came from for treatment to be successful, although it can obviously help understanding.

What is clear is that OCD didn't just emerge randomly; like all the other little Is, it evolved in response to something – in the case of OCD, usually to something experienced as inconceivable, yet which we think we are somehow responsible for, or would be if we didn't do the ritual. If you want to explore the origins of your OCD more, you may wish to revisit Chapter 7 on schemas, but don't spend too much time there! Also see the section on OCD and Big Mind further on.

When is it, and when is it not, OCD?
Especially if you have been troubled by OCD for a long time, you may need some help in distinguishing between an OCD-type thought or course of action and a 'normal' thought. There are two ways of dealing with this:

1. Act *against* what the thought is saying and see if it makes you anxious. If it does, it's probably OCD. If it doesn't, then it probably isn't.
2. Imagine you have an identical twin who acts just like you in every way, except s/he doesn't have OCD. If you have a middle name that you like, sometimes people call their OCD-free twin by that name. What would your OCD-free twin do or think in this situation?

Why do I believe it?
Even while people often recognise the OCD nature of their thought and behaviour, and see its irrationality, somehow it still has a hold. It has been established that people make a correlation between the strength of the physical sensations of the anxiety they feel and the truth of the thought that triggered it. So if I'm feeling really anxious, then that must mean the thought is true! When we look at it like that it is easy to see that there is no necessary connection between these two things, but that this is a case of *arbitrary inference* – another thinking error. Although of course it is important to realise that to *primitive brain* this is how we have survived up till now – the strength of our physical reactions has been our main sign of danger (better safe than sorry) and the need to take evasive action.

Medication
Sometimes, sufferers from OCD are reluctant to take medication. Beware all-or-nothing thinking: sometimes you need some help from medication in order to enable you even to do the experiments. The SSRI group of antidepressants has a good track record with OCD, but some

have side effects; if after a reasonable period you are still suffering from said side effects go back to your GP and see if another type works better for you.

"It's not me, it's my OCD"

Jeffrey Schwartz's celebrated book *Brain Lock*, on using mindfulness to treat OCD, has some areas about which I have concerns, but one place where there is definite agreement is in his phrase "It's not me, it's my OCD." It is helpful to see OCD as an interloper who has taken over too much of the brain, and is lording it over the other parts. If you think of yourself as a bus, do you really want OCD to be the driver?

And in fact this is the first step to becoming free of OCD – to recognise that this is a rogue program that is giving you unhelpful directions which take your thinking and behaviour to places you really don't want to go. But we need to think about what being free of OCD would look like – "To be free of all these horrible thoughts!" I hear you say.

Wrong!

In a survey of people who didn't have OCD, Paul Salkovskis and his team found that 90% of people have intrusive thoughts – nasty stuff in their mind that they'd rather wasn't there – and my belief is that the other 10% are probably lying! I think we all have unpleasant thoughts that come into our minds from time to time. The difference between OCD sufferers and the rest is *what we do about these thoughts*. For most people, the presence of a particular kind of thought in your head, by itself is no big deal. "That was a mad thought," you think, and move on. But if the presence of the thought *is itself* a problem, then you (think you) have to do something about it – just like worrying.

Taking a thought for an event is *thought-event fusion*, a kind of thinking error. Just because I think of something, it doesn't mean it will happen. It may or it may not, but it's not dependent on my thinking. I used to commute to work by train, and would ask the disaster-mongers in the OCD group to try and bump me off with thoughts about my train crashing. Not so much as a squeak!

Mistaking a thought for an action is *thought-action fusion*, also a kind of thinking error. If I have an image of me doing something, that is not the same as doing it.

Thinking that an object is dangerous/contaminated is the same as an object *being* dangerous or contaminated is *thought-object fusion*, also a kind of thinking error.

In short, what OCD and worriers have in common is in taking the thought for reality. "Because I've thought about it/seen it on TV/ something reminded me of it, I've got to apply deliberate thinking to it."

No.

We don't need to apply deliberate thinking to anything that comes in automatically (whether intrusive or not). Unless we *want* to, and if it's genuinely in our own best interests.

So recovery won't mean that the thoughts disappear! But they don't need to, because it's not the thoughts that are the problem. Take some time to let that sink in.

Recovery won't mean that the thoughts disappear.

Of course, if you try to make a thought disappear, what happens? Old campaigners will know the answer to this one.

Try not to think of pink elephants...
...or white bears...
...or spotted gerbils...

See, it doesn't matter which sort of wildlife you try not to think about, making that effort to make it go away keeps it right in the forefront of your mind. So if you try to suppress or banish particular kinds of thought, they will become louder and more prevalent. "We don't want to be disowned," they say.

So recovery won't mean that thoughts disappear, but if you stop trying to make them go away, they may well decrease in frequency and intensity – they are no longer shouting to be heard. Remember, *intrusive thoughts are only intrusive if you don't let them in!* And as they're 'in' already, it's a bit pointless trying to keep them out...

RADIO OCD AND MINDFULNESS

One way of thinking about OCD in a suitably detached way, and which helps us to know what to do and what not to do about it, is 'Radio OCD'[18]. If you go to visit a friend and there's a radio playing music you don't like – suppose you don't like heavy metal, and that's what's playing – you probably wouldn't be personally upset by this music, even if it's not to your taste. You wouldn't make a special effort to block it out – you'd just

---

18   Developed jointly with Rob Willson. Thanks Rob!

ignore it, and have a conversation with your friend. You might find it slightly irritating, but most people wouldn't be very strongly affected – you just accept it as a fact that this music is what is playing. You certainly don't blame yourself for the presence of this music.

This is the attitude that we want to encourage in relation to intrusive thoughts: you *didn't have any control* over their coming into your mind, you recognise that they are OCD-ish in origin (rather than your freely chosen understanding), and because of the elephants, bears and gerbils, you can't turn them off – in fact the volume control is on backwards, so the more you try not to think of them, the louder they get!

Another characteristic of the radio is that it is automatically preset to the particular OCD station that upsets you (so, for example, checkers who aren't bothered about contamination don't get 'dirty' intrusive thoughts.)

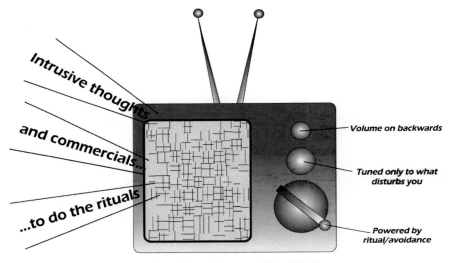

"...you're listening in stereo to Radio OCD..."

So Radio OCD broadcasts intrusive thoughts, but it also broadcasts advertisements – it's a commercial station. The adverts are promoting the use of ritual or avoidance or neutralising, and say something like, "If you just do this thing (wash, check, repeat etc.), just this once won't hurt, then I'll stop giving you a hard time with these nasty thoughts and images."
Quite reasonably, you are tempted to carry out the ritual – anything to stop these damned intrusive thoughts.

Stop! Just say no! Because what Radio OCD doesn't actually tell you is that it is actually a wind-up radio (in both senses of the term), and what is keeping the intrusive thoughts at their current level of mind-tearing intensity is the use of ritual. While in the short term you can't do anything to turn them down (and anything you do attempt will simply have the opposite effect), in the longer term *abstaining* from the ritual, so you don't reward the commercials, will reduce both the frequency and intensity of the intrusive thoughts. In short, you may have to listen to the commercials, *but **don't** buy the product*, because you don't want to give it power for the future. Remember, doing rituals recharges the battery of Radio OCD, so don't.

MINDFULNESS

This is, of course, a mindful strategy – seeing I am not my thoughts, I am free not to believe them, and I don't have to do what they say.

The concept of mindfulness is used for two different things, and so it can be a bit confusing. One is really an attitude, or insight. We could describe Radio OCD as an example of that: the sense that, as Buddhist monks are taught to remind themselves: "This am I not, this is not mine, this is not myself."

The other is what Jon Kabat-Zinn calls the 'scaffolding': the practices you do to help you get into or stay in that awareness. So on the one hand we use a mindful attitude to see that we are not the OCD, and on the other we can use (e.g.) mindfulness of breathing to help us stay with the feelings that come up when we don't do the rituals. After all, a good part of why people do the rituals in the first place is because they find the anxiety 'unbearable', right? Yet by using the breathing to help stay with the physical sensations, and not being taken in by the rantings of Radio OCD, we can learn that while the sensations may be deeply unpleasant, they are in fact bearable, and in the end we learn to become *comfortable with discomfort*.

So, to prevent us from getting too theoretical, and to practise what we have learned, you might like to do a little mindful breathing. Take a break from reading this chapter and do some now.

Sitting comfortably upright, begin to notice that you are in fact breathing (if you're not, go and see a doctor...). Allow yourself to notice what is going on in thoughts (hallo intrusive thoughts, welcome), and emotions (hallo anxiety, how do you do) and body sensations (feeling, feeling). Remind yourself they're all allowed to be here. Listen to what they have to say, they're your honoured guests. When you've heard them, do a mental bow to them, and take your attention to the breathing. Imagine them coming too if you like.

See where you notice the breath, perhaps coming and going in the nose... or following it down to wherever it goes down to, and back up again... or just in the expanding and contracting of the lower belly... wherever you notice it, just letting it do its thing in its own time and rhythm, and gently attaching your awareness to it. Of course from time to time your awareness will wander off – that's all right, minds do that!– but when you notice, just gently bringing your attention back to the breath...

Sitting comfortably upright, begin to notice that you are in fact breathing (if you're not, go and see a doctor...). Allow yourself to notice what is going on in thoughts (hallo intrusive thoughts, welcome), and emotions (hallo anxiety, how do you do) and body sensations (feeling, feeling). Remind yourself they're all allowed to be here. Listen to what they have to say, they're your honoured guests. When you've heard them, do a mental bow to them, and take your attention to the breathing. Imagine them coming too if you like.

See where you notice the breath, perhaps coming and going in the nose... or following it down to wherever it goes down to, and back up again... or just in the expanding and contracting of the lower belly... wherever you notice it, just letting it do its thing in its own time and rhythm, and gently attaching your awareness to it. Of course from time to time your awareness will wander off – that's all right, minds do that!– but when you notice, just gently bringing your attention back to the breath...

I hope you weren't doing that to make the intrusive thoughts go away!

Big I, little I

Another way of helping ourselves to remain detached from OCD is to view it as simply another little I in the 'Big I, Little I' model. This is the 'thoughts and feelings as my children' attitude. OCD is a little I; a particular program or schema formed over time in reaction to a particular set of circumstances. Like every little I it has something to say, and as we can't shut it out it's a good idea to listen to it (at least at first), but we don't have to do what it says. We can instead think of it as Radio OCD, let it broadcast, and use mindfulness of breathing to help us tolerate the feelings that come up.

What comes up

One thing that is often surprising, and sometimes discouraging, to people is what happens when you do this – allowing the feelings to arise without doing anything to close them down or make them go away. You may have had a fantasy that you would start to feel better if you did this. In one ongoing OCD group, we used to write a little motto at the top of the flipchart:

> *Feel better, get worse;*
> *Feel worse, get better.*

Horrible, isn't it? Of course in the longer term you will feel better (although not 100% blissfully happy all the time), but in the short term you will have to deal with what comes up when you don't do the rituals/neutralising etc. So you will probably feel worse! Most commonly this unwanted feeling is anxiety, but sometimes there are others as well, like anger or sadness.

As with all the other conditions in this book, we need to go through certain stages in working with OCD. After formulation, and reminding ourselves that we are not the contents of our minds *and* that we don't need to believe them or do what they say, it is nonetheless a good idea, especially if we want to avoid falling down this hole again, to find out what they want. Then you no longer have to use OCD to suppress whatever it is. Having done this, we can then bring other aspects to the fore to restore some balance.

The Big Mind Process and OCD

You will recall that the Big Mind process is a technique that comes from a synthesis of the sudden enlightenment doctrine from Zen with a kind of therapy called voice dialogue. Basically it is a technique to let all the little Is have a say but also to discover the bigger voices, like that of awareness itself. Remember, the 'big I little I' diagram has no edges.

One of the basic tenets is that it is important not to try to suppress any little I. If we do manage to do that, what can happen is that it pops up somewhere else. In voice dialogue, from which the big mind process is derived, we talk about a voice (a little I) becoming 'disowned'. (These are not voices in the sense of auditory hallucinations). If this happens, we talk about the voice going undercover and causing trouble. Of course we do not have to do what any particular little I is telling us to do, we simply have to let it have its say, like on a committee.

Actually, it can be helpful to view OCD as an already 'disowned' voice of something else – often anxiety, sometimes anger. Performing the compulsion is after all what we have been doing to keep the anxiety or other unpleasant emotion at bay! Naturally, you find out which emotion has been disowned by not doing the rituals and seeing what happens.

So let's suppose that there has been enough in this chapter to persuade you that doing the rituals is a bad idea, and you've taken the plunge; whatever normally happens to make you do the ritual has already happened and you're having the intrusive thoughts. You resist your usual compulsion. Now what?

We need to find out what is happening in there! If you have access to a therapist who can facilitate Big Mind then you can ask the OCD directly what it's afraid of, or use 'empty chair' (put an empty chair in front of you, imagine your OCD sitting in it, and just ask it what you want to ask it); or just breathe into the place where you feel the anxiety or other suppressed feeling the strongest. What is the feeling? Do you remember when you first felt like that? Was it in response to a particular difficult situation? What decision did you make (like "I'm never going to let myself go through that/ feel like that again")? Allow the feelings to be there with the body sensations. Cry if you need to. Be nice to yourself. Tea, chocolate biscuits, that sort of thing.

PUTTING IT ALL TOGETHER

Hopefully, if you've got this far you will now be aware of your OCD in a rather different way than you were at the beginning. So you know that OCD really isn't giving you correct information, but because of the imagined penalties (to yourself or others) you've kept on doing the rituals, mentally or physically. Now that you can see it's just Radio OCD, you definitely don't have to do what it says.

So now we can go back to behavioural experiments and even to exposure and response prevention, but in a new way. But we need to think, as with all behavioural experiments, about what it is we are testing. Fortunately, as we have noted, most people with OCD recognise that the intrusive thoughts are not rational. You cannot usually do a behavioural experiment about the content of an intrusive thought unless it refers to something predicted in the immediate future – like, if I think of somebody having a crash on Tuesday, will they actually have a crash on Tuesday? But you can do an experiment about what happens if you don't do what it says! "If I don't wash my hands (check/neutralise etc.), then does my anxiety go down anyway (after a while)?" Of course if you keep *looking for* the anxiety you can bring it up again, but that's another story.

Think of your behavioural experiment, and write it on the blank form on the next page. Look back over Chapter 5 on behaviour if you like, to help remind you of the principles.

Behavioural Experiment Record Sheet

Theory you want to test	Planned experiment	Safety Behaviours you might use	What happens when you carry it out	Results	What can I do now?

EXPOSURE AND RESPONSE PREVENTION REVISITED

OCD is sticky, there's no doubt about it. Doing your rituals, whether physical, like washing or checking, or mental, like neutralising or counting in your head, gives you temporary relief from your discomfort. This is what we call negative reinforcement, and it is understandably very powerful. It is like an addiction – if I take this, I don't have pain now.

Apparently the brain physiology of OCD *is* very similar to drug addiction. So although we discover that, in any particular instance, the intrusive thought may not be true, years of habit have created powerful patterns in the neural pathways, and the default reaction will be to revert to doing the ritual. Fortunately, this doesn't have to be an obstacle to effective treatment.

The process of working with these persistent patterns means employing an effective and well-targeted combination of behavioural experiments and exposure. So CBT practitioners no longer suggest dumping you in the situation that you fear in the hope that you will become habituated to it! Rather, we advise:

1. Unpicking *what it is* about the situation that particularly frightens you.
2. Testing it out.
3. And once you are happy that the fear is unfounded, going through a well-targeted exposure and response prevention programme so that the anxiety *discovers it is no longer needed.*

As we mentioned in Chapter 5, another way of looking at what you're doing in exposure, as compared to behavioural experiments, is that you're training *the body* or *the animal.* Behavioural experiments by themselves may convince rational mind, and sometimes intuitive, poetic mind as well, but often the body mysteriously remains untouched, so you still get the body sensations of anxiety, which can then start the cycle all over again. The frightened animal has to be deconditioned.

You will remember also that exposures have to be done repeatedly, consistently and without exception. If you occasionally reinforce the thing you're afraid of, that is like the occasional reward you get on a slot-machine game – it keeps you playing! And in this case we want to stop the game, so ideally we need to face whatever it is daily, *allow the anxiety to come up*, stay in the situation long enough for the anxiety to come down *by itself,* and repeat until the situation provokes no further anxiety. Of course the response-prevention bit means we don't do any rituals or safety-seeking behaviours.

Remember also not to undermine the exposure by distracting yourself while it's happening. That won't work, because although this is about training the 'body-mind', the 'mind-mind' needs to be there too. And if you're saying to yourself "I need to be distracted" then at some level you're telling yourself that the situation must be really scary – or why would you need to be distracting yourself? It is also important to emphasise that, for exposure to work, the anxiety needs to come up! The body can't discover that anxiety isn't needed unless it's there.

Finally, don't get caught up in the belief that, "I shouldn't feel anxious." This unfortunately is the red rag to the proverbial bull. It is as though you are saying to your (vital, necessary, helpful) alarm system, "You shouldn't be there, and I'm going to ignore you if I can." Of course the Protector isn't going to wear that, because as mentioned previously, there is often a deeper layer of meaning in the feared situation; a much earlier association, perhaps, of some traumatic event and something about the situation that's giving you trouble – the 'glue' in that case being the emotional charge attached to the original event. This is akin to what the Buddhists call *samskaras* – mental formations[19]. Whether you access this mental formation/schema/program by breathing into it mindfully or asking it directly what it wants is up to you, but it is a good idea to be open to it, although successful treatment does not necessarily depend on finding what's underneath.

Uncovering whatever may have given rise to the OCD may be painful, but it can take a lot of the 'heat' out of it . It is, however, important not to make the mistake that sufferers sometimes make, which is to say that, "I know where it comes from now, so I don't need to worry about doing the exposures." Unfortunately that won't work, because even though you may understand the origins of your OCD in some childhood situation, perhaps remembered somewhere in the body, the OCD itself has had a lot of time and practice to build up its own momentum and neural pathways. So even though your head or 'mind-mind' may know the connection, we still need to get to a place where the 'body-mind' no longer gets anxious in the situation.

Here is the form you can use for a hierarchy. There is a blank one for photocopying in the appendix at the back of the book. If you have some different areas you are working on, you may wish to have a different hierarchy for each one:

19   Which, interestingly, they consider to be located in the body!

Hierarchy			
Situation	How scary? 0-100	Working on it? (Tick)	No longer gives anxiety (Tick)

TIPS FOR SUCCESSFUL EXPOSURE WORK AND RELAPSE PREVENTION

As we have said, possibly *ad nauseam* by now, exposures need to be done repeatedly and consistently – daily if possible. The more you're really there in mind and body, the better they are likely to work. If you slip, and do the ritual/neutralising, then you need to do an **anti-ritual!** So if you wash your hands after an incident of 'contamination', then re-contaminate immediately, so that there is no benefit in ritualising.

If you check the door after leaving the house, then go back inside and come out and leave it unchecked (if that's where you are on your hierarchy). Sometimes it's good to do an anti-ritual at the time: one client I knew used praying as a ritual, so I suggested that she close each prayer with "Bollocks to God, Amen!" (I'm sure He understands!) She stopped using prayer as a ritual.

Sometimes, rather like an old Laurel and Hardy comedy, you manage to get one OCD aspect under control and another one, formerly minor, pops up with the severity of the first one! So you just have to keep on turning towards whatever it is, experiencing the feelings, not doing the ritual/neutralising, and carrying on. If this is happening a lot, then I'd be tempted to ask whether there's anything cooking underneath? Are you using ritualising of one sort or another to suppress something that is trying to come to the surface? Any clues in what we've been talking about earlier in the chapter, or in the chapter on schemas? Allow yourself to really *feel* whatever is present in the body sensations that come up when you don't do the rituals. It might not be anxiety, but could be another emotion you have disowned, like anger, for example.

Often, once the anxiety starts up, people get caught up in the whole secondary anxiety thing – the meaning of what it is to be anxious: 'I'm never going to get better"; "I'm a lost cause" etc. Try instead just to focus mindfully on the *physical* side of the feeling, rather than adding yet another layer of problems with a lot of futile speculation.

Of course you would expect the symptoms to be worse in times of stress, and they usually are. So don't give yourself a hard time if you have slipped back a bit for whatever reason (because that just triggers the threat/self-protection system which will only make it worse), but do take whatever steps are necessary to break the loop, including going to your medical practitioner to get your medication reviewed if necessary.

Finally, remember that the criteria for getting better don't concern the presence of the thoughts, but rather *how you react to them* and *what you can now do that you couldn't do before*, and the (hopefully reduced) severity of the anxiety, or at least greater tolerance of it. Once you've worked through the OCD section, it may be helpful to go back to the previous chapters on panic and worry. If you're no longer running from the OCD, and you've reached the top of your hierarchy but still have high levels of anxiety, then it may be that a mindfulness course is what you need to complete treatment.

RELAPSE PREVENTION

What is needed to deal with OCD is a thoroughgoing change of attitude, and the changes in behaviour that follow from that. This means *going on turning towards* whatever the thing is that's making you feel uncomfortable. I know that's difficult.

Unfortunately people sometimes get to a place – we call it the OCD plateau – where they've overcome it to some extent, got it a bit under control, so they're doing fewer rituals (or at least it interferes less with their daily functioning) but it's still dominating their lives. My understanding of this is that it's like a pair of weighing scales. On the one side you have the thing that threatens to come up if you *don't* do the OCD rituals: anxiety or other unpleasant stuff, maybe from the past. On the other side is the OCD itself, which if you give way to it too much will also seriously disrupt your life. So you play the balancing act, trying to do the OCD enough to stop the doo-doo rising to the surface, but not so much that you can't function in the world. I'm afraid it's not going to work, because sooner or later something of a stressful nature will happen, and before you know it, you'll be right back in the grip of full-blown OCD. No – if you're doing a bit of OCD to stop 'stuff' rising to the surface, please stop and let it come up and say its piece. It almost certainly won't be as bad as you fear. Get the help of a therapist who knows what s/he's doing, OCD-wise, and see what happens. Good luck!

Further Reading

Hyman, B. R. and Pedrick, C. (2005), *The OCD Workbook*, New Harbinger
Veale, D. and Willson, R. (2005), *Overcoming Obsessive Compulsive Disorder*, Robinson
Schwartz, J.M., with Beyette, B. (1996), *Brain Lock*, Harper Collins

CHAPTER 20: HEALTH ANXIETY

Fear I might catch something – Sickness and death – Fear I've already got something – Safety behaviours – How will they cope? – Who dies? – Mindfulness – Death – Hierarchy

Anxiety about health, formerly called *hypochondriasis*, has so much in common with OCD that if you suffer from it, it is worth going through the preceding chapter because you can work with it in exactly the same way. There are of course some particular characteristics, which we will feature here, but essentially this chapter is an add-on to the previous one.

We can divide up anxiety about health in various ways – for example you may have a *fear of* catching or contracting some kind of illness (this is particularly like, and overlaps with, OCD); in this case you are probably already aware that this is really a psychological problem. On the other hand, you may be troubled by the fear that you *already have* some kind of illness, because you have symptoms, but the doctor has given you the all-clear. In fact 'hypochondriasis' is the only diagnosis that includes a statement about what the doctors have done ("persists despite medical reassurance")!

There are also two other related conditions: anxiety about health where there *is* an agreed medical problem, and somatisation, which is where the psychological issues are only felt *through* the mechanism of physical illness. Inevitably there is some overlap between all these variants.

FEAR THAT I WILL CATCH A PARTICULAR DISEASE

In recognising that this has become a problem, we have acknowledged that this is an issue of psychology rather than medicine. It is of course understandable, especially when (at the time of writing) there is so much media attention given to various kinds of flu that purport to come from animals. ("What do you get when swine flu meets avian flu? Pigs might fly.")

Here the most effective strategy, assuming that you have become overly cautious in your behaviour, is probably the cost-benefit: *if* you caught whatever it is you're afraid of, your life might be restricted in various ways. But how restricted has it become because of the avoidant behaviour that you are currently adopting? Not going to shopping centres or crowded places could mean a restriction on your social life, for example.

And one thing that we all have to acknowledge, whichever version of health anxiety we are troubled by (or not), is that we are all going to die, sooner or later. We all have to face the perennial question, "Since the fact of death is certain, and the time of death uncertain, how should we live?" (Stephen Batchelor, summarising the Buddha).

SICKNESS AND DEATH

It will be obvious to those who have read this far that the ideas from Buddhism have had a profound influence on this author. The question of how to deal with sickness and death was the question that led the young Gautama to run away from the life as a prince that his father had planned for him (funny how children do that), and into the forest to learn the spiritual technologies of his time. In a sense the great question of life and death is the most difficult question any of us has to deal with. So I am sometimes relieved when death is revealed as the question that somebody has really come to see me with – there is a sense of "Ah, now we can get right down to it!"

In this society however we don't talk about death much – even our meat and fish comes neatly packaged so that we are removed from its origins as dead creatures. A friend of mine was shocked watching a cremation in India by the riverbank – as the corpse (openly visible on the top of the pyre) started to burn, the muscles and tendons contracted, causing the body to sit up! And round the bend in the river, people dive in to extract the gold fillings from the teeth. Nothing wasted...

If we are brought up in a religious family, we are taught a perfectly normal children's story about death – heaven if we're good, hell if we're bad – which may be as much about social control as anything. This is deeply unsatisfying later on. The only other version we usually get is a physicalist, pseudo-scientific story that says that mind or spirit is simply an epiphenomenon – a by-product if you like – of physical existence, and there is definitely nothing after death. This is as unscientific as saying that definitely there is something. So often the process of therapy for anxiety about death, if that is what it comes down to, is about getting a mature, intelligent perspective on death, which helps us to come to terms with it. More on this below.

FEAR THAT I HAVE AN ILLNESS ALREADY

If the worry is not so much about the fear that I might catch something but rather that I may already have something, then the first line of investigation is provided by our old friends Theory A and Theory B. I think of them as a sort of professorial Tweedledum and Tweedledee.

Theory A, when applied to this fear, defines the problem as, "You are really suffering from x disease; undoubtedly terminal or at the very least permanently debilitating." He is a bit of a pessimist.

Theory B says, "You are really *worried that* you might be suffering from x disease, which if you had it would be undoubtedly terminal or at the very least permanently debilitating."

Now if you say to Theory B, "So you're saying I *haven't* got x disease?" he will reply, "No, that's not what I said. I don't know if you have x disease or not. I'm not a doctor; I'm a theory. But it may be that your symptoms, which undoubtedly exist, are better explained by your worrying about the disease and the things you do because you believe that your worries are true."

So there we have them, Tweedledum and Tweedledee, standing before us, with their different opinions as to what is the case. You may recall that when we had this problem with panic, it was quite easy, if a bit scary, to find out which one was true, because the feared consequences were immediate and we could test them out. But if I've got the awful x disease, and it's there in my bloodstream, waiting to manifest in six months, and I don't do anything about it...eek!

The clue, I think, is in the very precise way that Theory B answered us: "...your symptoms, which undoubtedly exist, are better explained by your worrying about the disease and the things you do because you believe that your worries are true."

So what *do you* do because of these worries? There are a number of things – safety behaviours – that are commonly done:

Selective attention: you keep focusing on the part of the body or some aspect of the symptom or sensation, to the exclusion of all other parts of the body or indeed anything else much at all.

Checking: you keep interrupting whatever you may be involved in to check the status of or feelings around the part. "Has it got worse? Is it swollen or inflamed?" This can then be 'upgraded' to prodding or poking the affected area, which in turn can exacerbate the problem

Reassurance-seeking: as we noted, this actually forms part of the diagnosis. According to DSM-IV, the condition persists *despite medical reassurance*. It is pernicious, because the reassurance appears to satisfy, but the satisfaction is short-lived. It also takes up a lot of GPs' time. People become addicted to reassurance much like cigarettes: because it's so temporary you want another one ten minutes later. The solution is therefore to expose the temporary nature of the satisfaction: "If I reassure you now, how long will it last?"

Information-seeking: closely related to reassurance, the old version of this was to keep thumbing through some medical textbook; the modern variant is to trawl the internet for examples of symptoms like the ones you're experiencing in order to find out all the terrible things that can happen, and then to try to find ways of curing them.

It's worth doing a vicious daisy around these safety behaviours: what is the belief at the centre? What would be a more helpful belief (even if you don't believe it yet)? What happens to the need to do these things if you put the new belief at the centre of the daisy (and therefore make it into a 'kindly daisy')?

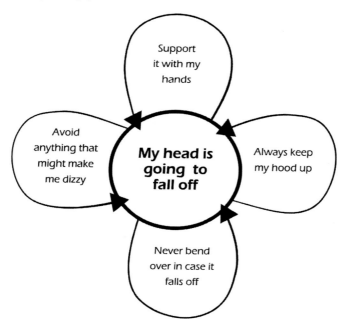

Although this seems ridiculous, it may be easier to see the process when you take an example like this. Apparently Tchaikovsky had a similar fear. So what happens if you substitute (in the central part) *My head is perfectly adequately attached?* That's right: you can bend over, let your hood down, go on a fairground ride or have a few beers, and take your hands away from your head! So let's take a more serious one:

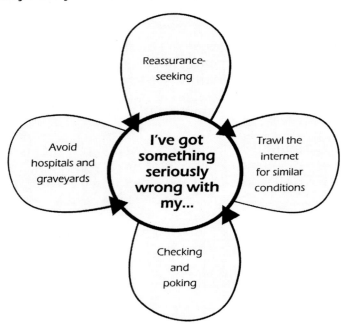

Does this look anything like yours? Of course you can't put in the centre: *There's absolutely nothing wrong with me and there never will be because I'm immortal* (unless you're in Big Mind!), because in fact we're all dying from the moment we're born. What has a beginning has an end. But you can put something like: *I'm good enough for now* or *There's no reason to focus on my health.* What happens if you put that at the centre? (No, you don't have to believe it yet!) What are the petals then? You can go back to visiting Granny's grave if you want to; you can use the internet for more interesting investigations; you can stop pestering your doctor and your body. So this is the experiment: make your kindly daisy and *act as if it is true,* which is the same as taking Theory B's approach. No, I'm still not asking you to believe it – just act in this way and see what happens – *then* you can decide which of our theories is right.

Use a blank daisy or two (from the back of the book) and do both your vicious (theory A) and your kindly (theory B) daisies.

How will they cope?

Sometimes it is not so much the inevitability of death and the question of what happens to oneself after that that is the problem; often, especially for parents, it is a worry about what will happen to the children, or how the newly bereft spouse or partner will cope.

Here we need to think about what will happen – but only once! Because we also need to think about *the effect of thinking about* what will happen – do people who *don't* have a lot of anxiety about health spend inordinate amounts of time working out what will happen to their children in the event of their death? Obviously not. Do people who don't have a lot of anxiety about health take routine precautions (writing a will; taking out life assurance, perhaps) about what might happen to their children in the event of their death? They most probably do.

So, once you have taken care of the necessary, spending too much time thinking on the post-death situation confirms, in a vicious daisy-type way, the 'truth' of the belief that there's something wrong with you.

However, as a one-off, it may be useful to do the movie-projection exercise: first (and you probably won't have much difficulty doing this) run the nightmare scenario – you know, the one in which your spouse becomes an alcoholic and neglects the children who end up begging on the streets or working as prostitutes in an undesirable quarter of Valparaíso. Then run the *Care Bears* version – equally unrealistic, but in a good way, where every neighbour who's ever met your family wins the lottery and festoons their path with £20 notes while ensuring that they all fulfil their potential (and talk to your photograph daily).

Obviously this wouldn't happen either. So what would be the likely outcome? After the horror movie and the *Care Bears* version, what's the documentary? Certainly, they'd be sad if you died. Probably relatives, friends and/or neighbours would help out a bit, in the short term at least. There might need to be some downsizing, depending on the economic impact of your death. Would they get over it? Almost certainly (although they'll still be sad sometimes). Might your death lead to some useful re-evaluation in terms of their priorities and their own mortality? It's possible, isn't it? (I'm not just talking about "You're gonna miss me when I'm dead and gone" as the song has it.)

So now you have a workable version of what would probably happen to your family in the event of your death, how about getting on with living? How much fun can you have/good stuff can you do *before* you die, so that your tombstone doesn't read, *Spent her/his life worrying about what would happen afterwards, and missed it?*

WHO OR WHAT DIES?

If we go back to the 'I am not this piece of furniture' game, you will remember that we came to the conclusion that if I can be aware of something, I am not it. That is the logic which we learn very early and helps us not to trip over things – I see it, so I go round it rather than trying to walk through it. Very useful.

So, likewise, in becoming *aware* of our thoughts and feelings we can discover that we are *not* our thoughts and feelings, and so don't need to identify with them, or indeed be bothered by them at all unless we want to, because they don't necessarily say anything about us. This can be helpful in anxiety about health as it can with any other emotional disorder.

But of course we can do the same thing with the body: can you be aware of your body? If you are reading this chapter, then the answer is most definitely yes! Actually I'm sure that everyone can be aware of their bodies. Well, if you can be aware of your body, are you your body, or the one who is aware of your body? I hope the answer is, 'the one who is aware of my body', or we could say, 'the one who lives in this body'. OK. So who or what becomes sick and dies? The body, of course. So, 'I' am not my body. Does that mean that 'I' won't die?

It is not up to me to tell you what to believe about life after death. You may well have your own religious viewpoint, which is helpful to you. But if you're happy with the analysis so far, then at least we can say, "I don't know what happens to the one who is aware." And in fact the 'don't know mind' is a very good place to hang out, especially if, as the worrying kind, you struggle with tolerating uncertainty. I mean 'good' in the sense of exposure, but also because when you get used to it, it's such a relief not having to know everything!

SCANNING VERSUS 'AWARENESS OF THE BODY IN THE BODY'

As we saw, and you know already, the tendency with anxiety about health is to be constantly on the lookout for any variation or unfamiliar sensation, which you then start to investigate from an anxious viewpoint. ("Is this a threat to me? What will it turn into? I'd better get it checked out" etc.) So the anxious body-radar is constantly scanning, and what you seek, so shall you find. There is always some weird sensation to be worried about if you look hard enough. If you like, try this experiment: take a part of your body that doesn't concern you (if you can find one) – let's say your left knee. Close your eyes and focus on it – try to see if everything seems to be OK with it. Are there any unexpected sensations, or a faint tingling that you hadn't noticed before? Oh my God, what's that? Is it a cartilage injury? Maybe I played too much football when I was younger? Or perhaps it's a ligament...

Do you see what I'm getting at? If you scan in a concentrated enough fashion, you will probably find something, but that doesn't necessarily mean there's anything there.

On the other hand (or knee), we can, with training, experience the body in a totally different way. The Buddha talked about becoming mindful of the body *in the body*. What I understand this to mean is where you locate the awareness. So when we scan – looking for trouble, as it were – we are 'in our heads' with a specific brief – the amygdala-style, "Will it hurt me?" agenda.

Dealing With Supplements

Sam is a health-conscious, formerly health-anxious businessman with a keen interest in keeping himself fit; he takes part in various activities ranging from boxing training to tai chi. He also takes vitamin supplements.

Away on a trip, he was unable to get his regular brand of supplement, and bought a cheaper brand, as that was all that was available. Some minutes after taking them, he felt a burning sensation envelop his body – and he went bright red, the change not a product of his imagination but clearly visible to his wife. His T-shirt felt as though it was burning against his chest.

Recognising that this might be an allergic reaction, he had the presence of mind to put the packet of pills in his pocket, so that if he did pass out or get taken to hospital, the medical people would know what he had taken. He then lay down on the bed. What he thought, as he described it later, was: "OK, this is what is happening in my body right now." He didn't panic, although he definitely felt some anxiety. "My heart fluttered a bit," he said. He just stayed with the sensations, and then drifted off to sleep. He slept for an hour, and when he woke up, the sensations and the red colouration had gone. Previously, he said, the anxiety and panic he would have felt in a situation like that would have been overwhelming.

But if we do mindfulness of the body *in the body*, we actually take our consciousness into the tissue, the bone and so on, rather than viewing it from 'upstairs,' which is the view of the 'head-dictator', and instead explore it *non-judgementally*. To the extent you can do this, I promise that you will find quite different results. The example on the previous page is an incident that happened to someone who had previously suffered from health anxiety and panic; this event occurred towards the end of the eight-week mindfulness programme.

But if you've been stuck in the health-anxious way of being aware of your body for a while, it may be difficult to do mindfulness of the body to start with, so in the short term, it will probably be more helpful to take your awareness away from your body and see what the effect is on your anxiety. So if you find yourself scanning or checking, say to yourself, "Scanning; checking" and return your attention back to whatever you were doing. That is also a sort of mindfulness.

My guess is that when you don't check or poke, trawl the internet, seek reassurance or do anything else about your bodily symptoms, your anxiety will reduce *even if there's something wrong with you*. Because let's face it, there's something wrong with all of us; the seeds of our own demise are present in our birth. Or at least, the seeds of the demise of our *bodies*; about the rest, perhaps "it were better to say nothing".

I HAVE AN ILLNESS ALREADY AND AM ANXIOUS ABOUT IT: WHAT TO DO ABOUT DEATH?

This brings us to the related category of the person who has a diagnosed, possibly fatal illness and is worried about it. First and foremost, as always, cut yourself some slack. No wonder you're worried about it. Take the necessary care of yourself to maintain whatever quality of life is possible, but don't focus any more on it than is helpful; if, as Jon Kabat-Zinn says, you are still breathing, there is more right with you than wrong with you. The question is, how can I most appreciate the life I have left?

But of course, like every single person on the planet, you are faced with the main question: how do I come to terms with my own death? Philosophers, scientists, mystics, poets and other curious people have been struggling with this one since prehistory, and they haven't all come up with the same answer. So it's not surprising you are at least apprehensive.

To begin with, we need to start thinking about it in a constructive adult way. In western societies most of us are brought up with a story to placate and control children, which says that we go to one place if we're good, and another if we're bad. This is deeply unsatisfying to anyone who can think, because you know that time and place are properties of the material life, which is the one we presumably leave when we die. So we can let go of ideas, like in the UK TV commercial of a few years ago: "When my hamster dies, will he go to Devon?" So when we die, we are liberated from time and space. Does that mean we no longer are? That's the materialist position, and to some extent can be a relief: "No further suffering," we say. But of course the truth is that we don't know that for sure.

Is there some kind of soul or spirit that somehow re-enters physical existence – our awareness becomes once again encased in a physical body? Well, that's the position, roughly, that is adhered to by large numbers of people, particularly in the eastern half of the planet. Does that mean it's true? We don't know.

Does the soul or spirit go 'somewhere' else? We're in danger of falling back into time and space metaphors here, but this view is held by a lot of people, not all of whom are simply repeating childhood indoctrination. We don't know.

One version of the Buddhist interpretation which is more or less compatible with a scientific outlook (which of course doesn't necessarily mean it's right) is that we disintegrate into our component parts. These parts, because matter can be neither created nor destroyed (the first law of thermodynamics), recombine in different ways; a scientific view of reincarnation, if you like. So our hard stuff goes back to being hard stuff, like calcium and so on, our liquid seeps away and reverts to being liquid, our gases float up into the atmosphere, and so on. So far so good, but what happens to consciousness? The materialist position is that consciousness is simply a product of physical existence – an accidental by-product, perhaps – and some Buddhist views are like this. But if we reintroduce a sense of Big Mind, then, being undying, it is as present after the death of the individual as it was before. So then *death doesn't matter*, if you are able to be at one with Big Mind. This, I suggest, is why the Tibetans take such trouble at the moment of death to say helpful things to the dying person, so that they can feel that identity at that moment, which in the Tibetan cosmology, will therefore prevent rebirth and further suffering.

Of course if one has practised meditation extensively during one's life so that one has a genuine confidence from experiencing Big Mind more or less at will, then death ceases to be a problem. This then makes sense of what is otherwise an outlandish story:

Death Is Sweet?

A Zen master was taking a walk along a cliff path. Suddenly, a tiger appeared and trapped him so that he had no choice but to jump over the cliff. He reached out his hand and, by chance, managed to catch hold of a shrub in the cliff-face. He held on with one hand, dangling over the rocks below, upon which he would surely be dashed to death if he fell. Two mice appeared and started to gnaw away at the root of the plant, thus inevitably presaging his death. He noticed that the plant was a wild strawberry; with his other hand, he reached for a ripe strawberry and popped it into his mouth. "How delicious," he thought.

So much for death; what about sickness? Is there anyone who is free from any affliction at all? We've all got something wrong with us. We could see our organism as the site of a thousand or more ongoing battles as white blood cells go to places of potential infection, as cancer cells repeatedly get wiped out and bacteria yet again fail to overwhelm the immune system. Sometimes the 'baddies' get through. And of course the beauty of the system is that there is nothing deliberate we can do which will help directly, beyond abstaining from that which is harmful, and giving ourselves appropriate nutrition and exercise. Although we know that to live mindfully with awareness and appropriate expression of emotion probably gives us a better chance of resisting cancer and heart disease etc., **_there are no guarantees_**. There are things that are beyond our control.

In a way, this is the mantra which those who are overly worried about sickness and death should repeat to themselves regularly. And if you can't control it, what is there to do but accept our inevitable degeneration and vulnerability to illness and mortality?

Sometimes excessive concern about health stems from a lack of control in another area of our lives. Most obviously, the death of somebody close can be a trigger – "Oh, I must take better care so that I don't end up like them." But sometimes it may be something that is not directly related to health, like an unexpected and negative turnaround in financial matters or or the end of a relationship, and the unconscious reasoning seems to be something like: "Well, I can't control that; I can't prevent bad things happening outside my physical body, so I'm going to make damn sure that I take control of what's inside my body." The irony of course being that this isn't actually under our direct control either, any more than you can prevent your car breaking down by force of will.

PAIN VERSUS SUFFERING

One of the principles that is as true in the physical as it is in the mental or emotional spheres is the relation between pain and suffering. A certain amount of pain is just inevitable and is part of life. In western societies we have come to regard any pain as avoidable, and tend to see it as a sign of something wrong. So straightaway we take a pill, or alternatively, adopt the 'stiff upper lip' option and do our best not to feel it, but tough it out. That way leads to numbness. Either way the goal is the avoidance of feeling.

As we mentioned in the section on mindfulness, a more useful approach is to 'work the edge' wherever possible. That doesn't mean you shouldn't ever take a painkiller! You may have an important task to perform, and that headache is going to get in the way. But otherwise, see if you can allow yourself to feel a little pain if that is what has presented itself. Is it really unbearable *in the present moment?* Pain is nonetheless a messenger. Is it just telling you to slow down? Is it in your best interests to carry on doing what you're doing? When we want to get selected for a sports team, we may be quite happy to endure the pain that comes with training to a more intense level. On the other hand, there are of course occasions when you need to get help, just as you would take your car to the garage if you thought that strange noise was a sign it was about to blow up!

SOMATISATION

If you suffer from the condition known as somatisation, it's very unlikely you'll be reading this book! Because you most likely wouldn't accept that there is any problem psychologically, even though the doctors have said that there isn't a physical cause for your symptoms. But unlike people with health anxiety, you'd actually be glad of a physical diagnosis, because it would make sense of what's happening to you, and to be physically ill would be infinitely preferable to accepting a diagnosis that is psychological, because to you that means your character is flawed, or you're weak or something like that, and somehow it seems that a bodily symptom is more controllable because it is less nebulous than a 'mental problem'.

However, if by some bizarre coincidence you might be reading this, then to start with I would ask you to work at the place where body and mind do overlap – perhaps do some yoga or tai chi – as a way into looking at your 'stuff' that isn't so threatening for you. One of the most basic thinking errors is all-or-nothing (also known as black-and-white) thinking. This applies to body and mind as much as anything else. We know that there are all kinds of ways in which they influence each other; and some would say that mind is just the subtle end of body...

PUTTING IT ALL TOGETHER: TREATMENT

Having read the above – and perhaps going on to read some other (intelligent) stuff about death, like Stephen Levine's work, for example – you now, I hope, have a more workable understanding of what it's about. But as so often, the new understanding remains a competing theory until it's tested out or put into practice in behaviour, and for this the twin tools of the Vicious Daisy and Exposure and Response Prevention will serve you very well.

So, if you haven't already, do a vicious daisy around your health-anxious belief ("I've got x disease"), and make sure you list *all* the safety behaviours – one person I worked with said his daisy was more like a chrysanthemum there were so many petals. Now make your kindly daisy around a statement like "I have a fear problem which is about having x disease." Notice how the petals are different!

Hierarchy			
Situation	How scary? 0-100	Working on it? (Tick)	No longer gives anxiety (Tick)
(Not avoiding) watching TV hospital drama	40		
Visiting my elderly aunt Jenny in hospital	55		
Not checking particular parts of my body all day	75		
Not trawling the internet about my symptoms	80		
Not consulting medical encyclopaedia for a whole week	80		
Sitting in a graveyard, thinking about my own death	95		

Now list all the safety behaviours on your hierarchy, rating them in order of how anxious it would make you feel not to do them, where 100 is so anxious you may need to change your underwear, and 0 is not anxious at all. Starting at the point at which you can manage, step by step, drop the safety behaviours and see what happens. Of course everyone has different fears, but I will put in a hierarchy below including some of the common safety behaviours and avoidances to help remind you. Remember: do them repeatedly and consistently – perhaps daily if possible. One tick means you're working on it, two that it no longer makes you anxious. I don't recommend having too many things at the one-tick stage at any one time – maybe three or four maximum.

Now do yours! Good luck, and remember, we're all going to die soon enough...

Hierarchy			
Situation	How scary? 0-100	Working on it? (Tick)	No longer gives anxiety (Tick)

The Summer Day

Who made the world?
Who made the swan, and the black bear?
Who made the grasshopper?
This grasshopper, I mean –
The one who has flung herself out of the grass,
The one who is eating sugar out of my hand,
Who is moving her jaws back and forth instead of up and down –
Who is gazing around with her enormous and complicated eyes.
Now she lifts her pale forearms and thoroughly washes her face.
Now she snaps her wings open and floats away.
I don't know exactly what a prayer is.
I do know how to pay attention, how to fall down
Into the grass, how to kneel down in the grass,
How to be idle and blessed, how to stroll through the fields,
Which is what I have been doing all day.
Tell me, what else should I have done?
Doesn't everything die at last and too soon?
Tell me, what is it you plan to do with your one wild and precious life?

From Mary Oliver, *House of Light*

Further reading

David Veale and Rob Willson, *Overcoming Health Anxiety*, Robinson
Stephen Levine,(1989) *Healing Into Life and Death* Gateway and
(1988) *Who Dies?*, Gateway
Elizabeth Kubler-Ross, (1970) *On Death and Dying*, Tavistock/
Routledge

CHAPTER 21: SOCIAL ANXIETY

*The plumbing diagram – Safety behaviours – The orange juice story –
Social anxiety thought record – Attention training – Other techniques*

Social anxiety, known in its most extreme form as social phobia, is
something most of us know to some degree. If we think of it as a family,
it has different members, including performance anxiety as experienced
by musicians and actors, stuttering or stammering, and what we might
think of as ordinary shyness.

As we progress through this book, many of the techniques and ideas
that related to other problems will apply here: identifying what the
safety-seeking behaviours are and using behavioural experiments to
see what happens when we don't do them applies to social anxiety
as it does to all the anxiety disorders. What is peculiar about the use of
safety behaviours in social anxiety is:

*   They tend to work spectacularly badly.
*   The main one involves the way our attention is focused. For this
    reason Chapter 6 on attention will be of particular interest, and
    you may want to look at that now.

But let us start, on the next page, with the classic CBT 'central heating
diagram' for social anxiety, based on the work of David M. Clark and
Adrian Wells, two leading cognitive therapists.

We enter any situation with a set of beliefs and assumptions. In entering
a social situation, people who suffer from social anxiety will be carrying
beliefs such as "Other people will judge me"; "If I feel anxious, they will
see it"; or "I have to have something interesting to say."

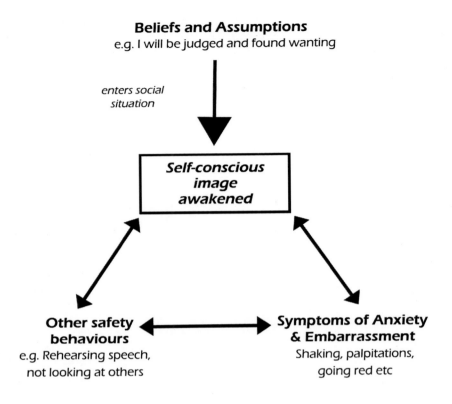

Beliefs and Assumptions
e.g. I will be judged and found wanting

enters social situation

Self-conscious image awakened

Other safety behaviours
e.g. Rehearsing speech, not looking at others

Symptoms of Anxiety & Embarrassment
Shaking, palpitations, going red etc

Cognitive model of social anxiety after Clark & Wells (1995)

Unsurprisingly, the core beliefs underlying this problem often relate to questions of lovability or acceptability to others, and may derive from early experiences of bullying or humiliation. It is as though the Protector decided, "We're never going to let *that* happen again" and as a result resolved to make sure that the way the self presented to others always had to be 'right' in order to avoid any further punishment. Of course the closer the situation seems to the original humiliation, the worse the anxiety is.

So, on entering the social situation of whatever kind, these beliefs and assumptions are activated. The immediate response is to check how I look or am coming across, and an image appears in my mind where I look like (e.g.)the worst kind of blithering idiot, exactly as I did in some horrible situation from my past. So I (think I) have to make sure I don't come across like that, and in checking to see whether I do or not, I am already engaging in the most profound of the social anxiety safety behaviours: ***going self-focused.***

The other things I may do to prevent myself resembling that original image are many and varied: checking what I am going to say before I say it; listening to the sound of my own voice as I speak to make sure it sounds 'right'; going over what I just said in order to check that I didn't make any mistakes; doing a mental check of how I think I look to 'make sure' it's OK, etc. So now fill in your formulation in the blank version below.

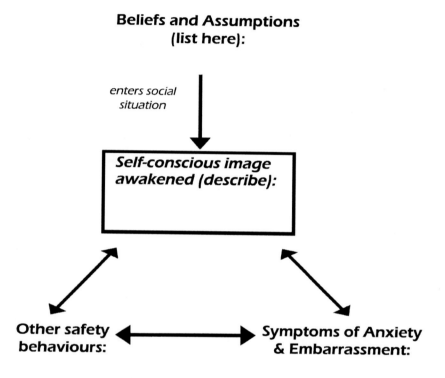

Beliefs and Assumptions (list here):

enters social situation

Self-conscious image awakened (describe):

Other safety behaviours: ⟷ **Symptoms of Anxiety & Embarrassment:**

Self-consciousness and threat

One of the most basic points about social anxiety that tends to get overlooked is what going self-conscious actually does. It may be easiest to think of this by thinking about its opposite: when do we feel most *un*selfconscious? In the most extreme cases, we might even talk about 'losing our self'. Isn't that interesting? Another way of putting it is 'being absorbed' in whatever we're doing. Musicians talk about being lost in the music; horse-riders may become 'at one' with their animal, and in fact here we are back at the hot dog joke. (You can't have forgotten it already! Oh, all right then: what did the Zen student say to the hot dog man? "Make me one with everything".) So when we are completely in the zone, we are not thinking about ourselves. *But we have to feel safe to do that!*

Imagine you are working on a painting, completely absorbed in it, when suddenly, out of the corner of your eye, you notice that there is a tiger looking at you *and* it appears to be drooling slightly. How long do you stay absorbed in the painting? "Oh, I think I'll just add the finishing touches to that tree" – I don't think so.

Suddenly you are acutely aware of the difference between self and other, in this case the tiger. So we can only lose our sense of self when it is safe to do so, but the converse is also true: *the more we focus* on the sense of (separate) self, the *more anxious* we get – because why would we do that if we weren't in danger? So the more we see ourselves as separate from (= opposed to?) those we are in company with, the more threatened and anxious we will feel.

Anxiety about anxiety

In social anxiety, as in other sorts of anxiety, we can get into a pickle when the self-critic pipes up and tells us we shouldn't be anxious. Especially in social anxiety, the question of shame and embarrassment looms large, and that can attach itself to anxiety as well. So sometimes it can be helpful as a behavioural experiment to *admit* to feeling anxious in a performance-type or social situation. In fact, it often just makes you seem more human.

Dropping safety behaviours

Now we have a formulation, the next step is to drop the safety behaviours and see what happens. The main one – going self-conscious – we will look at below, as this is an area where we need to develop particular attention-training skills. But for the others, we need to treat them just as we did with the other anxiety disorders: list them, discover what is the particular purpose of each one, perhaps using a vicious daisy (why do I do it?) and experiment with not doing whatever it is and noting the outcome. Use the hierarchy form (if you like) to grade the exposures.

Monitoring and rehearsing/replaying speech

This is one of the safety behaviours that is so clearly unhelpful. A conversation between two people has to involve reciprocity: if I am playing tennis with someone, then at any given time one person is focused on hitting the ball while the other is focused on receiving it. If the one who should be looking to receive it is too busy thinking about whether he hit the last one right or not, or thinking about how he is going to hit the next one (before it arrives), then sure as eggs is eggs he's going to miss the ball coming in. And this is how it is with the socially anxious person rehearsing the next sentence or replaying the last one: s/he misses the feedback from the other person. Or even if not, the extra time taken to do the rehearsing or replaying makes them seem wooden and unspontaneous, thus contributing to the very image they were trying to avoid.

Feedback
More generally research has shown that, contrary to what one might assume, people with social anxiety don't spend their time concentrating on every nuance of how the other people in the situation are reacting to them, because they are too busy concentrating on how *they* are coming across, and trying to make sure they don't look like the blithering idiot in the image. But paradoxically, because of this, they *never find out* whether other people are seeing them like that or not. So the unhelpful belief (e.g. "I look like an idiot") can persist despite a lack of any evidence to support it. Dropping this safety behaviour would mean deliberately checking out the cues that others are giving you, both verbally and non-verbally.

Eye contact
This leads us to an area that becomes problematic as soon as you start to think about it! If when you have a conversation you think about how much eye contact you should have, then it becomes really difficult to be natural. In fact, at least in the UK, when you are speaking to someone, you don't usually fix them with a stare, but just look at them intermittently – in order to check they are still engaged in the conversation, I suppose. But if you are on the receiving side, then you usually do stay with your eyes focused on the speaker. Sometimes this does become a problem; if you feel too shy to have as much eye contact as you would like to, one trick is to focus instead on the *ears;* the other person probably won't notice, and you won't feel quite so exposed.

Stammering and stuttering
We can think of stammering or stuttering as a particular form of social anxiety related to self-expression. Like other types, it often relates to an experience of humiliation around what was said or how it was said; there's sometimes a core belief about being 'stupid', which (remembering the first law of core beliefs) isn't true, any more than a fuzzy radio broadcast says anything about the quality of the programme's contents. Exactly the same approach can be used for this kind of problem as for the other types of social anxiety.

Shame-attacking
Of course one way of cutting to the chase in relation to feeling embarrassed or ashamed is to deliberately provoke the reactions one fears: if you are convinced that the only way you are acceptable is if you

are wearing the most stylish and co-ordinated clothes, go to a charity shop and buy (and wear) an old-fashioned and clashing combination of attire. You may have the thought that "I look a complete prat" but what actually happens? Do people publicly ridicule you? Do they notice at all?

And here's another thought – do you want to surround yourself with people who are so superficial they judge you according to your clothing, before you've even opened your mouth?

Shame-attacking (a technique from Rational Emotive Behaviour Therapy) doesn't have to be limited to appearance. If your fear is about making a fool of yourself, wouldn't it be interesting to see what happened if you did? How bad could it feel? Wouldn't there be at least something of a relief that "OK, that's what it feels like. Nobody died. Now at least I don't have to worry about it any more"?

Seeing commonality
If shame-attacking solves the problem by deliberately bringing you 'down' to the level you fear, another way of working provides a way of bringing the other people down to an ordinary level too, so that you no longer feel intimidated. We are all human. Imagine them on the toilet, or in unflattering underwear! There is a downside to this – I once mentioned it to a friend who was going to an interview, but as she pointed out, it's very hard to concentrate on the questions you're being asked if you're thinking about the interviewer's underwear...

But both of these techniques are designed to undermine one thing – the notion that somehow we are inferior to those we are in the presence of. Actually we all screw up from time to time, and what shows on the outside isn't necessarily any guide as to what the person's like underneath. The more anxious we are, the more we exaggerate the difference between ourselves and our 'audience'. The 'Big I, Little I' diagram (and of course the Big Mind process) is a useful reminder not to judge ourselves as a whole.

Thinking errors
The main thinking error in social anxiety is of course *mindreading*, although others (like catastrophising, labelling and demands) come along in its wake. The truth is that we can't know what is going on in somebody else's mind unless they tell us – and perhaps not even then.

It was for the problem of worrying too much about how you think others see you that the orange juice story was devised:

The Orange Juice Story

So, we're sitting together in a room. There's a jug of orange juice on the table. The orange juice is just perfect – freshly squeezed, organic, from the best orange trees, in a nice jug, maybe some ice... as it happens, we've both just had a drink, we're not thirsty, so we don't drink the orange juice. Does that say anything about the quality of the orange juice? Of course not.

Perhaps we are thirsty, but because of when and where and how we were brought up, we choose to drink some fizzy concoction in a can which has no nutritional value, instead of the beautiful orange juice. Does that say anything about the quality of the orange juice? Again, of course not.

Suppose there's some equally fine pineapple juice, freshly made, organic, etc., and we choose to drink that, instead. Does that say anything about the orange juice (Am I labouring the point here?)? Seeing that, for some reason we prefer the pineapple juice, should the orange juice try to turn itself into pineapple juice in order to get itself consumed? No! The orange juice can only ever be orange juice! Even if it tried to be pineapple juice, we'd pick it up and taste it, and say, ugh, this pineapple juice tastes like orange juice...

So we can just be what we are, and if someone else prefers fizzy pop or pineapple juice, well, that's up to them. Either way, there's no necessary relation between actual quality and preference... just be the best orange juice you can be!

It can be helpful, if you like them, to work through your social anxiety scenarios using a modified thought record which includes the safety behaviours. I reproduce it on the next page:

Of course you can't be getting out these forms in the middle of a party or something like that! So at first it will be about reviewing what happened in a situation after the event. But as you practise – and again you can use a hierarchy to grade different levels of scariness – you will find that you can do the process in your head while in the situation.

Attention techniques

If we don't ever think about it, we probably assume that our attention is more or less a given – that is, it is determined by what is happening to us, although many may remember teachers saying (or shouting) "Pay attention!" without ever giving us any training in how to do it. The treatment for social anxiety rests at least as much on how our attention is focused as it does on challenging the content of your socially anxious thoughts.

Social Anxiety Thought Record   Date:

Situation	Emotion	Negative Automatic Thoughts (NATs)	Meaning
What was I doing or thinking about? Who was I with?	*What emotion? How intense (0-100%)*	*How much did you believe them (0-100%)?*	*What did the NATs mean to you? What's the worst thing about that?*
			What would that say about you if it were true? How did you see yourself in that situation? How old did you feel?
Thinking errors?	**Safety Behaviours & Effects**	**Alternative Thoughts**	**Results: What can I do now?**
*Check the NATs **and** the meaning against the list*	*What did you do to prevent others seeing your anxiety or who you 'really' are?*	*Is there another way of thinking about this that isn't distorted and is more helpful? How much do you believe the new version?*	*How could you test out which version is more useful? If you drop the safety behaviours, what happens?*

As we mentioned, the main safety-seeking behaviour in social anxiety is often going self-focused. This may be triggered by your thoughts about what will happen in the social situation, but it is not primarily a matter of mental content. Like rituals in OCD, after a while it becomes a pattern; a sort of neural habit that just happens automatically whenever you're in that situation.

So in addition to answering the content of what you believe about what others may be thinking, you also need to recognise that your attention *is in the wrong place* and do something about that. Adrian Wells' Situational Attention Refocusing (SAR) is designed to do just this. I (again) reproduce his instructions:

> *When you enter a feared social situation, you tend to focus your attention on yourself. For example, your anxiety symptoms become the centre of your attention, and because they feel bad you think you must look bad. Focusing on yourself prevents you from getting a realistic sense of the social situation. In order to overcome your anxiety, you have to go into the situation and allow yourself to discover that your fears are not true. To do this, you should observe other people closely in order to gain clues about their reaction to you. For example, when you are self-conscious and it feels as if everyone is looking at you, you should look around and check this out. By focusing attention on what is happening around you, you will become more confident and discover that your fears are not true. (Wells and Papageorgiou 1998 in Wells 2000 p152)*

However, I think that – while this technique is effective – it may be helpful to put the retraining of attention in a broader context. As I mentioned above, the sense of separateness increases the more we are in a threat situation, and this is functional: if your aim is to survive, then you don't want to be troubled by feelings of empathy for the tiger cubs who are going to go hungry if their mother doesn't get to eat you up (although the Buddha, in a previous life, is said to have gone down precisely that route!). Or, perhaps more commonly, if you're a soldier, you don't want to be thinking about the welfare of the enemy you're aiming your rifle at – such hesitation could cost you your life. So where the threat is real, then separateness is appropriate.

But here's the rub – if your anxiety is of the social kind, not only do you feel more separate ('outcast'; 'reject') but you locate yourself *outside yourself.* The technical name for this is 'observer perspective'. Of course sometimes observer position is not bad – it can be useful if you're too caught up in self-criticism and are trying to imagine (compassionately!)

how someone else might see the situation. But in a situation where you're feeling socially anxious it is definitely unhelpful for a number of reasons, not least because you don't get the accurate feedback from others that you need to make good sense of the situation.

I think it's worth clarifying what you are trying to do here: if observer perspective is 'outside looking in' where do you want to be? Well, if you feel your house is under threat and you want to defend it you had better be inside the house, right? So how about taking a stance of 'inside looking out' instead? That way you can see the 'enemy' and decide for yourself if they really are out to get you!

There are two ways to do this. One is the deliberate external focus as in the SAR technique above: if you look out, then automatically you must be 'in'. But you can also do it by using mindfulness: if you deliberately relocate your awareness in the body, non-judgementally (because there may be some anxious sensations there that you don't like), then again you are 'inside looking out', and again following the tried and tested principle of facing your fears. Also, being more in your body than your head, you may be less caught up in, and thus better able to see, the mindreading distortions for what they are.

Task Concentration Training (TCT) is also useful in learning to direct your attention so that you cope better in times where you have been socially anxious. But it is a slightly different attentional shift: SAR works by going from 'outside (the self) looking in' to 'inside (the self) looking out' – the boundaries between self and other are maintained at the same level of firmness, at least until the threat is seen to have passed or been revealed as unreal. Task concentration works by moving us along a slightly different continuum, from 'self-conscious' to 'absorbed'. Most people have something that they can 'lose themselves in' – I use the phrase deliberately – and we can start with that.

For a start, especially if the social anxiety has brought some depression in its wake, you may have stopped doing the things that give you pleasure (see the chapters on behaviour and depression above). So start again with the country walks or playing the guitar or dancing or whatever it is, so that you remind yourself of what it is to be lost in what you love. Really get a feeling of that and notice what is different in your body. Make some notes shortly afterwards – you'll probably find that you don't have so much of a sense of separateness, but that you are relaxed and your senses are more alert, but not in a 'scanning' kind of way. Just write how it is for you. In particular, note how much attention was on your self, how much on the activity, and how much on the environment. Presumably, if you *were* really absorbed, very little will have been on the self. If you like, you can use the Task Concentration Training (TCT) form below. Using it helps you to see this as a parallel process to doing an ABC or thought record – just as re-evaluating the thought content can affect feelings, so can shifting the focus of your attention.

Now try being *in that (absorbed) state of mind* in a relatively non-threatening situation. Give yourself a task as you go on a walk; to notice how many kinds of bark you can discover on the trees you pass, for example, and feel them if you like, to help you stay tuned in to your senses. Again, note what proportion of your attention was on the self, and how much was on the task and the environment.

When you have done a number of these, see if you can retain something of that state in unchallenging *social* situations, and again record the proportions of your attention. Finally, try it in more challenging situations. Remember that you are not powerless in this! If you find yourself slipping back into self-consciousness or observer perspective, then try either deliberate focusing (SAR above) or relocating in the body and then looking out through your 'windows'.

People have used TCT in group therapy, working in pairs, in which case you might start interacting back-to-back to make it less threatening.

Task Concentration Training form   Date:

Situation	Attention	Mood/Feeling	Exercise	Outcome
Who were you with? What was the task?	What were you mainly focusing on?	How did you feel? (describe emotions and rate how intense 0 - 100%)	How did you try to redirect your attention to the task and environment?	How did the situation turn out?
				How did you feel? (describe emotions and rate how intense 0 – 100%)

	How much attention (%) was directed at:
	
	1. Self
	   %
	
	2. Task
	   %
	
	3. Environment
	   %
	
	(total should equal 100%)
			How effective was it?	What did you do?
				
				What did the other people do?

(Based on Sandra Mulkens et al., Task Concentration Training)

We can summarise the process of dealing with social anxiety in the diagram: on the next page

Dealing with Self-Consciousness in Social Situations

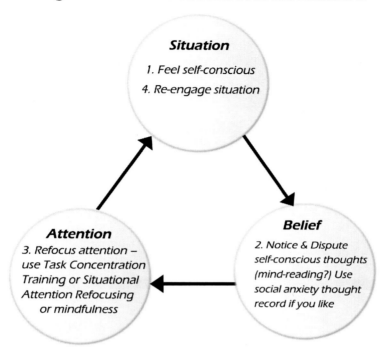

What to do if it doesn't work

Sometimes following the above advice doesn't hit the spot, or does so only partially, because as soon as you try to enter particular kinds of situation you find that the anxiety shoots up beyond a bearable level. In that case it is worth noting what is going through your mind at that point. The chances are that the self-conscious image has got fired up and is jumping up and down, and won't let you disregard it! In which case we need to pay attention to it and work it through in a constructive way. There are (at least) two ways of doing this, which kind of overlap: imagery rescripting and voice dialogue or Big Mind. These both need to be done with help from a suitably qualified professional.

Whichever way we go, we need to find out more about the image to start with. One question that is often useful is, "How old are you in the image?" It usually turns out that the self-conscious image is like a flashback to a particular traumatic event from childhood. Through questioning we can discover more. Sometimes it's a conflation of a number of different events which were similar in kind.

One way or another we need to get three things out of working through this situation:

1. We need to take the emotional charge off it.

2. We need to find out what the decision was that got made here, which might be something like, "I'm never going to allow myself to go through anything like this ever again" which was probably a very necessary decision at the time.
3. Validate that decision for then, but modify it from now on.

The first can be done through imagery rescripting. This is described in detail in Chapter 10, but we can briefly go over the stages here:

1. Create a sense of a safe place that you can go back to if necessary at any stage in the process.
2. Visualise the situation, but run it as a movie with a frame around it, and see your younger self going through whatever you went through. Stop or pause the movie whenever you need to.
3. Decide who you want to intervene in this situation: it could be you as an adult, if you feel the perpetrator (the person who humiliated you) would respect you as an adult; if not choose somebody they *would* take notice of.
4. When you feel ready, replay the movie, but have the rescuer come in at the right time to prevent the humiliation or abuse. Enjoy the look on the perpetrator's face! If *you* are the rescuer, enter the movie so that you, as the rescuer, are in it.
5. Give the story a better ending: take the younger you out of the horrible situation (s/he's been there long enough!) to somewhere you know they'll like and feel safe, their grandma's place or the play-park or wherever.

Some people object to this technique on the grounds that it's rewriting history. No! Of course whatever happened is what happened, and it was damaging at the time. But the *continuing* trouble is not being caused by the original incident itself, but rather by the *memory* of the original incident, which is what we're attempting to work with here; to see perhaps that there might have been some other way it could have turned out, which perhaps enables you, as the one who was given a hard time, not to blame yourself for it.

Another way of working with this is through the Big Mind process. Having done the necessary introductory process (Protector, Controller etc.), you then access the self-conscious image – the little you from all that time ago – by asking, "Can I speak to the young (name), please?" and finding out what s/he wants; what is still needed. While working in this way, you can also find out what the decision was and do the validation, but ask if perhaps now that part would be prepared to relinquish its hold if it feels safe enough.

It is also possible to work through the same material (again with the help of someone who knows what s/he is doing!) using empty chair: Leslie Greenberg's Emotion Focused Therapy does just this.

The objective is to take sufficient charge *off* the memory of the original situation so that you are able to enter current social situations with the anxiety reduced enough for you – with the help of SAR or TCT if necessary – to start getting back into your (social) life.

SUMMARY

- To start with, notice what you are doing that is different from someone who doesn't have social anxiety: your safety behaviours (use a vicious daisy).

- Practise identifying what thinking errors are going on in social situations – mindreading? Catastrophising? Use a thought record if necessary; in any case discount the contents as a symptom of social anxiety.

- As well as mind-contents, take note of what you are doing with your *attention*; practise refocusing from outside-looking-in to inside-looking-out, using TCT, SAR and/or mindfulness.

- If you are aware of a self-conscious image, ask yourself how old you feel in it, and cut yourself some slack about it! If you can, get help to rework it. If you can't, see it as the expression of a particular little I (probably quite little), and feel compassionate towards it, while shifting into another mode to operate in social situations. Think of it like changing hats or costumes.

- Remind yourself that lots of people don't feel *that* comfortable in a whole range of social situations, and don't give yourself a hard time for feeling anxious.

Further Reading

Gillian Butler (2009) *Overcoming Social Anxiety and Shyness,* Constable Robinson

CHAPTER 22: BODY DYSMORPHIC DISORDER

Definition – Possible origins – Beliefs – Disgust – Theory A & theory B – Working backwards from safety behaviours – Vicious daisy – Department store – Attention training – Comparison - Experiments

Body Dysmorphic Disorder (BDD) is one of the most under-recognised and therefore least diagnosed conditions in the world of psychiatry. Thus many sufferers get no treatment or the wrong kind of treatment, being misdiagnosed as having depression or OCD (although both of these often partner BDD). When I was new to working with this condition, a colleague described it to me as "the illegitimate child of OCD and social phobia". That certainly captures something of its flavour, but essentially it is an *excessive preoccupation with one's appearance*. Sometimes it is known as the 'imagined ugliness syndrome' but that takes us just where we don't want to go: into evaluating whether you are 'really' ugly or not.

BDD can be a problem to people with Adonis-like looks or to people with deformities, although if you have BDD, you'll almost certainly put yourself in the second category. But the nub is that your looks (or some aspect of them) have become the *default preoccupying concern of your life*. The object of treatment is to get to a place where that is no longer the case.

So what leads people to get caught up in this way? Like any other condition, there will be a number of contributing influences. Two of the most important are:

1. Some incidents of humiliation or ridicule earlier on in life, which may or may not have been about appearance directly.
2. An aptitude for or leaning towards aesthetic matters: art, design, photography etc.

To say a little more about these: parents or significant adults (perhaps teachers) earlier in life may have acted in ways that made you feel very bad about yourself at the time. This is very similar to the origins of social anxiety. But for some reason you connected this to your appearance. This may have been, and often is, because of the words the person used when mocking you. But it may also have been because the situation seemed so horrible, and the implications of what the person said or did were so awfully out of control, that you were desperate to get some control back, and so to reassure yourself that you weren't genuinely unlovable or bad or worthless, you thought, "If only I looked better they wouldn't treat me like this" or something similar. Because it seems that my appearance, being to do with my body, is somehow closer to being under my control – at least in theory, I ought to be able to do something about it – and that's better than accepting the terrible possibility that the reason they treated me like that is that they really hate me and I'm bad or worthless, about which I think I can't do anything. So not surprisingly people develop beliefs like:

a) My worth is defined by how I look.
b) My lovability/likeability is defined by how I look.
c) I feel disgusting in myself, and this shows in my appearance (if I don't do something about it).
d) My appearance will lead to further humiliation.

One of the reasons why people develop BDD rather than, say, social anxiety (and some people have both) in response to the humiliating early episodes are to do with how highly developed their artistic sensibilities are – although this is a bit of a chicken-and-egg situation in that the focus on their own appearance may have *contributed* to this development. People with BDD often work in occupations like graphic design, advertising and so on. Artists have often been encouraged to be self-critical about their work, so they have maybe spent years learning to discern whether something is just slightly askew; to focus on the single flaw in an otherwise perfect painting or design and make it invalidate the whole thing. Small wonder then that they (you) do the same to them- (your)selves...

The emotions that are triggered by this mental behaviour are various, but almost always include disgust and anxiety. This is a very pernicious combination. If you have OCD, it usually still seems like there's something worth protecting; in BDD it is often others whom you think need protecting from the sight of you! There is variation here; for some it is more like social anxiety, but for others the problem might even be there if they were alone on a desert island, so deep is the repulsion the person feels for whatever aspect of their appearance they are worried about.

Unlike in Obsessive Compulsive Disorder, people with BDD don't usually think they have a psychological problem: it's just that I look horrible, right? So to start to think about this in a more helpful way there are three CBT techniques which can be helpful: Theory A and Theory B, working backwards from safety behaviours and the vicious daisy.

You will remember our Tweedledum- and Tweedledee-like friends from the chapters on panic and health anxiety. If we apply their formula to this it could run something like:

Theory A: "The problem is that my nose is too big."
Theory B: "The problem is that *I worry that* my nose is too big."

Notice that Theory B is not saying anything about the size of the nose, either negatively or positively! He is just saying that it is a worry problem, not a nose problem, whether your nose is half a millimetre or two metres long. So, going with Theory B, we work out what paying attention to the worry leads us to *in terms of what we do*, and what would happen if we didn't.

There is a whole raft of safety behaviours that go with BDD, of which the most famous and probably the most common is *mirror-checking*. But if I accepted that the problem was one of excess *worry* about my appearance, rather than my *appearance itself* (or some aspect of it), then I wouldn't need to check, would I?

So what are your safety behaviours around your appearance? How much time per day do you spend doing them... and wouldn't it be nice not to have to?

Safety behaviour	Time spent on it/frequency
Mirror checking;	Half an hour x 10 times a day
Looking in reflective surfaces	Whenever I pass one
Re-applying make-up	20 mins, whenever I go out the door
Stay indoors	Whenever possible

As we mentioned, many people with BDD don't think there is really a psychological issue. One way of getting through this problem is to use the strategy of working backwards from safety behaviours. Use the blank form on the next page. There is a filled-in one below which you could use as a guide.

Working Backwards from Safety Behaviours

START HERE!

5. Early Experience	4. Core beliefs	3. Rules and Assumptions	2. Thoughts & Feelings if I didn't do it	1. Safety Behaviours
Artist parents. Didn't pay much attention to child. Father left mother for model. Mother contemptuous to child, called me 'funny-face'. Bullied at school for not having the right 'look'	I'm unlovable, different, a freak. I don't matter. Appearance is the most important thing. Love is everything	You have to look good to be accepted If people notice me they'll pity me If I feel it, it must be true	I'm disgusting I'm a freak My face is an odd shape Anxious Depressed	Mirror checking Excess make-up (disguise) Staying indoors Wear hat or headscarf
6. Compassionate View	7. Alternative Beliefs	8. Helpful Guidelines	9. Thoughts and Feelings	10. New Behaviours
These were very unpleasant experiences. It's not surprising you developed these ideas. Your parents weren't very good at making you feel wanted. Children can be cruel to those they see as different	Just because my parents didn't love me doesn't mean I'm unlovable. I matter just as much as anyone else, no matter how I look. Love is good, but I don't have to have it to lead a fulfilled life.	If people accept me for who I am, rather than how I look, they'll be better friends Most people don't care about appearance as much as I do, so I don't have to worry so much If I feel something, it may or may not be true	I may feel disgusting, sometimes, but that may be my faulty feelometer. Faces can be all kinds of shapes, it's not the most important thing. More confident!	Just use the mirror to get a brief overview Go out when I want to Only wear hats for the weather Reserve make-up for special occasions or work Go out sometimes without it to see what happens

Working Backwards from Safety Behaviours

START HERE!

5. Early Experience	4. Core beliefs	3. Rules and Assumptions	2. Thoughts & Feelings if I didn't do it	1. Safety Behaviours
6. Compassionate View	7. Alternative Beliefs	8. Helpful Guidelines	9. Thoughts and Feelings	10. New Behaviours

So we start at 1 (top right) with all the different things that you do to try and fix the problem relating to appearance that you have listed above. Then, working from right to left across the top of the form, put in the thoughts and feelings you think you would have if you *didn't* do the behaviours. Then think about whether those thoughts come from a particular rule or assumption you may be holding about, or related to, appearance. Put that in the next column. Next, what are the *underlying* beliefs that you have and that you think might emerge if you didn't carry out those rules? If you're working with a therapist, s/he may be able to help you uncover them.

Put the underlying or 'core' beliefs in column 4. It may be helpful to go back to the chapter on schemas (Chapter 7) for this one. So what were the experiences, as far as you can remember, that gave rise to these beliefs? Was it at home, or at school, or both? How important was how you looked to your parents; teachers; school friends? Were there episodes of humiliation? Put this in column 5.

Now take a compassionate view of all this stuff. If you were looking in on, say, your family of origin or perhaps your school, would you *really* say, "Yes, that little boy or girl is disgusting"? My guess is that you would say something closer to, "No, s/he's having a really hard time in there; the parents are focusing on the wrong things" or "The children have just focused on appearance as a way of getting at him/her." Think of the younger you as a suffering individual. What could you say *now* to the you *then* (the younger you) to comfort yourself in a way that is helpful? Put that in column 6.

So, leading from that, what could you put in as alternatives to the unhelpful core beliefs that you put in 4? Again, look at the schema chapter if you need to so that you come up with really helpful alternatives. Put the new beliefs in 7.

Now that you don't have to follow the rules in 3 (because you can see that you're not really unlovable/bad/worthless etc.), what guidelines would be more helpful, particularly in relation to the amount of time and energy that you put into your appearance? Put the new guidelines in 8.

While following the new guidelines, what kind of thoughts and feelings are generated? You may need to hold off filling this in for a while, or you can put in what you guess will happen once you make the changes. And what would those changes be? How much time is it *really* helpful to spend in front of a mirror? How many times do you need to check your appearance before going to the cornershop to buy a newspaper? What is the purpose of make-up?

THE VICIOUS DAISY

Now that you have some understanding of what the thoughts and beliefs are that are driving the BDD, we can use the vicious daisy to see how you are (unwittingly) keeping the problem going. Put a key belief at the centre of the daisy (e.g. "I'm ugly" or "My nose is too big"). Then, just as we did in Chapter 2, put around it as petals anything that you do to try and take care of this problem (e.g. mirror-check, don't go out in the daytime, wear excess make-up etc.). Notice how all these things have the unintended consequence of confirming your central belief, just like Asterix and Obelix's actions made them convinced the sky was going to fall on their heads.
Fill it in here (blank overleaf).

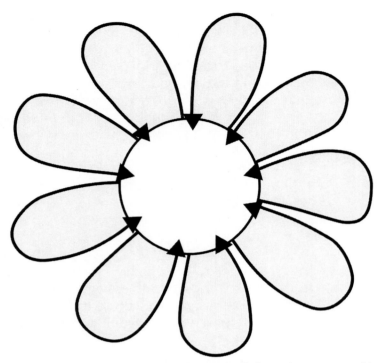

Now do another one with a healthier belief at the centre. No, don't put "I'm beautiful" or "My nose is perfectly shaped." Firstly, you'd never believe it, but secondly (and much more importantly), it keeps you focused on your appearance! So how about something like, "My looks are not the most important thing"; "My worth/lovability isn't dependent on how I look"; "People are more interested in who I am than how I look"; "People don't care about the shape of my nose" or even "I can have more fun if I don't focus on my looks"?

If you put whichever one at the centre of your new 'kindly' daisy, what are the new petals that confirm the healthier belief? Do they correspond with the new behaviours in column 10?

MORE ON SAFETY BEHAVIOURS

There are a number of ways in which people with BDD restrict their lives because of the safety behaviours that they do: not going out, or in some way camouflaging their 'deformity', or spending so much time checking their appearance that they never get out. All of these are bad enough, and can and often do lead to an agoraphobic lifestyle.

There is unfortunately a further stage that people get into because their distress is so intense and they haven't found a better way of thinking about the problem yet. This is where the person deliberately tries to make it better by physical intervention: either themselves, or with the aid of a cosmetic surgeon. These efforts are often doomed to failure, and make the person feel even worse because they then feel responsible for making the problem worse – even when the results may look perfectly acceptable from the outside! That stuff is almost never undoable, and sufferers can become suicidal. So please, if you have BDD, don't consult a cosmetic surgeon. There are enough people out there with more money than sense without you adding to them.

COMPASSIONATE MIND

BDD sufferers can be the most self-critical, self-hating people that I have ever come across. For this reason compassionate mind training is both one of the most important and one of the most difficult interventions. It may be that it is only possible once the original incidents of humiliation have been addressed, perhaps using the imagery rescripting technique described in the previous chapter and in Chapter 10.

"How can you be nicer to yourself when you've got a nose/hairline/forehead etc. like this?" I hear you say. Well, for the time being, let's go with "Be nicer to yourself even though you've got a nose/hairline/forehead like that." Jon Kabat-Zinn says, "Act as though your life mattered", so how about "Act as though your life mattered more than how you look"?

This leads us to the question of what does really matter. Do you want your tombstone to read, *Missed life while looking in the mirror*? Of course not. So, putting aside your appearance, what would your department store look like? This time it's not about how well you're doing in each department, but more about what you would like to achieve in each area. I'll put in 'Joe's' again from Chapter 7 and then a blank for you to fill in.

Joe's Department Store

Relationship	Children	Work
Spend more time with my partner doing nice ordinary things – walks, etc.	Take them to the park at least once a week	Take up the offer of further training to make it more interesting
Social life	**Church**	**Sport**
Go out with our friends in the daytime to country pubs	Help out on the committee	Go back to the taekwondo class
Fishing	**Gardening**	**Holidays**
Catch the biggest trout I can!	Re-do the front garden that I've been promising to do for ages	Allow ourselves to have a holiday that isn't 'educational'

My Department Store

Of course you are not Joe (unless you are), so the departments in your life may be different: you may be single, for example, or not working at the moment. That doesn't mean you can't have valued goals! If you're struggling to think up your goals then you could do worse than start from the Activity Window: devise goals in relation to the different areas of:

1. Physical activity
2. Nature (walks, gardening, animals?)
3. Social
4. Creative

Add more departments if you need to!

Attention
Particularly (but not only) for those of you whose BDD is close to the social phobia end of the spectrum, attention training can be really helpful in a number of ways:

1. Using the Situation Attentional Refocusing (SAR) or Task Concentration Training (TCT) techniques described in the previous chapter, your attention is automatically focused away from your appearance. Just as you'd be more concerned about some scruffy paintwork on your house if you spent your time walking round and round the outside than if you were inside it looking out through the windows, so remembering to focus outwards both takes your attention away from the perceived issue and enables you to get accurate feedback on how others react to you.

2. Mindfulness practice over time enables you to see the stuff about your appearance as just stuff that is passing through the thoughtosphere. You are the one who is aware of that stuff, not the stuff. You don't need to act out the movie.

3. You don't want to have to avoid mirrors (or other reflective surfaces) for the rest of your life! So you need to be able to look in them as others do, and this requires a broadening of your focus. You can learn to do this with your hearing using Attention Training Technique (see Chapter 6), but it may be just a little more difficult with vision. Nonetheless, try sitting and noticing just what's in front of you: a speck of dust on the carpet, or a particular bit of the pattern. Now expand it to include an area about a metre square...now the whole floor...now imagine the whole house or flat...now move your attention swiftly from one to another, randomly. Doing this will increase your attentional flexibility. Now when you approach a mirror, just get a whole person view. Only focus on a particular bit if it's about tucking something in, removing spinach from your teeth or making sure the tie's inside the shirt collar! You know, *functional* stuff.

Comparison

A problem that sometimes happens when BDDers try the attentional refocusing techniques like SAR is that as soon as their gaze falls upon another person, the dreaded demon of comparison chirps up. The only thing to do in the moment is to keep refocusing back to *inside looking out*, but I do know it's hard to break long habits.

In principle of course comparison is not just odious, it's *impossible* in relation to appearance because no two people are alike, and more symmetrical *doesn't mean better* in any meaningful sense of that term. It is a truism, but perhaps a necessary one, to say that in judging somebody by their appearance we are doing the part-whole error – overgeneralising.

The whole of a person's appearance is just one little I; more often in BDD we will be comparing just one aspect of someone's appearance with the bit of ourselves we don't like – and how unrepresentative is that? It would be like judging someone's worth on the basis of their intelligence, and judging their overall intelligence by how well they can do puzzles! Some quite intelligent people aren't good at puzzles! More importantly, no one quality, neither intelligence nor appearance, can be used to measure overall worth (or lovability etc.).

Behavioural experiments

We can describe behavioural experiments for BDD as being basically of two kinds:

1. What happens if I don't do my safety behaviours: mirror checking, comparison, staying indoors in the daytime, checking my appearance, etc., and what happens to my mood if I live as if my appearance isn't so important.

2. Discovery experiments about how other imperfect-looking people get along.

The first kind is fairly self-explanatory: review your list of safety behaviours, rank them according to difficulty as on the hierarchy form, and start acting against them to see what happens. Of course you may feel more anxious in the short term, but I suggest (and of course it's up to you to find out if I am telling the truth) that this will be outweighed by the gains you make later on in terms of getting your life back.

The second kind, finding out about other people, can often take the form of a survey. I know you think your particular 'bit' that you're worried about is worse than anyone else's has ever been, but just for the moment, accept that this is not really a universe of physically beautiful people. Then, remembering this, go and have a look in your local shopping centre to see if it is only the pretty ones who ever wear a smile, or are wandering hand-in-hand in relationships. Even in your bank, or other places where customer-facing staff obviously make an effort with their appearance, are they all Adonis-like? Is it always the prettiest ones who seem happiest? Record your conclusions.

Relapse prevention
In essence, relapse prevention will be about keeping the above going. Notice the first signs if you are back spending more time in front of the mirror. Be aware that for you, increased stress may well lead to increased preoccupation with appearance. To remind yourself, deliberately make one thing not quite right, and go out into the world without a second thought.

SUMMARY

BDD is a disorder characterised by excessive concern with appearance. The way out is not about expending more effort on how you look, but rather reducing the time and energy spent on how you think you seem from the outside. A combination of unpicking any early humiliations, dropping rituals and safety behaviours, learning to shift your attention, and exploring how others (who don't have this problem) operate in the world, will help you to refocus on what is really important in life.

Further reading

Katharine A. Phillips (2005), *The Broken Mirror: Understanding and Treating Body Dysmorphic Disorder*, Oxford University Press
Fugen Neziroglu (2012) *Overcoming Body Dysmorphic Disorder A Cognitive Behavioral Approach to Reclaiming Your Life* New Harbinger
David Veale, Rob Willson and Alex Clarke (2009), *Overcoming Body Image Problems*, Constable Robinson

CHAPTER 23: ANGER

Anger and aggression – Acceptance, compassion & mindfulness– The anger record – Cost-benefit of rules – Chaining – Physical effects and not making it worse

I wish the world would get offa my case and get on to one of its own. (Little Feat)

Anger, or its expression, is a serious problem in western societies (and some eastern ones too). On the one hand, we are taught that it is a bad thing – if our children get angry at school, they are told off (often angrily) by the teacher; on the other we see all sorts of examples in our movies and on the TV of our heroes getting angry and achieving what they aim for, so maybe we think it's OK to be angry if we are on the 'right' side. Yet in our city centres, we are horrified by what we see when people consume large quantities of alcohol and then start attacking each other, sometimes with weapons.

So how can we make sense of this? First, I think we need to make a clear distinction between the *emotion* of anger, and aggressive *behaviour*. Because we all feel angry sometimes – this is, after all, the 'other half' of *fight-and-flight* that we looked at under panic. If we feel under threat, we will respond in one of three ways: fight, freeze or flee. Which of these we do will be less about choice and more about instinct or early programming, at least to start with.

Courts wisely make a distinction between a *crime passionelle*, something done in the heat of the moment, and a premeditated action. Sometimes people, through a simple process of learning what worked in the situation where they grew up, use aggression (coldly, though often with a 'show' of anger) to get what they want. This is not an anger problem – this is an aggression problem, and these people have to discover better ways of getting what they want, although this may be difficult in the particular environment in which they live. This is less a psychological and more a social and educational problem.

In working with anger, we need two things: motivation to change, and a preparedness to be in for the long haul; after all, we are apparently trying to go *against* our basic equipment. We are back to lizard brain again, but less timid gecko and more T. rex. It is hard to retrain that which has been instinctually programmed into us for zillions of years with the upstart front brain stuff that has only been around for a short while, especially when showing anger and acting with aggression has been so successful in terms of our own survival.

So how do we go about it? First, we need to learn to notice it just as it begins to kick off – this is where *mindfulness* is very useful, because at first it seems as if it arrives instantaneously (and sometimes it does). After all, if anger was too slow, we'd all have been killed and/or eaten by now.

Second, we need to *accept its presence*. This stage is often missed out, and that leads us into all sorts of trouble. Remember, acceptance doesn't have to include liking or resignation, but means that we accept that what has already happened *has happened*. So if anger is here, anger is here. If we get on our own case about it, saying to ourselves "You shouldn't be angry!" then *that* seems like a threat (to our inner T. rex) and guess what happens then? You've got it: we get even more frustrated and angry.

At a conference on Buddhism and psychotherapy some years ago with the mindfulness teacher Thich Nhat Hanh, many psychotherapists seemed to be asking versions of the same question: "What do I do with my anger and my clients' anger?" Thich Nhat Hanh replied, "Do the same as you would with anything else you've got locked up in the basement – invite it up into your living room and give it a cup of tea!" And, as with the panic, we need to learn to ask it, "What do you want?"

So there is what anger wants, and what it is worried about. To find this out, we need (third) to *evaluate the threat*. If there is anger (as opposed to 'cold' aggression), then there is some kind of threat. Anger is there to prevent me losing (for example) the gazelle carcass – that I have risked life and limb for, and which will keep my family and me alive – to you because you think you can take it off me.

Of course most threats we experience in our modern lives are not like this, but this is the drama that is being played out. Apart from anything else, is reacting with anger really going to be helpful in this particular circumstance? Anger is usually seen these days as a sign of being out of control; nonetheless, it has its valuable protective function, even in 'modern' contexts.

Anger as a Line of Defence

Some years after the break-up of a relationship, Sam found himself unable to get close to people. In therapy, we noticed that he could sometimes get angry on behalf of others, but never on his own account. Further questioning revealed a core belief: 'I don't matter'. Using the Big Mind process, we spoke to the Protector, who said that it wasn't safe to allow people in, because Anger wasn't there as a back-up in case things went wrong – Sam would have been too vulnerable. Re-owning Anger meant Sam could start to allow intimacy again.

Fourth, we need to begin the *reconditioning process*. Having decided that we no longer wish to get so angry so easily, we need to change the threshold at which anger kicks off. This is done through a combination of mindfulness (or other relaxation techniques) for the arousal levels, an anger record for the cognitive re-evaluation, and the technique known as *chaining* for retraining behaviour.

For more on the eight-week programme and mindfulness in general, see Chapter 9. But if you don't want to or can't do the full programme, I recommend at least practising twice a day for 20 minutes or so, especially if you find, say, the 40-minute bodyscan too hard to endure at first. Twice a day is good anyway. We are attempting two things here: one, to reduce the levels of arousal, and two, to learn to respond rather than react to anger-provoking situations. That is, not to make anything of them, as in "You want to make something of it?"

In fact, Thich Nhat Hanh suggests treating the anger itself with compassion. If there's anger, then there is suffering. So he advocates treating the anger as a mother would her baby in discomfort: find out what is troubling it and take care of it. It is dealing with what I call the 'sore spot' in the Anger Record below.

COGNITIVE RE-EVALUATION

The anger record is like an ABC specifically for anger. As with ABCs, it is always useful to refer to the thinking errors: three that will often figure prominently are mindreading, demands and low frustration tolerance: "Looking at me like that means he thinks I'm a *****; he absolutely shouldn't think that, and I can't bear it if he does (so I'm going to lamp him)."

Here's the anger record:

Situation: What was I doing and with whom?	First signs: (body sensations, negative (hot) thoughts)	Meaning: Threat, rule of mine that was broken or sore spot touched	Emotion Anger (0-100) and other emotions?	What I did
Where did this meaning come from?	Is it still useful to believe this?	Different meaning?	Re-rate emotions	New behaviour

On the next page is a filled-in one to give you an idea.

We see from this example that it is often because a situation carries some markers from a particular or repeated situation in the past that it carries so much more intensity than is appropriate in the present, *especially* if it was impossible or unsafe to show or express anger in the original situation (because you were a child, or smaller than the bully etc.).

Situation: What was I doing and with whom?	First signs: (body sensations, negative (hot) thoughts)	Meaning: Threat, rule of mine that was broken or sore spot touched	Emotion Anger (0-100) and other emotions?	What I did
With Fred at the bowling alley	Tense, sweaty. "He's cheating" "He's always trying to put one over on me"	"It's not fair" "Just because he's bigger than me, he thinks he can take advantage"	Anger 80 Fear 75	Dropped the bowling ball on his foot and stormed out

Where did this meaning come from?	Is it still useful to believe this?	Different meaning?	Re-rate emotions	New behaviour
My Dad was always like this, trying to make me feel small. It was the same with the sergeant in the army	Just because Dad did it, doesn't mean everyone else is. If I always feel like I'm at war, my anger is going to be easily triggered	I don't know if Fred was cheating. At other times we're good friends. It's not worth getting upset about even if he was. My self-worth doesn't depend on how I do in the bowling alley	Anger 30 Fear 0 Empathy 60 (for Fred and me – how easily we get hooked up in this stuff!)	If I get upset, go off to the drinks machine to cool down; don't say anything until it no longer seems to matter so much. And now, go and visit him in hospital (if he'd like it)!

This is one of two elements at the heart of anger: a sore spot or hurt place that has been touched. The other is a rule that has been broken. Usually they link together in that a sore spot is a reminder of a past injury – rather like a bruise which is still sensitive – and the rule is the protective strategy you put in place to stop it getting bashed again. This will probably have come in the form of a decision: "I'm never going to put myself in a situation where I can get hurt like that again." It will usually have some *shoulds* or *shouldn'ts* in it. In Big Mind terms, it is as though the little I of anger was unable to do its (right and proper) job of protecting you in the initial situation, and is now going to make damn sure it never slips up again – by kicking off at the very first signs of trouble!

It may be useful, again, to do some imagery rescripting or role-play exercises with a therapist so that you are no longer trying to right hurts, wrongs or slights from the past in every potential conflict situation that you find yourself in. That way the past stays more in the past (although of course you don't forget it), and you can take the present more on its own terms.

Then, having at least to some extent defused the original situation, you can have another look at the rule you have been carrying, using a cost-benefit analysis. First, identify the rule; it is clearest if you can express it in an *if... then...*format, like: "If somebody looks at me funny I have to challenge them, or that means I'm weak, and they'll push me around."

Then, using the cost-benefit analysis form below, re-evaluate the rule. What you will probably find is that the rule makes perfect sense in terms of the original situation where you got hurt, and it's important to validate it for then. But what I hope will also become clear is that it is less helpful for you now!

Cost-benefit analysis

In what ways does this rule make sense?	In what ways is this rule illogical?
How realistic is it to follow this rule?	How unrealistic is this rule?
What advantages are there for me or those I care about in following this rule?	What disadvantages are there for me and those I care about in following this rule?
Why would I recommend this rule as a guideline to those I care about?	Why wouldn't I recommend this rule as a guideline to those I care about?

Please refer back to Chapter 7 on schemas for more on questioning rules.

ALCOHOL AND DRUGS

It probably goes without saying that the expression of anger can be exacerbated by drug and alcohol use and abuse, either because the alcohol or drug reduces inhibition, or because you're strung out and getting desperate about trying to get hold of whatever is your particular poison. If that is a significant problem for you, then you need to seek specialist help for your addiction. If it is a lesser problem, then it's probably still worth monitoring your drug or alcohol use and seeing if there's a correlation with the times you get angry and lose control and do stuff you regret.

CHAINING

I want to come back to the issue of what is the major problem with anger, and that is **the expression of it in behaviour**.

Actually of course that's an overstatement, because too much anger – even unexpressed – can give you ulcers, and is there waiting to kick off, given the right trigger. We all have the seeds of anger within ourselves, and can benefit from cognitive and mindfulness work to deal with them. But nonetheless, most people's problems with anger are really problems of *unwanted behaviour* and its aftermath. To work with this, I recommend the technique called 'chain analysis': this is where we follow the chain of events that led up to the unwanted behaviour, and see all the different points at which we could have done something different.

The first step is to start keeping a basic anger diary: this should include incidents of anger, but also whether you had consumed alcohol and other important factors. On the next page is an example, which I have borrowed from Maggie Stanton, Christine Dunkley and Sara Melly.

Of course this needs to be tailored to what is helpful to you: if you don't use alcohol or other mind-altering substances then that column can be omitted; similarly if you're not working, you might want to substitute 'engaged in normal activities' or something like that.

Day & Date	Intensity of Anger 0-10	Alcohol Units	Unwanted Behaviour	Went to work? Y/N	Minutes of Relaxation	% effort on new response
Mon						
Tue						
Wed						
Thur						
Fri						
Sat						
Sun						

The 'new response' is whatever you have identified, perhaps with your therapist, as a better way to go on than the explosions which were happening previously.

The anger diary is a useful tool in itself. Notice the effects of how much relaxation (or mindfulness practice) you do on a given day and whether you 'blew' or not. But it is also the first step in chain analysis, because it enables you to identify when an unwanted behaviour occurred and the context of that behaviour.

Having done that, and identified a particular behaviour and its location in time and space, you can then back-track it to where it came from in a chain of events:

Type	Chain	Solutions

Type' refers to what kind of a thing it was: thought, emotion, behaviour, vulnerability factor, event etc. 'Chain' describes what happens. 'Solutions' is what you could have done differently, so that you can learn to see a whole heap of different options when something similar pops up in the future.

Below is a fictional example:

Type	Chain	Solutions
Behaviour	Having a few drinks on Sunday night	Don't go out drinking on nights before workdays
Body sensations	Feeling hung over on Monday morning	a) Take whatever helps: vitamin C, water, etc b) Remind self this is a temporary feeling
Behaviour	Not having breakfast	Eat something even if I don't feel like it
Behaviour	Getting in late to work	Get in on time
Event	Being told off by my line manager	Accept the specific criticism without making it say anything about me, even if he does remind me of my father
Thought	"He's a pillock"	He's doing his job as he sees it, it's not about me
Emotion/Behaviour	Sitting at my desk seething for 2 hours	Focus on the work
Body sensation/ vulnerability factor	Feeling hungry	Be aware that this is a danger situation, take care of it
Event	Discovering I've left my money at home	Borrow some money or even find a way to get some
Event	Watching a colleague eating	Focus on the work even though it's difficult, leave calmly if you have to
Thought	"To hell with today"	Just because I'm hungry and tired doesn't mean the whole day's bad
TARGET BEHAVIOUR	Overturning my desk	Leave calmly
TARGET BEHAVIOUR	Storming out of the office	Leave calmly, make excuses
Emotion	Shame (10)	Shame (4)
Thought	"She'll throw me out this time"	I'll get some money and buy some food and offer to make up any lost time

Here you can see a whole range of different possibilities for acting differently at earlier stages. Of course, the drinking is in a way the prime cause (although we don't know why he had more than a couple), but even after that, there were alternative possibilities before he got to the stage where he blew.

If you're using chain analysis with a therapist, then try rerunning the series of events and getting the therapist to coach you with alternative possibilities at each stage. Role-play it so that your body gets a feeling of the new way of going on – that way it goes deeper than if you just remember the instructions intellectually.

PHYSICAL EFFECTS

There are differing views about what to do about the physical symptoms that are present once anger has been awakened. In the 'bad old days' of the 1970s, we were encouraged in some therapy groups to beat pillows or even have fights to 'get it out', on the 'toothpaste tube' analogy of emotion. As Thich Nhat Hanh points out, this only trains you to become angrier.

On the other hand, it is indisputable that, once aroused, anger remains present for a while – a few hours at least. This is right in evolutionary terms: if we have just been attacked by a marauding rival tribe, we need to be on the alert in case they come back to attempt rape and pillage again.

So we're left with the aftereffects, even if we've managed not to act on our original impulse. Our body has been primed with the chemicals designed to turn us into terrifying warriors. The animal side wants to fight; indeed, competitive sportsmen of a certain kind are geed up to try to get them into this state before a big match. Usually afterwards there is just relaxation and exhaustion, but also a tendency at other times to get into fights. Remember: however you train your mind in work, so will it operate at leisure. So there is something in both sides. We need therefore to pacify our animal side ("It's OK, we're out of danger now"), but there may also be a need to go for a run, or do something energetic but *non-violent* to calm down.

It is also true that when troublesome boys (it's usually boys) take up martial arts with a strong moral and ethical emphasis, they get into trouble a lot less. But this is not about hitting something or somebody when they're angry – it's about learning appropriate control, to the point where physical expression is more a matter of choice than reacting to perceived threat when there isn't any. In other words, mood is no longer in control of behaviour. It also has a lot to do with being part of a disciplined group that has self-respect, rather than being a vulnerable outsider who thinks that nobody loves him...

Not compounding anger in thought, word or deed

To summarise, anger is there as a protective emotion. In prehistoric times, such as the Stone Age and earlier, if you felt angry, that mostly meant you needed to fight – either another species or someone from another clan – in order to hang on to your life or your dinner (and thus your life). This is re-enacted in inner-city gang life.

Today, as with anxiety, the threats are different, and the overt expression of anger in aggressive behaviour is rarely the best option.

We need therefore to be aware when anger rears its head, but not to follow it up with aggressive action. Rather, practise assertiveness, stand your ground if necessary (though sometimes we do need to ask if it is necessary to protect *this particular* ground), but stop short of trying to impose your will on another, especially by physical or intimidating means. One way of thinking about the difference between assertiveness and anger is that assertiveness says "I'm OK; you're OK" while anger says "I'm OK; you're not OK." This is ironic, because as we have seen anger is hurting so much it's not OK at all...

If it is a persistent problem, do an anger record to unpick it and discover a more helpful route. Try to find out what it really wants – what is the Protector afraid will happen if you don't act on this anger? Which bit is hurting? Can you instead apply the healing balm of mindfulness – Thích Nhat Hanh suggests mindful breathing and mindful walking outdoors in particular – to the way you're feeling right now?

Keep an anger diary to see when and under what conditions you get most fired up, and then carry out a chain analysis to identify alternative courses of action. It is of course important to be compassionate to yourself, but don't make that into an excuse for justifying unwanted behaviour: "S/he made me do it" isn't an option. *You are responsible for your behaviour.*

Similarly, while your automatic angry thoughts are just thoughts, and need to be noticed and no more, don't make the mistake of winding yourself up by ruminating over what may have happened and what sort of a two-faced idiot he was to do whatever he did. This *compounds* the anger and leads to you justifying behaviour which you know really isn't going to be helpful.

Good luck with your lion-taming...

Further reading:

Thich Nhat Hanh (2001), *Anger: Buddhist Wisdom for Cooling the Flames*, Rider
Gladeana McMahon (2007), *No More Anger: Be Your Own Anger Management Coach*, Karnac Press

CHAPTER 24: STRESS AND PTSD

Stress and stressors – Reducing the frequency – Processing the backlog – Living the life you want – PTSD – four parts to treatment: Helping yourself to feel safe again – Reducing arousal – Stopping any safety – Seeking behaviours – Unhooking the glitch – Acceptance

Stress, as defined by the man who coined the term, Dr Hans Selye, is both a physical and mental phenomenon. It is what happens in the body and mind when there is more pressure than the organism can cope with. However, the pressures (the *stressors*) are not the same as the response (the state of *being stressed*). Unfortunately we tend to confuse these in everyday speech, which obscures the difference, and therefore our effectiveness in doing something about it. The stressors can be external, like money or relationship issues, or internal, like the presence of certain thoughts or memories which we find stressful. So everyone has situations where stressors are present, but there are obviously differences in people's ability to deal with these. That is, some people are more stress-hardy than others.

As with physical constitutions, it would be foolish to rule out some genetic variation. Some people are just more sensitive, and this obviously has costs and benefits. However (and fortunately), there are things we can do to increase our own stress-hardiness. But what are the qualities we are trying to gain or increase? Various studies have reviewed the differences between those who cope with stress better and those who struggle to do so.

Those who cope better have a greater sense that life is *meaningful* and that they can to some extent influence how it turns out (*self-efficacy*), and that it is worth engaging in that process (*commitment*). They also display a greater sense of *acceptance of change* and a *willingness to take on challenges*. These are preventative qualities in relation to stress. But what about when it has already happened? The most extreme version of that is of course Post Traumatic Stress Disorder (see p. 340), but most of us have at some time had a sense of 'being stressed to the max'.

What I suggest has happened then is that, due to overloading (i.e. stressors have presented themselves and for a variety of reasons we have not been able to make sense of or deal with them), the residue of these events has become somehow stored in the body. This can be because there has been much too much to process in a short period, or chronically over time. The bodily tension that results is actually a sort of physical 'pending tray', in which the difficulties are encoded.

One of the contributions of mindfulness is that we can both reduce how often this happens and process the backlog.

REDUCING THE FREQUENCY

If we go back to some of the qualities of stress-hardiness, we can see how mindfulness, and the attitudes associated with it, can be beneficial. Some of these can seem a bit paradoxical. So, 'life is meaningful' doesn't necessarily mean engaging in some kind of philosophical discussion – actually, you only tend to do that if you are afraid it isn't!

And I want to distinguish *imposing some kind of meaning on life* from coming to see that *life is its own meaning*. There is nothing extra that we need to add. What a relief! So now we are free to commit to whatever we care about: child poverty, the environment, taking care of those who need taking care of, or whatever matters to you. That is, we can now *single-mindedly and wholeheartedly* engage in our lives. We are now 'on board'.

As such, we are more likely to be able to see what is actually happening *as it happens*. So we can ride the waves of change, rather than being submerged by them because we think life should always stay the same. Remember the bit about acceptance in the section on mindfulness: if our inner representation of what is happening matches what is happening, then we are much less likely to get stressed. We are seeing things as they really are. But that is only possible in the present – if what we are seeing is actually in part a memory of a past event which is emotionally colouring the present, then we are not in reality and so we don't catch the ball, whatever it is. We have to *be here* to process what is happening – if our mind is elsewhere, any of the brown stuff hitting the fan will get stored in the pending tray of our bodies and come back to haunt us later with nightmares, ulcers, high blood pressure and so on. Yuck...

PROCESSING THE BACKLOG: THE POND METAPHOR

So let's just say that we've learned (however imperfectly) to deal with present stress. Like most people, though, we've got a history. What we find, as we sit regularly, is that as we calm down and stop trying to fix things by thinking, the muddy water clears. Previously all our scrabbling around kept it murky and we couldn't see what was going on.

But as we settle down and become kinder to ourselves; less caught up in our own dramas, then sometimes old stuff starts to make itself felt. This can be a problem as it tends to send people back into mental fix-it mode, which muddies all the water again. However, if we can stay grounded and aware, then we can allow the stuff to rise to the surface and evaporate – a bit like a gas bubble from deep in the silt of the pond. Sometimes there's a bit of a bad smell!

The first sign that something needs to emerge may be a lowering of mood or an increase in negative automatic thoughts, but sometimes it may be an awareness of bodily tension (which may in turn provoke panicky feelings, if that's your 'style'). Learning to breathe mindfully into the tension, often in the belly or chest, can allow the long-suppressed pending tray to release its material, and thus the tension. But of course, you have to process what comes up. What does that mean? Sometimes no more than simply witnessing it in full awareness and feeling whatever the feelings are that come with it. But sometimes it will mean needing to take some action to clear whatever it is – saying something to someone (either in reality or simulated in therapy), or perhaps reviewing the life rule that came from the initial incident, or doing one of the 'vertical' techniques like imagery rescripting or Big Mind.

BALANCE YOUR LIFE

Naturally we need to strike a balance between giving ourselves so much to do that we can't process it, and being knocked off our stride by any little thing that comes up. I once co-ran a many-session-long CBT group for depression, and at the end of it one of the remaining participants said, "I get what this is all about now: it's about making the hurdles the right height!"

So all the material on activity scheduling and the activity window becomes relevant here. Is your life *optimally* challenging? That is, challenging enough to keep it interesting, without feeling like you're going to blow a gasket?

Jon Kabat-Zinn's distinction between problem-focused coping and emotion-focused coping is relevant here. If this stuff (whatever it is) is difficult, how much of that is down to the situation itself, and how much is it down to the schemas that are getting triggered? (Which means that it's partly about something else – i.e. whatever the initial situation was that led to the formation of the schemas.) Again, see the chapter on schemas for a review.

To summarise: we all expect to encounter situations in our lives that are stressful: birth, sickness or death of loved ones; getting divorced or married; being made redundant or starting a new job; moving house and so on, and it's very important to cut ourselves some slack at these times. But if our lives seem like one long period of stress, then it's probably necessary to make some structural changes. I have been astonished, for example, by the number of people who continue in high-powered jobs they hate because they 'have to' keep up the payments on some grand property that they hardly ever see because they're too busy working. A cost-benefit analysis is in order here! Sell the house and go live in a yurt, maybe...

But whatever your physical circumstances, ask yourself the tombstone question: what do I want written on my tombstone, and if I carry on as I am, will I get that? Or, to put it another way, am I living the life that expresses who I really am? This isn't always about what I *feel* like doing, necessarily – that can be a powerful red herring. Instead, try thinking something like this: if there were a purpose in my being on this planet – let's just suppose a purposeful universe for the moment – what might that purpose be? What might be the *contribution* that I am here to make?

That may or may not be in relation to work – for some it's about being a good parent, spouse, church member or activist. It's really about what the best part of you knows, deep down, is why you're here. And if you don't know, fine! In the sweet shop of your life, what flavours do you *really* want?

Once you are clear about this, much of your remaining *excessive* stress is probably down to an overactive, seeking, grasping mind. Doing mindfulness and Big Mind to learn to spend more time in non-seeking, non-grasping mind helps put things in perspective. After all, beyond the basics needed for living, what do we really need to 'get'?

Learning to *walk the razor's edge*, as Charlotte Joko Beck puts it, means that we are trying to experience, physically, the difficult and painful stuff as it happens, and then there's no residue. Because we can't do this perfectly, we give ourselves regular time out in meditation to process the backlog. Mostly if you sit well, that just happens by itself – bubbles rise, and we cope with the stink. Sometimes you need to see someone about it – maybe just a chat with a friend, or a therapist if it's more serious – to help you make sense of it and complete the processing.

PTSD

Post-traumatic stress disorder (PTSD) is classified as one of the anxiety disorders, but is unique among them in that it refers to something that has already happened, rather than something which is about to happen. But the prime fear is that *it will happen again,* or even that *it is happening again.* So it is something from the past which is experienced as something which is going to happen again. Quite naturally, this then provokes a whole raft of safety behaviours and avoidances to prevent that happening, as well as increased anger and/or panic in reaction to the perceived threat.

It is important to note that this part of the chapter can only give some pointers to the process to be followed. If you are suffering from PTSD you should seek professional help, preferably from someone qualified in CBT or EMDR (eye movement desensitisation and reprocessing – this 'unhooks the glitch' in a different way).

So why should something that has happened in the past be coming back to haunt us? We can look at this as a glitch in our processing. We know that if something happens to us to make us less aware of what is going on, then it may be hard to put our mind at rest about it. An obvious example is the shady memory of what happened at the office party: because we were a bit too drunk, we can't clearly remember (perhaps) how intimately we came onto that colleague…we're not quite sure, hence it continues to bother us, particularly in the days leading up to going back to work after the Christmas break! The mind *can't put it away.*

In PTSD, the reason we can't put it away is because it was too much – either there was too much going on, suddenly and at the same time, for us to be able to process it (like in a car crash) or the import of what was going on was too much (like in battle). Either way we are left with unprocessed material floating about causing trouble, especially whenever any situation occurs that *carries any markers* of the original one. The more severe the incident was, the less exact the markers have to be. To soldiers traumatised in Iraq or Afghanistan, a banging door can sound like a mortar bomb. They are suddenly transported back to the hell of the battleground, and their military training kicks in to help keep them alive. But they are in the supermarket, so the consequences can therefore be extremely troubling, both for the soldier and sometimes those nearby.

The main goal, then, for therapy in PTSD is to help the person put away the incident; to find a cupboard where it can be safely stored and taken out and looked at again if necessary, without it provoking a traumatised reaction – flashbacks, nightmares etc. This doesn't mean it disappears from memory. If we have been through horrific situations, it is healthy (if unpleasant) to be able to remember what happened. With any luck, that will help us to avoid getting into a similar situation again. But we won't think we're in that situation again when we remember it – that's the difference between an unpleasant memory and a flashback.

The core beliefs that we hold – about the world and sometimes other people as well as the self – are important here. This can go two ways: people who have had a rough time in their upbringing, to the point where (perhaps unconsciously) they hold the belief that the world is hostile and other people are out to get you, may suffer from PTSD following a traumatic incident partly because it seems that their worst fears about life, the universe and everything have been confirmed. Conversely, people who were brought up in some version of 'Care Bear world', and to whom nothing bad ever happened prior to the traumatic incident, get PTSD partly because their illusions have been shattered.

We can also develop PTSD 'second-hand' by witnessing an event happening to somebody else – particularly (but not only) if it is someone we love or loved. This may in addition provoke feelings of guilt and shame, if we feel (however irrationally) that we should have been able to stop it happening.

The treatment for PTSD has four parts:

- Helping yourself to feel safe again.
- Reducing arousal.
- Stopping any safety-seeking behaviours.
- Reworking the incident in such a way that it can be put away in safe storage: 'unhooking the glitch'.

Of course there may well be other conditions which have developed from the PTSD and need to be dealt with in their own terms (panic, anger, depression etc.) – for these see the relevant chapters.

Regaining safety

Initially this may mean taking yourself away from the situation. Leave the battlefield. We know that layers of PTSD are more difficult to treat, so be compassionate to yourself. Work gradually to restore normal functioning, and use a hierarchy to re-enter situations that resemble the one that bit you. Sometimes people find it useful to do things to help them feel safer in their bodies, like practising a martial art, for example. To start with, be with people whom you trust and who can be unconditionally supportive if you can.

Guilt and shame can take on a life of their own here, both in relation to the incident itself (you blame yourself in some way for it having happened) and for having the condition of PTSD ("I should be over it by now.") Again, use compassionate mind (see Chapter 10) to help you cut yourself some slack.

Reducing arousal

Using mindfulness or relaxation techniques in a regular rather than reactive way can help you to systematically lower your arousal. In other words, don't do it just when you're feeling anxious – do it at a particular time of day, whether you're feeling anxious or not. (See Chapter 9 for further guidance.)

Dropping unhealthy behaviours

Do a vicious daisy (see Chapter 1).

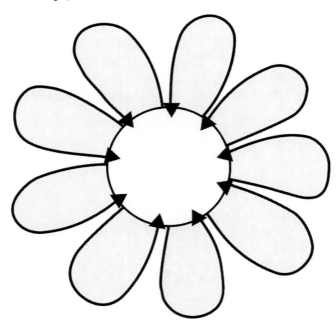

At the centre, put some version of your fear, e.g. "It'll happen again." Around the outside, put anything that you are doing to confirm that belief: any safety behaviours, avoidances and anything else that makes you think your fear is true. One PTSD client of mine had so many we called it a vicious chrysanthemum. But however many there are, it is still a *finite* amount and can be written on a hierarchy and worked through. Drivers need eventually to revisit the site of their accident, probably as a passenger at first...

Once you have the vicious daisy, write out the petals as a hierarchy and work your way through, starting with the easiest and dealing with each one until it no longer generates (disproportionate) anxiety. Again, you can use the one tick/two ticks system – one means you're working on it; two means it no longer causes you anxiety and you can move on to the next one.

Hierarchy			
Situation	How scary? 0-100	Working on it? (Tick)	No longer gives anxiety (Tick)
Sitting in the car	40	>	>
Driving to the local town, not via the accident site	60	>	
Not checking in my wing mirrors more than usual	60	>	
Driving fast when conditions allow	75		
Driving by the site of the accident (as passenger)	80		
Driving by the site of the accident (as driver)	95		

Now fill yours in using the blank form on the next page:

Hierarchy			
Situation	How scary? 0-100	Working on it? (Tick)	No longer gives anxiety (Tick)

Unhooking the glitch

It seems that PTSD remains because our minds cannot process what has happened to us: too much was going on, or it was too intense, or what happened went beyond the bounds of how we thought the universe worked. So recovery involves telling the story in such a way that it has a beginning, a middle and an end. Thoughts and emotion need to be reintegrated, and above all, what happened needs to be *accepted*. Then it can be stored in such a way that it no longer interferes with our life, and we have 'unhooked the glitch'.

Preparatory work

The first steps are what we have just described: formulation, using the vicious daisy; exposure to situations which carry some markers of the original trauma; relaxation or mindfulness practice to reduce arousal; and if you have withdrawn, a gradual re-entry into the world. Many of the generic CBT skills from the first half of the book will be useful here – ABCs, behavioural experiments and so on. Particularly helpful will be the discovery that "I am not my thoughts; feelings etc." Developing that standbackability enables you better to allow difficult stuff to come to the surface without being caught up in it.

Once you have learned the basic skills to the point where you recognise that just because something is passing through your mind doesn't mean it is necessarily significant or true; but equally you can tolerate the presence of pretty much anything in your mind without being knocked off your perch, *then* you are in a position to begin the focused work on the traumatic material.

Telling the story

The first step is just to tell the story – to give it a rough beginning, middle and end. You may or may not notice that there are some bits missing, but there usually are. Now try writing it out in detail – put it into segments or chapters if you like. Working with your therapist (I can't imagine this is a situation you would want to re-enter alone), read what you have written to him or her. S/he will be looking to see if there are any emotional 'spikes' as you recount the story. These may indicate that there is some hidden material in there, which will be worth digging into. As you go through the account, other bits may come to the surface to fill in any gaps. If they don't, obviously you can only work with what you've got.

It can be very helpful to use some kind of voice recorder to record either yourself or your therapist reading the account. One client said he found it worked better when he listened passively to the story, whether the tape was playing or I was reading notes I had made from what he was saying.

The story may need to be retold time and again; often if you do that, new material will surface to fill in the gaps, until you have an account that is complete chronologically – has a beginning, middle and end – and also emotionally. Sometimes the account reads as a very factual, cold and detached account, in which case you may need to do 'once more, with feeling'. Working with military personnel, their training was very helpful in enabling them to give a good factual account of events in chronological order. Equally, their training had also driven them not to feel the feelings which might have been natural in such circumstances, but simply pausing every so often (and when there was an emotional 'spike' which I could see from their body language, facial expression, etc.) to allow the feelings through seemed remarkably effective in getting them to a point where the story could be told from beginning to end with appropriate, but not excessive, emotion. In other words, the event can be relived without the client being re-traumatised.

Acceptance

What is often at the heart of PTSD seems to be a level of non-acceptance that the event or some part of it actually happened. When talking to the client, the key phrase uttered at the time (and repeated in therapy) is often something like, "I can't believe this is happening to me", which another part of the brain seems to be picking up as, "Well then, it didn't happen, did it?", with the consequent storage problems: if it didn't happen, it can't be stored anywhere.

Sometimes giving clients a thorough course in (group) CBT skills and the eight-week mindfulness programme has resulted in the number of reliving sessions being reduced to two, of which one was a follow-up. In each case the non-accepted part of what happened came to the surface in the first reliving session, and the symptoms never came back after that.

My theory is that the greater detachment or (better-functioning) metaperspective learned beforehand means that the client is more at ease with the scary stuff coming up, and can tolerate it better when it does (it's not so personal), so it doesn't take so long (the client is understandably less resistant), and re-traumatisation is much less likely. The object with acceptance is to get to a place where the inner representation of the event matches what actually happened, and the whole lot is contextualised in time, space and order.

A word on EMDR
Eye Movement Desensitisation and Reprocessing (EMDR) is used on its own or with CBT to work with PTSD. It seems to speed up the treatment, and can be effective with clients for whom CBT has not always worked, as well as complementing the CBT where it has.

CONCLUSION: TRAUMA IS NOT BLACK AND WHITE

We have seen that, while there are definitely extreme situations that can result in particular sets of symptoms that we call PTSD, there are many 'lesser' versions, which, while they would not be seen as PTSD, can result in our being troubled by unwanted memories or even flashbacks.

These may date from early childhood as a result of physical or sexual abuse, or from schooldays as a consequence of bullying or humiliation. Unhooking the glitch is a necessary part of treatment in a much wider range of disorders than just PTSD. In fact, to be as free of our past as we can be could be seen as a legitimate goal of all psychotherapy. That is not to forget, however – that would prevent us from benefiting from our experience – but simply to be able to look back on whatever happened with a degree of equanimity: "It was tough, *and* I can cope with the fact that it happened to me."

CHAPTER 25: BODY REGULATION DISORDERS: CHRONIC PAIN AND CHRONIC FATIGUE

Relationship with the body – Wisdom and compassion – Formulation – Pacing and records – Sleep – Physical exercise – More on pain – More on fatigue – Identification or disidentification

I have grouped these two conditions together because they are similar, both in presentation and in how they need to be treated. There are of course differences, although they can both exist in the same person. Two excellent books exist in Constable Robinson's *Overcoming...*series, and I will not try to go over everything that is covered in those useful guides. Rather, while covering the basics, I will try to show how a more mindful/Big Mind-type approach can give some added value.

To state the obvious, chronic pain is about 'physical' hurt, while chronic fatigue is about tiredness. But the point is that both hurt and tiredness are physical conditions which can seriously restrict our activities, our achievements and our enjoyment of life. In both cases you may have been told, hopefully not by a health professional, that "It's all in your head." I would say, rather, that the *relationship with* your body (or a particular aspect of it) has broken down, usually for quite understandable reasons, and needs attention. Of course the symptoms are real!

A useful philosophy?
In both chronic pain and chronic fatigue, because of the extent to which they get in the way of you doing what you want to do, they become the most important thing in your life. "How will I manage to cope with the pain/tiredness today?" and "How can I go on like this? It's ruining my life/work/relationships etc." are common thoughts sufferers may have.

Understandably, as the difficulty increases, so does the pre-eminence given to body matters, and we just try to do whatever we can when the pain/tiredness will let us. In fact *It's* in charge, and we just do what we can when it's dormant. Or, from time to time, we battle with it and try to overcome it by force of will. You don't need me to tell you what happens then. Either you manage it in the short term but then it bites you back the next day, or you can't manage it and feel defeated and hopeless.

Jon Kabat-Zinn's Mindfulness-Based Stress Reduction (MBSR) course was originally designed to reduce stress for people who were suffering from chronic physical conditions. Not surprisingly, the pain clinic sent him many referrals! And year after year they found considerable improvement in pain levels and how much the participants were able to do after taking the eight-week programme.

Much of this book has been about learning to be in your body in a helpful and present way. That may seem like the last thing you need to do when it's giving you so much trouble, but to paraphrase a well-known saying, I am encouraging you to be *in* your body, but not *of* it. Just as you do with thoughts and feelings, try taking the view that "I am the one who is aware of the body", rather than the body itself. You are the one who is *in* this vehicle, or in this animal! Jon Kabat-Zinn puts it this way:

> It may also strike you at a certain point, particularly if there is a moment of calmness in the midst of the inner turmoil, that your awareness of sensations, thoughts and feelings is different from the sensations, the thoughts and the feelings themselves – the part of 'you' that is aware is not itself in pain or ruled by these thoughts and feelings at all. It knows them, but it itself is free of them. When practising the bodyscan or any of the other mindfulness techniques, you may come to notice that when you identify with your thoughts or feelings or with the sensations in your body or with the body itself for that matter, there is much greater turmoil and suffering than when you dwell as the non-judgmental observer of it all, identifying with the knower, with awareness itself. (*Full Catastrophe Living*, p297)

Likewise with tiredness: the part of 'you' that is aware of the tiredness is not itself tired. In Buddhist terms this is the *wisdom* side of things: understanding that "This am I not, this is not me, this is not myself."

But we also need the *compassion* side: this poor body (which is not you) has been hurting or tired *for so long.* Poor animal! How can I take care of you and nourish you back to greater health and fitness? Remember, as Mary Oliver says: "you only have to let the soft animal of your body love what it loves" (*Wild Geese*). But if, through no fault of your own, the animal has been on the receiving end of some bad treatment, it may not respond naturally to ordinary requests to go for a walk. You will have to coax it, be nice to it, but also not let it bully you! If it doesn't seem too barmy to you, try talking to it as you would a reluctant beast of burden. But try not to take it personally if it doesn't want to play. After all, you are you, and your body is your body. Be in it (rather than dictating from the head!), but not of it.

Formulation: cycles

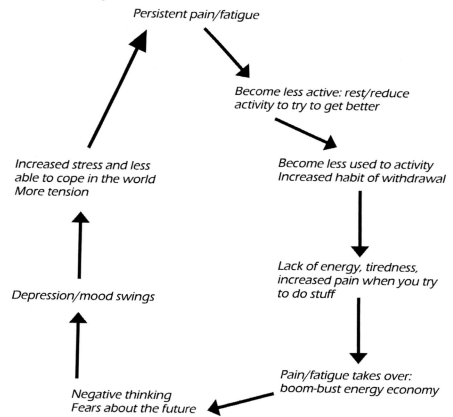

Persistent pain/fatigue

Become less active: rest/reduce activity to try to get better

Increased stress and less able to cope in the world
More tension

Become less used to activity
Increased habit of withdrawal

Lack of energy, tiredness, increased pain when you try to do stuff

Depression/mood swings

Pain/fatigue takes over: boom-bust energy economy

Negative thinking
Fears about the future

We can see from the above example that we are stuck in a loop. But this can change if we can bring four things to the situation:

1.   Acceptance: at this moment, things are as they are.
2.   The wisdom to know that I am not the pain and the tiredness.

3. The compassion that sees that this poor animal is suffering and needs help.
4. The patience to work with it slowly over time.

Then we can start, slowly, to make a difference. In a way it is the (entirely understandable) non-acceptance that things are as they are that keeps us stuck. How is that? Well, if the pain is less or you feel less tired on a particular day, don't you run around and try to do all those things that you couldn't do yesterday or the day before? And then what happens? You are laid up for the next few days, barely able to move. That's the 'boom and bust' energy economy.

So, we are starting where we are starting. That is however it is, and never mind "It shouldn't be like this." That's a *demand*, remember, and sadly there is no law in heaven that says it is not allowed for you to be in this much pain or fatigue. (But it is you *in* it; you are *not* the pain or fatigue.)

Pacing and records
This is where the tried and tested CBT technique of keeping records is helpful. Without at this point trying to change anything, keep a diary of your pain or tiredness over, say, a week. Notice the range of activities; of how much what you are able to do varies between good and bad days. This is the first step in learning *pacing*, an invaluable technique for coping with these conditions. If we live our lives in *reaction* to our pain or fatigue, then the pain or fatigue is the boss. That's like the horse deciding where and for how long we should ride. And a poor, confused and frustrated horse at that.

However, this animal is trainable, but not by 'breaking' – you tried that, remember? No, we need to do 'body-whispering'. Within an achievable framework, coax and kindly cajole your body to a level of activity which you can manage and which, to switch metaphors, leaves at least a little something in the tank. No more boom-and-bust – it's as bad for our bodies as it has proved to be for the economy! *Gradually* increase the average level of activity over time, taking rests on a regular basis as you need to without giving up altogether. But just as with anxiety and depression, we are working with a faulty feelometer, and cannot rely on how we feel as the best indicator of what and how much we should be doing. Instead we need to act AIYOBI! (Act In Your Own Best Interests!), which in this case means keeping within the bounds of our scheduled plan or the deal that we've made with our suffering animal. The sections in the self-help books already mentioned Chapter 7 (*Planning activity and rest* in 'Overcoming Chronic Fatigue*) and

Chapter 8 (*Understanding pacing skills* in *Overcoming Chronic Pain*) are invaluable here.

Action and non-action

Because we have been prevented, by our pain and/or fatigue, from doing a lot of things that other people do, we tend to focus on what we think we need to achieve. And while we don't want to retreat into the total wipe-out that may have characterised our condition so far, we do need also to think about scheduled non-action, both in terms of rest and relaxation. Mindfulness in particular (as we saw above) can be really helpful in reminding ourselves that we are not our bodies – paradoxically, that seems to make it easier to treat them more compassionately.

Perhaps it would be useful to consider the Chinese concept of *wu-wei*, 'acting without acting' or effortless action. This is (probably) the origin of the cliché 'going with the flow'. This often misrepresented as taking the easy option. In fact it is more like a musician who manages not to obscure the pure Mozart s/he is playing, or the athlete 'in the zone' or any other activity which is selfless, in the sense that one is no longer aware of the self; instead just being absorbed in whatever it is. A similar sense derives from tai chi, where the effort is minimal and the effect is maximal. It is as though one is carried along in or by the sequence of moves.

Goals and targets

But in order to get this plan going we need to have a sense of where we want to get to, and again, an acceptance that it can't all be done at once. So we need to think about goals and targets. What are the things that your condition is preventing you from doing? List them. Try ranking them in order of difficulty (as in a hierarchy): start working towards the easier ones at first, and use the confidence you get from that to progress towards the more challenging ones. Don't compare with some ideal state! If, for you, walking to the first lamppost on the street is what you've got to work on, congratulate yourself (and your animal) when you get there! Congratulate even at halfway, or for trying! Use the daily activity schedule on the following page, if you like, to plan your days.

Daily Activity Schedule and Presence Gauge   DAY:

Time	Event or Activity (What was I doing?)	Sense of mastery or achievement (M = 0-10)	Sense of pleasure (P = 0-10)	Which senses? Did I see, hear, smell, taste, touch or think about it?	Creative? Social? Physical? Nature? (C, P, S or N?)	Was I there in my body as it was happening? (yes, no, a bit)
4-7 a.m.						
7-9 a.m.						
9-11 a.m.						
11a.m.-12noon						
12 noon-2pm						
2-4pm						
4-6p.m.						
6-8p.m						
8-10p.m.						
10-12midnight						
12midnight-4a.m.						

Thoughts and feelings

You are probably also struggling with any amount of thoughts and feelings *about* the pain or fatigue – mostly not about how it is *now*, but whether it's going to get better or not; the imagined effect of your condition on other people etc. I suggest you treat these according to the techniques laid out in the first half of the book: ABCs, behavioural experiments, schema work and so on.

Particularly important will be to look at the rules you may have about rest, pain, laziness, achievement, worth and so on. Often people with chronic pain and/or fatigue have viciously high standards which would be impossible for most people to maintain even if they didn't have symptoms of pain or fatigue. Remember compassionate mind and cut yourself some slack!

Sleep diaries

Irregular and interrupted sleep is a characteristic of the lives of sufferers of both chronic pain and chronic fatigue. There are some key practices here:

1. Try to have a regular bedtime, and more importantly, a regular getting-up time.
2. Keep a sleep diary: record how much you slept, any daytime sleep and any other factors which may have affected how you slept.
3. Wind down before going to sleep: nothing either mentally or chemically stimulating.
4. Do some exercise, but not immediately (within an hour) before bed as that can be stimulating too.
5. If you are having trouble with sleep, practise the bodyscan daily.

Use the blank sleep diary form on the next page.
Also note down any periods of sleep that were not in your bed or during time you had allocated for sleep (in your chair in the living room, for example), and any times you woke up at night for more than a few seconds.

Sleep Diary

Time	Mon	Tues	Weds	Thurs	Fri	Sat	Sun
6-8am							
8-10am							
10-12 noon							
12-2pm							
2-4pm							
4-6pm							
6-8pm							
8-10pm							
10pm-12am							
12am-2am							
2am – 4am							
4am-6am							

PHYSICAL EXERCISE

Physical exercise is the *bête noir* of the chronic conditions: it is one of the things that people do, and overdo, when they have these sorts of conditions, or alternatively avoid completely.

Let's examine what happens under both conditions:

Overdoing it

So you find yourself with some energy, or the pain is not too bad today; you notice that, through prolonged inactivity, you've got a bit flabby and you think, "Great! Today I can really do something about this" and off you go to the gym, or for a 12-mile run. Or it might be much less than that, but still it uses up *all* the available juice, or you push it till it really hurts – partly due to an entirely natural wish to be able to use your body, which has been unavailable for so long.

And the consequences? If the condition you suffer from is pain, your body really starts screaming at you: "Why did you do this to me? You know you can't treat me like this and get away with it!" You can barely get out of your chair for days.

If it's fatigue, you're empty again. Just making a cup of tea seems like running a marathon, and it's ages before you can start on your hierarchy again.

So what about the other approach?

Avoiding exercise altogether

Particularly if you've had a few experiences like the above, you'll probably be tempted to give it up altogether. But listen:

"Reduced activity leads to muscles being less efficient (reduced in strength, tone and size), and consequently less effective in squeezing the blood back to the heart; this causes blood to pool in the lower part of the legs.

Pooling of blood can cause pain both during activity and at rest.

When muscles are not used regularly, they become unfit or deconditioned. When these muscles contract during activity, uneven stresses are produced.

This may result in a feeling of weakness and unsteadiness followed by delayed pain and discomfort.

In respect of the last point, it is important to note that for everyone muscle pain and stiffness are natural consequences of beginning a new exercise programme, or taking exercise to which they are unaccustomed. They are therefore not an indication that the exercise should be halted; only that it should be built up gradually."

(Mary Burgess and Trudie Chalder, *Overcoming Chronic Fatigue* p11, italics in original)

So the message is clearly, "Use it or lose it." The less you exercise, the tighter the muscles become when you do, and then even reaching for the kettle can seem like – and have the after-effects of – doing a pole vault.

Devising a healthy exercise programme
Of course, we have to start from where we are. If the pain or fatigue – or both – is extreme, then it may be a case of walking across the room twice a day. What's needed is for you to stick to that, even when, on a good day, you *could* do it three times – but then you'd have nothing left in the tank. But try to do it twice *however you feel*. Naturally there needs to be some accommodation for whether it's a 'good' or a 'bad' day pain- or fatigue-wise, but in general, we're trying to get away from the pain or fatigue being the boss, and instead making an effort to gauge the level of activity at a manageable degree. The insights from mindfulness are invaluable here. This is Mark Williams et al. on doing yoga in the mindfulness course:

> Let's imagine we have our hands above our heads, we are stretching upward with our whole bodies, and it is beginning to feel uncomfortable in our shoulders and upper arms. One way to react (the avoidance option) is to back off as soon as we feel any discomfort, perhaps immediately lowering our arms and turning our attention to some other part of the body or even out of the body altogether, maybe into a stream of thoughts or images. Another possibility (the unkind option) is to grit our teeth, tell ourselves we just have to put up with the increasing pain and discomfort, and not make a fuss, as if this were the aim of the practice. We would then put even more effort into pushing ourselves to stretch further. Here, too, we are likely to numb out, removing our awareness from those regions of the body experiencing the discomfort.

> But there is also a third option, one that strikes a balance between withdrawing at the first sign of discomfort and forcing ourselves to meet some self-designated standard of endurance. This mindful option *calls for approaching the situation in a spirit of gentle nurturing, using the stretch to extend our ways of relating to discomfort. We direct our attention right into the area of discomfort as best we can, using the breath as a vehicle to bring awareness right into that region, as in the body scan. With a gentle curiosity we then explore what we find there – physical sensations and

*feelings, coming, going, and changing. We sense them directly, perhaps focusing on any changes in intensity over time...We can play with the intensity of sensation by actually varying the stretch itself, experimenting with **working the edge**[20] of our discomfort and our acceptance, exploring for ourselves just how the body responds directly to every tiny change we introduce. This approach gives us some sense of being able to modulate the intensity of unpleasant sensations...*" ('The Mindful Way Through Depression' p144–145)

We have met 'working the edge' before, in Joko Beck's approach to feeling our emotions in the body, although she calls it 'walking the razor's edge'. But both are about staying with what is going on; a kind of emotional (in the first case) or bodily surfing of our inner world – and of course we fall off from time to time!

In a way, exercise is just doing what we are programmed to do. Stone Age people didn't need to go to the gym: they probably never got to overeat much, so they didn't have any excess to burn off, but more importantly, their life of hunting and gathering (and avoiding predators) kept them fit – or dead! Our more sedentary lives mean that we need at least to mimic what our ancestors did.

Probably, our ancestors also concentrated on what they were doing. It would have been dangerous not to. But how often do we exacerbate our pain by moving carelessly? As Jon Kabat-Zinn says:

Doing things on automatic pilot can lead to serious setbacks. As you probably know, it is particularly important to avoid lifting and twisting simultaneously, even very light objects. First lift, always bending your knees and keeping the object close to your body, then turn. Are you twisting and standing up simultaneously when you get out of the car? Don't. Instead, do one first, then the other. Are you leaning over at the waist to push up a window? Don't. Instead, get in close to it before you attempt to lift it. Mindfulness of little things like this can make a big difference in protecting yourself from injury and pain.
(*Full Catastrophe Living* p304)

Not only is it essential to stay mindful when performing physical tasks, but you also get more benefit from the physical exercise if you do. Just running on the treadmill while thinking of something else will not help as much as really focusing, non-judgmentally, on how it feels in your body as you do it: putting the mind where the body is.

20   My emphasis.

Frances Cole et al. (in their chapter on exercise in *Overcoming Chronic Pain*) recommend using a range of techniques to improve stamina, flexibility and strength. There is a further step which some of you may like to take – and this demands a bit of a leap of faith, at least temporarily – and that is to take seriously some of the claims of the gentler exercise systems from the east.

To a practitioner of chi gong, it is *chi*, or energy, that drives the whole thing: it makes the nerves work better, the blood flow more easily and so on. By doing this sort of exercise regularly, you are not only performing a mindfulness exercise and taking care to some extent of stamina, flexibility and strength, but if the principles of chi gong are to be believed, you are addressing the central driving force; the interruptions in which (again, from their point of view) may well be seen as the root of your pain or fatigue issues in the first place. Obviously, although I 'happen to be' a practitioner of such arts, it is not my role *as a therapist* to make claims for the truth of the traditional Chinese system. But neither is it my job to dismiss them! What I can say is this: if you are attracted to that style, then I encourage you to take an experimental attitude to the practice of chi gong and see what happens. You may be favourably surprised. However, and this is most important, you still need to avoid boom-and-bust! In tai chi, it is suggested never to use more than 70% of your available energy or stretch in carrying out a move. This seems a very good principle for sufferers of these conditions whichever form of exercise you are doing. So, if you like, practise chi gong within the context of your overall exercise and activity programme, and don't become extreme about it: "If only I do six hours of chi gong a day then I'll never get tired or have pain again." Believe me, you will!

Bruce Frantzis, one of the west's leading exponents of the internal arts of China and who has also studied yoga, considers that while chi gong works to regulate a steady flow of energy, yoga works on an energy build-up-and-release pattern. If that's true, then chi gong would seem to be more helpful as it works against the boom-and-bust pattern. That said, it is *not* my experience that *hatha* yoga works like that, when practised lightly for exercise and flexibility, and if you are more drawn to yoga than chi gong or tai chi, then I think that is far more important in this context. For example, Jon Kabat-Zinn's 'Mindful Yoga 2' CD (in his Guided Mindfulness Meditation series 1 collection) is very gentle, and you can certainly start by listening to it and visualising yourself doing the postures. Then, next time you play the CD, just attempt the ones that seem manageable considering where you are starting from. Yoga is of course best known for its effects on flexibility, but it certainly develops strength and stamina, too. It also has its understanding of internal energy flow (*prana*), and if you are interested in following that up you should consult a suitably qualified teacher.

SUMMARY ON EXERCISE

Exercise is not an optional extra, either in the treatment of chronic pain or fatigue, but gauging the level is very important. It should happen within the context of your daily activity plan, and should never be at a level where you've got nothing left at the end of it. When you are beginning to get up and running, so to speak, then you need to take care of developing strength, stamina and flexibility. Try to exercise mindfully – you will be far less likely to injure yourself, and you will be more likely to notice healthy limits as you listen to your body.

If you choose you may wish to adopt a non-western discipline like yoga or chi gong, but don't get carried away! Remember the 70% rule. Keep it within your overall activity programme, and at manageable levels. Then you may be pleasantly surprised at how transforming it can be.

More on pain

Ronald Melzack and Patrick Wall developed a theory of pain in the 1960s called the 'gate theory'. The gate theory notes that we can do things that make pain more or less present in our consciousness: distraction, absorption in something else, athletes not feeling the pain of injury until after the game is finished and so on. This was the first step away from seeing pain as a purely automatic reaction to a painful stimulus, which of course would not have any way of accounting for chronic pain (as the stimulus is no longer there).

The gate theory is very useful to those of us who are prepared to take an experimental approach, because we can, by trial and error, discover what opens the gate to our pain (e.g. ruminating over it, worrying about how long it's going to be there, blaming ourselves for whatever caused it in the first place etc.) and what closes it (doing things we enjoy, being with loved ones, being absorbed in a hobby or good movie etc.). Although it is worth noting, as Jon Kabat-Zinn does, that:

Several laboratory experiments with acute pain have shown that tuning in *to sensations is a more effective way of reducing the level of pain experienced when the pain is intense and prolonged than is distracting yourself. In fact, even if distraction does alleviate your pain or help you to cope with it some of the time, bringing mindfulness to it can lead to new levels of insight and understanding about yourself and your body, which distraction or escape can never do. Understanding and insight,*

of course, are an extremely important part of the process of coming to terms with your condition and really learning how to live with it, not just endure it.
(*Full Catastrophe Living* p291)

Melzack has since gone on to develop the *neuromatrix* theory, which takes it a step further. Based on the evidence that people who have lost limbs still feel pain in those limbs, he recognised that we have what amounts to an inner working model of the body that governs pain. This neuromatrix has many different aspects, and is partly genetic in origin (which could account for why some people seem constitutionally more susceptible to pain than others), but otherwise I would guess is put in place early in development. It also "produces the pattern that is felt as a whole body possessing a sense of self". (Ronald Melzack 2001, *Pain and the neuromatrix in the brain, Journal of Dental Education* 65:12; 1378–1382)

From a psychological point of view, this generates some helpful ideas: first and foremost, it confirms Paul Gilbert's assertion that "we all just find ourselves here" – we didn't design the pain equipment and are not responsible for how it works. Secondly, what we have here is a sophisticated and elaborate system that, at the 'sentient hub', thinks it's **who we are.** No wonder we identify with our bodies! Melzack also states that "the neuromatrix 'casts' its distinctive signature on all inputs (nerve impulse patterns) that flow through it" (ibid. p1380). It begins to sound very much like the biological, neuronal end of a complex of schemas.

So our animal nervous system, which thinks it's who we are, has a particular style of programming that strongly influences how we feel pain (among other things). Nonetheless, as we have seen, it's possible to transcend this limitation. Whether Melzack's 'sentient hub' is the biological source of awareness, or is simply the network through which awareness manifests, probably remains an unanswerable question.

What is clear is that the neuromatrix interprets – it 'thinks', for example, that an ex-limb is still there and feeling. Therefore, we can (again) learn to hold its messages as *objects of awareness* and *not the truth*. Again, to quote Jon Kabat-Zinn:

The system's approach to pain opens the door for many different possible ways to use your mind intentionally to influence your experience of pain...your body and mind are not two separate and distinct entities and that, therefore, there is always a mental

component to pain. This means that you can always influence the pain experience to some extent by mobilising the inner resources of the brain.
(*Full Catastrophe Living* p288)

More on fatigue

Inevitably the struggle, in the face of overwhelming tiredness, to find the energy resources to do what we need to do leads us to a view of energy as limited and within the boundaries of what we could call the 'bodyself'. When we think about it carefully, we can see that this isn't how it is.

Where does the energy come from? Literally? Carbohydrates in food. So at the very least it's a processing problem, rather than an internal resource problem. Of course I am not suggesting that all CFS sufferers should simply eat more, or take vitamins, although I'm sure that taking care of diet can be a helpful contributory factor in recovery. All I am suggesting here is that 'no man is an island'. There are all manner of things that can affect our energy levels, and quite a lot of them come from 'outside'. However, a belief that energy is limited – that we have, as it were, batteries – can be a very restrictive view that can get in the way of recovery. To carry the analogy on, we are in fact mains-powered – we are part of ecosystems, social systems, and if you like, energy systems. Often the problem with CFS sufferers is not with the source of energy (the sun is still there, food is still there, other people are still there, the earth is still there) but more with the 'wiring'. It is as though with just a little too much activity, the earth contact gets lost, the fuse blows and there is no more available juice. So we need to do things to earth ourselves, strengthen the wiring and gradually increase activity – as we covered above.

Identification or disidentification?

In both of the conditions covered in this chapter, there is underneath it all the question of identification with the body or not. I have advocated a position of compassion towards the body without being identified with it. It is important, however, not to mistake this stance for an intellectual position, or 'being in your head'. In such states we are so detached from our bodies that we don't know what is going on, and so the body just goes on doing the same old stuff. We need to be in it but not of it, even if that means being much closer to the direct experience of pain or fatigue. In the end, hopefully, we can graduate from "This am I not, this is not mine, this is not myself" – the detached but hopefully still compassionate stance – to: "The true human body is this whole universe", wherein our identification expands from awareness to include not just the limited physical body but all bodies and phenomena! If you are at ease with the Big Mind process, you may like to speak directly to the pain, or the tiredness, or the animal...but for now, just treat your animal kindly, please!

Further reading

- Frances Cole, Helen Macdonald, Catherine Carus and Hazel Howden-Leach (2005) *Overcoming Chronic Pain*, Constable Robinson
- Mary Burgess with Trudie Chalder (2005) *Overcoming Chronic Fatigue*, Constable Robinson
- Jon Kabat-Zinn (1990) *Full Catastrophe Living*, Piatkus
- Vidyamala Burch (2008) *Living Well with Pain and Illness: the Mindful Way to Free Yourself from Suffering*, Piatkus

CHAPTER 26: DIRECTIONS FOR PROBLEMS NOT ADDRESSED HERE

Eating disorders – Psychosis – The autistic spectrum – Smoking and other addictions – Personality disorders – Self-harming behaviours

In any book of this kind that attempts to say something about a range of problems, the author is going to come across the issue of specialisation: inevitably, there are going to be some areas where the writer's experience is too limited to be able to give an authoritative account of what to do. Nonetheless, it is important that these areas are acknowledged, and directions given as to where the reader may seek help.

EATING DISORDERS

Anorexia and bulimia nervosa are certainly treatable with CBT, but if the weight loss has become severe, then your cognitive functioning goes out of the window and it is very hard to do anything but the most basic behavioural work. While there are self-help books on the subject (e.g. in the *Overcoming...*series), it is important that you get medical input as well, and engage in a structured programme with a therapist who has experience in this area.

There are a few hints and tips I can give here that may complement a conventional CBT approach:

1. Not eating is of course an appropriate response when you are under actual physical threat: who needs to finish their dinner when about to be eaten by a sabre-toothed tiger? It is therefore important to treat the anxiety component so that you feel safe to have something to eat.
2. Often people with eating disorders have very poor engagement with their bodies! I have known people who appear to do really well using cognitive techniques, but

continue to lose weight. Body and mind are not talking to each other. Here mindfulness is helpful, not as a way of 'switching off', but as a way of putting the mind where the body is – the two need to be reconnected. Jan Chozen Bays has written a wonderful book, *Mindful Eating* (Shambhala 2009), which explores the seven kinds of hunger which are often confused or ignored[21] and how to deal helpfully with each one.

3. Related to this, the attentional stance of eating disorders often resembles that of people with social anxiety or BDD: outside-looking-in. And of course those prone to eating disorders are often very susceptible to the size zero nonsense in teen and fashion magazines about what is attractive. Inside-looking-out will of course work better.

4. While teenagers often experiment with their eating patterns, partly because of media influence, it doesn't always become serious. When it does, there is usually a *control* issue. If everything about the person's life is (or feels) controlled by someone else, then what goes into your mouth seems like the only thing left that you can have some say over. Obviously, then, what we need is for you to have more of a sense of participation in your life. This doesn't mean we can ignore the eating stuff, but if you feel that you are more involved in how your life is, and want to be (!), then that should help prevent relapse.

Overall, if this is a problem area for you, I would like to encourage you to seek specialist help: start with your medical practitioner and get a referral for some specialist CBT.

PSYCHOSIS

There has been huge controversy in the therapeutic world over diagnosis in this area. Perhaps the most useful work in CBT has focused on working with the most troubling symptoms: the voices or hallucinations. What we know is that these 'inputs' which seem to come from outside are actually products of the thinking part of the brain. Some approaches would see them as 'disowned' parts of the self.

The approach which most closely parallels the stance of this book is that of Paul Chadwick. He takes the voices or hallucinations as an A in the ABC model; it is not that these inputs themselves are harmful, but rather what we think they mean or what we think we have to do about

---

21 The seven kinds of hunger are: eye hunger, mouth hunger, nose hunger, stomach hunger, cellular hunger, mind hunger and heart hunger.

them. It is not that we can just dismiss them lightly! After all, as the Nazis knew, if you tell people the same lies for long enough, they come to believe them. The lies need to be exposed as lies.

Chadwick combines this ABC approach and mindfulness (horizontal metaperspective) with empty chair work (vertical metaperspective) to work with the negative experiences of self. Although Chadwick's book, *Person-Based Cognitive Therapy for Distressing Psychosis*, is a treatment manual for therapists, it is very accessible. I would suggest trying to find a therapist who works in this way.

THE AUTISTIC SPECTRUM

People with some version of autism will of course have the same problems as the rest of us! And most of the therapy will be just like that – working with whatever problems the person has. All the unfortunate stories that exist about people on the spectrum not being able to feel warmth etc. are just unhelpful. As with all good therapy, we need to build a good relationship, and this is perfectly possible. But if you have this kind of condition, you may find it more difficult to know what is going on in someone else's head. Mindreading is a thinking error for all of us, but for you it's a nightmare!

So we have to start by accepting that this is how it is. And if you can't tell what others are thinking, then you may be jumping to the wrong sorts of conclusions, which won't help you at all.

In my limited experience of working with people on the spectrum, I have found four techniques which clients have found particularly useful:

1. Thinking errors: how great to have a way of checking one's own thoughts to see if they're accurate or not!
2. Doing cost-benefits of rules: if you can't gauge what's going on in someone else's head, then it's helpful to have some rules as to how to behave in response to the cues in others' actions, as well as more general working rules.
3. The Big I, Little I model (as a committee!) and the Big Mind process: instead of getting upset by e.g. feeling anxious, say, "Ah, it's Mr Anxiety; what are you afraid of, Mr Anxiety?"
4. Mindfulness, and particularly the breathing and the yoga. There seems to be a tendency towards being uneasy in your body in this condition, and learning to be at ease through gentle exercise and non-seeking mind seems to work very well. In the one case where we did the whole eight-week

programme on a one-to-one basis, we took it a little slower and covered most of it in about twelve one-hour sessions.

Sometimes a diagnosis on the autistic spectrum is combined with Attention Deficit Disorder, although of course that is a problem in its own right. Actually most of us have Attention Deficit Disorder to some degree – who has perfect concentration? The solution is of course mindfulness, but the level and degree will depend on the severity of the problem.

ADDICTIONS

While there is a perfectly good CBT protocol for working with addictions – the master himself, Aaron T. Beck, with colleagues Wright, Newman and Liese (1993), has written the seminal text *Cognitive Therapy of Substance Abuse* – it so happens that the hospitals within which I have done most of my practice have a tradition of only using the 12-step model for the treatment of addictions. I have therefore tended to work with addicts in recovery (say, on self-esteem issues), and it would be somewhat hypocritical of me to advance a model of which I have very little experience. But as you would expect, a large part of the cognitive model looks at encouraging *helpful* beliefs about substance abuse (e.g. 'using' doesn't solve anything and it may be better to address whatever it is rather than using; look at long-term consequences of excessive use etc.), *discouraging* permission beliefs (it doesn't matter; just this one; I can't relax without a drink/joint etc.) and *facilitating* control beliefs. As always, especially in complex problems (and addiction is complex), a precise individual formulation is needed to get the best from therapy. I can, however, make a few general observations on the nature of addiction and the treatment of it, which can perhaps complement whichever style of treatment you may choose to follow.

The first question I would like to ask is: "What is the hole you are trying to fill?" and refer you back to 'the wrong kind of emptiness' (in *Self-esteem*, Chapter 14). But that may be too late if by now your animal is an addict. The addiction definitely needs to be treated in its own right, but that will be easier if the addict has accepted:

a) That it is OK, and in fact a good idea, to *feel emotions*.
b) That s/he has learned, or is prepared to learn, how to be in his or her body non-judgmentally ('at ease in your own skin').
c) Has some sense of who they want to be 'on the other side' – what are their valued goals?

D. Genpo Merzel talks about rehabilitating the addict – not in the sense of denying that part of him or her, but rather about changing the focus of the addiction. How about being addicted to working towards world peace, or (the Buddhist formula) saving all sentient beings?

Smoking

There is one particular kind of addiction that I can talk about, however, because I have been through it myself, and used it clinically too. I am not in any sense recommending that this advice can be transferred wholesale to other kinds of addiction. It works, partly, because smoking is a complex addiction. That makes it difficult, but also provides the opening to go beyond it. Cigarettes contain more than just nicotine, and I believe that the plan below, by initially cutting out the non-nicotine elements, makes it possible with only minimal effort.

It is a ten-point plan, I call it the 'Smotocol':

1) This happens before you even get to the treatment room. You have to want to do this: to stop smoking. It has to matter to you. I was concerned about my health, and there was a family history of lung cancer. I thought I might well get cancer if I carried on, and had (and have) things I wanted to do. You have to be prepared to put up with a little discomfort – but only a little!

2) If you like, find a buddy to do this with. It's great to encourage each other. If you want to, find a therapist to help you through this protocol.

3) Think of all the things you get out of smoking. In this approach, we don't agree with the view that you don't get anything out of smoking: of course you do, or you wouldn't do it – you're not that stupid! List them all and take them seriously. *Apart from* the nicotine hit, you need to find **behavioural alternatives for every one**. That means strategies for dealing with stress, but also strategies for taking time out or celebrating minor triumphs; it means remembering to go outside and look at the moon anyway, not just because you have to go outside for a ciggy. It's very important that you get them all, even if they seem trivial or stupid.

4) Use nicotine replacement therapy (NRT) to take care of the nicotine hit. I favour the inhalator or the chewing gum. Patches mean you're getting nicotine when you're asleep, and even at my worst, I never smoked when I was asleep. I liked the inhalator because one of the things I got from smoking was 'something to do with my hands'. Playing

with the inhalator was like rolling a cigarette, and you had something to hold. **Use it as much as you want, for as long as you want.**

5) Make a deal with yourself. Say: "I may be a nicotine addict for the rest of my life, but I'm never going to smoke another cigarette. But if I want nicotine, I'm going to have it. The only thing I'm doing is changing my mode of intake." What we have found is that if people try to combine NRT with reduced smoking as a halfway house, it just doesn't work. So once you make the decision, *just get your nicotine from the inhalator or gum*. For me the discomfort was only that the inhalator tasted like a menthol cigarette – always my least favourite option, but one which I'd always taken if that was all that was available. You can still get a hit!

6) Look at the beliefs you have around smoking being cool. It's not, but there is something about being an *ex-smoker*. For those of us brought up on positive images of smokers, the ones who never tried it seem to lack a certain sense of adventure. But to have done it and quit – now that really is cool. You tasted it, enjoyed it and decided that you cared about your body enough to stop doing it. And now you can run or swim or dance or do martial arts (this relates to point eight). Apparently it takes ten years from stopping before your lungs clear, but that's stopping smoking, not stopping NRT.

7) Ignore the instructions on the NRT packet. When I bought mine, it said something like, "Have as much as you want for three weeks, then reduce by half, then stop. If it's still a problem, see your doctor." On those instructions, I would have thought that I'd failed, and would probably have started smoking again. Go on using the NRT *until you don't want to anymore*. For me, it dropped away slowly over about a year. I kept the inhalator and some cartridges in my desk for another six months, and would have used them if I'd felt like it, rather than have another cigarette. Positively enjoy the fact that you can use it on the bus, in the train, in a pub, in the theatre...

8) Actively encourage possibility goals that you would struggle with if you smoked. For me it was swimming and martial arts. You cannot do a kung fu class like we do it in our club and smoke – or at least, I know I can't! And the pressure I used to feel on my chest while swimming, when I smoked, was enough to keep me out of the pool or sea. Now I can swim if I want to, with no pressure on my chest. What you want is to have things you value that you would lose if you started smoking again. Think about your increased chances of seeing your kids grow up, for a start.

9) Be prepared for an unhealthy transition period, especially if you've smoked for a long time. I had three years of bad chests, colds, coughs and bringing up disgusting gunk – but that was after nearly 30 years of smoking. But it did get better! Use vitamins, Echinacea or whatever you think will help you through it. Keep exercising.

10) Have evaluation points and give yourself treats when you reach certain milestones – although reaching them is great in itself. And as with any other treatment plan, if you slip in a moment of absent-mindedness or worse, don't beat yourself up, just start again. Once I found that you *could* get a hit from the inhalator, I never needed to smoke again. If I'd known how easy it was, I'd have done it years before...

PERSONALITY DISORDERS

The concept of 'personality disorder' (PD) is one that, not surprisingly, does not find much approval in certain quarters. According to the medical approach, it means the condition is not a 'mental illness' and is therefore untreatable. As I mentioned earlier, the wonderful Taizan Maezumi Roshi once said to me, "We're all mentally ill, it's just a matter of degree." I would like to say the same about personality disorders: we've all got a personality disorder, it's just a matter of degree. Actually, having a personality that is too ordered is also a personality disorder: Obsessive Compulsive Personality Disorder.

That said, it is my clinical experience that, when CBT hasn't seemed to be working with a particular client and I've gone to Beck et al.'s *Cognitive Therapy of Personality Disorders*, I have usually been able to find a solution. So, as with all diagnoses, *having* a particular kind of personality disorder doesn't mean that you *are* a personality disorder. Beck suggests that the personality disorders are evolutionary survivals of tendencies which in previous ages were extremely functional. It is a well-known cultural phenomenon that brilliant soldiers in combat don't always settle down easily in peacetime: does that mean they suffer from Anti-Social Personality Disorder?

Perhaps the most difficult aspect of all this is that while most therapists will admit to having had at least a taste of anxiety or depression, very few would admit to a personality disorder! And that sets the client further away from the therapist. In essence, the problem in personality disorders is that any anxiety or depression issues may be compounded by a difficulty with forming and maintaining relationships, yet it is in relationships that the problems are most acute.

It is not surprising, therefore, that it is often those therapists on the fringes of CBT who have the most helpful approaches. There is not space to go into it in any detail here, but the condition known as Borderline Personality Disorder (BPD) also makes it very hard for the sufferer to *stay with* strong emotions – whether positive or negative. Marsha Linehan has developed a very specific protocol for BPD, involving both behavioural and mindfulness elements, called Dialectical Behaviour Therapy.

Jeff Young has adapted CBT for the personality disorders – and included other influences –and called it Schema Therapy; cognitively, it is work on the schemas that is particularly called for in this area, in addition to the regular CBT techniques of thought records, behavioural experiments etc.

There are other therapists who straddle CBT and psychodynamic approaches like Jeremy Safran, who work specifically on the relationship issues by using the therapeutic relationship itself, in the psychodynamic style. So it may take you a little longer to find an appropriately experienced therapist, but they do exist!

If we come to the issue of personality disorders from a Big Mind perspective, we discover a radically different approach which at least doesn't distance the therapist from the client. Through Big Mind itself we discover that, as Big Mind, we contain all kinds of personality, and therefore all personality 'disorders'. Perhaps more parts have been disowned in someone with a PD diagnosis, but they're all there in all of us. How's *your* inner psychopath?

All of this is really to say that if you have been given a diagnosis of personality disorder, there is the possibility of treatment out there, but you may have to look a little harder to find someone who's willing and able to do a good job. Good luck! In the meantime, Jeff Young and Janet Klosko's *Reinventing Your Life* is a great place to start.

SELF-HARMING BEHAVIOURS

Many people self-harm at some point in their lives. Some of these behaviours are seen as more or less socially acceptable (smoking; drinking to excess), while others (e.g. cutting) are not.

People often do these behaviours to get a sense of relief or release from tension, or to feel real when the prevailing sense is one of numbness, or as the lesser of two evils when serious suicidal impulses are present.

While obviously self-harming is not great, it's a whole lot better than suicide. If it seems to be the best way you can deal with stuff at the moment, so be it. Beating yourself up about it, as we know, will simply exacerbate the problem. Often this is about allowing yourself to be open to difficult feelings, and I would like to encourage you to get help for that. You can learn that, with help, even difficult feelings are tolerable. The more you can feel the bad, the more you'll be able to feel the good.

SUMMARY

Some of the more complex issues are not really amenable to being worked with in a self-help book. Nonetheless, there are many techniques here which can contribute to recovery even with apparently intractable problems. But if that describes your situation, you will probably benefit by using the book with the help of a good therapist[22].

Further reading

Eating disorders:
Christopher G. Fairburn (1995) *Overcoming Binge Eating*, Constable Robinson
Peter J. Cooper (2009) *Overcoming Bulimia Nervosa and Binge Eating*, and (2007) *Overcoming Bulimia Self-Help Course: A Self-Help Practical Manual Using Cognitive Behavioral Techniques* (three volumes), Constable Robinson
Christopher Freeman (2009) *Overcoming Anorexia Nervosa*, Constable Robinson
Michelle Heffner and Georg H. Eifert (2004) *The Anorexia Workbook*, New Harbinger
Jan Chozen Bays (2009) *Mindful Eating*, Shambhala

Psychosis:
Paul Chadwick (2006) *Person-based Cognitive Therapy for Distressing Psychosis*, Wiley

Personality disorders:
Jeff Young and Janet Klosko (1998) *Reinventing Your Life*, Penguin
Matthew McKay, Jeffrey C. Wood and Jeffrey Brantley (2007) *The Dialectical Behavior Therapy Skills Workbook*, New Harbinger

Addictions:
Deirdre Bounds (2009) *Fulfilled*, Pearson/Prentice Hall/Harlow

---

22 See appendix: How do I get this stuff?

CHAPTER 27: RELATIONSHIPS

Trying to get what you want – Communication difficulties – Intimate relationships – Family relationships – The wider family – Friendships and work relationships – The therapeutic relationship

We are social beings. As Mark Rowlands has pointed out in *The Philosopher and the Wolf,* our relatively enormous forebrains grew out of the complexities of primate relationships – which, he claims, are all about scheming and deception! While perhaps we don't need to go quite that far, it is certainly true, once you think about it, that this is what a lot of our relationships comprise:

"How can I get what I want from that person?"
"If I get flowers for my spouse, will s/he sleep with me tonight?"
"How can interacting with that person or group benefit me (or my immediate family) in some way?"
"If I can sell them this idea/product/philosophy, how can I make sure I get more out of it than they do?"

I'm sure this sounds pretty normal, if unpleasant, to most of us, and we wonder why the news we hear isn't very joyful! In a way, this states the problem. Fortunately, it isn't the only way of relating. But as always, we need to accept our primitive – and in this case *primate* – origins, in order to be able to go beyond them.

Contracts

Therapist (to husband in couple group): "What's your contract with each other?"
Husband "We don't have one."
Therapist: "There's always a contract. If it's not explicit, then it's more difficult. We need to find out what the hidden rules are."

In Buddhism, suffering is subdivided into four kinds:

1. Not getting what you want.
2. Getting what you don't want.
3. Not being with those you love.
4. Having to be with the unloved.

Clearly the last two are about relationships, so it's worth examining them in some depth. You might still ask, "Why is there a problem?" And in response I am reminded of a scintillating talk I heard some years ago by the psychologist Dorothy Rowe on this very subject: why relationships fail. It was all about what we might call 'the pitfalls of communication'. She compared two aspects of what happens when you go to visit someone. The following is my memory of what she said:

The Pitfalls of Communication (after Dorothy Rowe)

'Your visitor might say, "Give me your coat". In that case there is a definite thing that can be handed over; but they might also say, "Give me your news". That turns out to be a different matter. Suppose you are relating an event to your friend. Before that event even happened, you had certain beliefs and assumptions relating to whatever it was, which will have influenced how you came to it, and what of it you were likely to notice; then the event happened and those preconceptions will have affected what of it you remembered. After the event you will have edited it, consciously and/or unconsciously, partly according to what you were trying to achieve from the event. Later when you meet your friend, you will edit your memory again, in terms of what you think s/he will be interested in/not offended by. And so you tell your story of what happened.

They on the other hand, will be bringing their own beliefs and assumptions to your meeting, which may be completely different from yours; they will receive (from what you say) only that which their programming allows them to receive (this is not mainly about choice); unconscious and conscious editing follows according to what their hopes and fears were about your encounter, or about whatever the event concerned.

Is it any surprise, then, that people have difficulty communicating (and thus living) with each other? All the above could have happened in a context of completely well-intentioned relating; when we factor in the 'scheming simian' influence that Mark Rowlands describes so pitilessly, then it's a wonder that there are any long-term relationships left standing!

So, guess what? We need to be *compassionate* with ourselves when we have trouble in our relationships. Yet again, we are trying to work with equipment from lizards, monkeys and our own childhoods, the combination of which is uniquely formulated, complex and likely to be unreliable and biased. By uncovering the biases, cultivating basic friendliness (to ourselves and others) and trying to be mindful of what is actually happening in any given moment, we can go some way towards having better interactions.

These are general principles; in addition there are points which relate to different kinds of relationship, which we will explore in the rest of this chapter. And in making the transition from the chapters on problem areas to the concluding chapters on the wider applications of the fourth wave approach, we will also look at the therapeutic relationship and group dynamics.

INTIMATE RELATIONSHIPS

'Marriage' from The Prophet

Then Almitra spoke again and said, And what of Marriage, master?
And he answered saying:
You were born together, and together you shall be for evermore.
You shall be together when the white wings of death scatter your days.
Aye, you shall be together even in the silent memory of God.
But let there be spaces in your togetherness.
And let the winds of heaven dance between you.

Love one another, but make not a bond of love:
Let it rather be a moving sea between the shores of your souls.
Fill each other's cup but drink not from one cup.
Give one another of your bread but eat not from the same loaf.
Sing and dance together and be joyous, but let each one of you be alone,
Even as the strings of a lute are alone though they quiver with the same music.

Give your hearts, but not into each other's keeping.
For only the hand of Life can contain your hearts.
And stand together yet not too near together:
For the pillars of the temple stand apart,
And the oak tree and the cypress grow not in each other's shadow.

Often clients come to therapy for depression or anxiety, and after a while, it turns out that there is an issue in their marriage or relationship. It may even be the principal cause of the problem. What is often interesting is that, while the person may have a perfectly healthy attitude to their friendships or workplace interactions, somehow their marriage is hedged around with all kinds of demands that the person knows are unhealthy, but somehow can't face the prospect of even confronting them.

For me the bottom line is described beautifully by Fritz Perls (the founder of Gestalt Therapy) in his *Gestalt Prayer*, which I quote in full:

> *I do my thing, and you do your thing.*
> *I am not in this world to live up to your expectations,*
> *And you are not in this world to live up to mine.*
> *I am I, and you are you.*
> *If by chance we meet, wonderful.*
> *If not, it can't be helped.*

From a CBT point of view, this takes all the demands out of a relationship, and I would like to see it read in every marriage service in the land, along with Kahlil Gibran's chapter on marriage from *The Prophet* (see box on the previous page):

At risk of labouring the point, I would like to draw out a few points from my understanding of this that might not be immediately obvious:

"You were born together..."
This is our innate interdependence; 'interbeing'. In my stick-drawing series it is the last picture: actually we are all waves on the same ocean.

"Make not a bond of love."
I don't *think* this is saying "Don't get married"! But there are things which can be reasonably promised, like behaviour – "I vow not to leave my socks on the floor" – and things which are beyond our control, and which may actually be prevented by vowing them. Love is the most obvious of these; forgiveness is another. In my view, we can try to create the conditions under which love may flourish, but like the wind, it "bloweth where it listeth". If we say to ourselves, or to the other, "You have to love!" then it will almost certainly disappear.

"Drink not from one cup..."
This is the main point! For there to be a relationship, there need to be two parties, and uniqueness is not in opposition to intimacy and harmony: "Even as the strings are alone, though they quiver with the same music."

Also the relationship, it is implied, will be more stable if there is some distance:
"...the pillars of the temple stand apart,
And the oak tree and the cypress grow not in each other's shadow."

Finally, we are exhorted to take responsibility for our emotional life, or to hand it over only to the Absolute ('the hand of Life'), and not to our partner. That doesn't mean holding back: "Give your hearts, but not into each other's keeping."

Give and take

This brings us to one of the commonly spoken assumptions about relationships: "You've got to have some give and take." This is usually taken to mean that both partners have to be prepared to compromise; but I wonder if it's worth exploring this little nugget a bit deeper. Perhaps one of the most helpful factors in making a successful relationship is if the partners can *both give and take*. That is, each one can accept what the other is giving: compliments, gifts, positive and negative feedback, *and* be able to offer selflessly what s/he perceives as being helpful and generous, perhaps even irrespective (sometimes) of one's own desires or preferences.

'Hollywood assumptions'

On the other hand, most of us carry around a number of assumptions about our romantic relationships that are, at the very least, questionable. Many of them appear to come from the Hollywood of the 1950s, or even earlier, with the 'happy ever after' endings of the fairy stories some of us were brought up on:

- If a relationship is good, it has to last forever (or at least until death!).
- If a relationship ends, it was never any good.
- We should do everything together.
- We should like all the same things.
- I should be able to get everything I need from my partner.
- I can only really love one person in my life.

When we look at these, we can see that, apart from anything else, these sorts of assumptions put a huge amount of pressure on a relationship. Most partnerships would be bound to disintegrate if they had to conform to all of them. I'd like to suggest some other ways of looking at these rules; what I suggest you do, however, is a cost-benefit on any that *you* think may be unhelpful (see the chapter on schemas), while (if you like) considering the points I make below.

Let us take them one by one:

"If a relationship is good, it has to last forever."
If human beings stayed the same all their lives, it might work, *if* the couple were totally compatible at the beginning. But people change.

Especially if the pair got together when they were very young, then they are likely to change quite a bit over time. Those changes may be manageable within the relationship, or they may not be. Some of the changes may have nothing to do with personal development, and more to do with life stages:

- The couple who meet when young, e.g. while travelling or at university, when they had a great time, but later struggle to cope with getting along in the everyday treadmill of work, children etc.
- The couple who are fine whilst actively involved in child-rearing, but fall apart when the children leave home.
- The couple who struggle to cope with the husband's retirement, or the wife's menopause.

Other changes may be more to do with the personal development of one of the partners:

- The couple who struggle to cope with one partner having therapy, going to university or having other transformative experiences, with the other feeling left behind or wanting the 'old version' of their partner back.

The Three-day Week

During the 1970s' miners' strike in Britain, the Conservative government of Ted Heath put in place, as a temporary measure, a three-day working week to save energy. Research apparently showed that productivity per day was much higher than it had been in the normal five-day week, and analysts considered whether it would actually be better to convert to a shorter working week in the long term. The story goes that this was rejected on social grounds – because the divorce rate went through the roof!

Allowing for a certain amount of caricaturing, we could portray the typical marriage of the 1970s as the husband going out to work, coming home with the pay packet and perhaps going shopping with the wife on Friday night, but then he's off to the pub with his mates. Saturday afternoon he's at the football, and while 'her indoors' is making dinner he's again at the pub on Sunday. Monday morning he's back at work. Evenings during the week he's either at the pub or they're watching the TV. Talk to each other? You're having a laugh...

Not surprising they didn't know what to do with all that extra time!

So for various reasons, couples (humans!) struggle to cope with change, and if one partner changes in a way that is difficult for the other, then it obviously puts a strain on the relationship.

What is more frightening to my eyes is where one member of a couple feels they cannot grow/change within the relationship, but inhibits their own development rather than put a strain on it, and so becomes depressed.

We should also consider that as people live longer, marriages are also expected to persist infinitely. In Stone Age times, 25 was a good age and 40 was positively ancient. These days, marriages are often expected to last a good deal longer than that.

"If a relationship ends it was never any good."
This is the other side of the same coin. But even if a relationship didn't last through some structural change, should we really devalue it for the period while it *was* working? Especially in the example of relationships that started young, it may have been what a friend of mine once called a 'growing-up relationship' – you had adventures together, and wonderful experiences, but it wasn't built to last. I think it's very sad if people devalue those good times. Some relationships have a long sell-by date and others have a short one. That doesn't mean the short ones are any less valuable (while they're still in date)!

"We should do everything together/we should like all the same things."
This seems to be quite typical of those kinds of relationships we've just been talking about, and sometimes I wonder if it's these very demands that provide the pressure under which the partnership disintegrates. Also, of course, sexual jealousy may well be stronger when young, and doing everything together seems to provide a way of not letting the partner out of your sight!

Of course this is not sustainable. Even if you share lots of interests, you both, as Kahlil Gibran says, need to have time and space to do your own thing.

"I should be able to get everything I need from my partner."
Do you think this might be slightly unrealistic? Assuming for the moment that you have a deal regarding sexual monogamy – which most people seem to espouse even if considerably fewer keep – is it really OK to expect all your (other) interests to be shared: tapestry, rugby, jazz, bingo, archaeology...not to mention the necessity of having friends outside the relationship! Being 'soulmates' (if that's what you think is going on) doesn't necessarily mean you can't have independence.

"I can only really love one person in my life."

There is of course the saying, "The first cut is the deepest", but there's another hidden assumption inside this one, like rather unhealthy Russian dolls; namely that all loves are the same. Yet if you consider the Big I, Little I diagram, what we are talking about is not really a one-on-one business at all, but a meeting of a number of little Is in one person with a number of little Is in the other. You may have a relationship when you are young which is all about excitement, sex, adventure, experimenting and so on, but which is a very different partnership from a later one, which may be more about homebuilding, children etc. (not that any of those things have to be mutually exclusive). In old age, relationships may be more about companionship (as well as excitement, sex and adventures!). The loves may be different; last for shorter or longer periods of time; may involve different little Is or departments, but as with the self, don't benefit from being judged as a whole.

SEX

Sex has become one of the most important matters in our society. Almost everything is advertised in terms of its ability to make you sexier or richer, or preferably both. In reaction to an earlier prudence, for a while in the 1960s and 70s it seemed as though any sex was better than no sex, and you were always supposed to say yes, especially if you were a woman. This sort of attitude, unfortunately, still has currency in some quarters, and obviously leads to exploitation. While not wishing to go back to the days when sex was only supposed to be for reproduction, surely it has become too important?

John Gray, among others, has pointed out that there is a difference in how men and women approach sex: the stereotype is that the woman needs to feel love in order to want sex, while the man needs to have sex in order to feel love. Is that how it is in your experience?

I suggest that if you as a couple are having trouble in this area, you examine what the contracts are in relation to sex. Maybe we are all prostitutes sometimes. I would also suggest that the bottom line is: "Don't do anything you don't feel good about (especially afterwards)." The Zen precepts, points of moral guidance taken by everyone who formally becomes a Zen Buddhist, include something on sex, which is translated in one version as: "No bad sex." I think this sums it up perfectly – don't sleep with anyone you shouldn't, don't do it when it doesn't feel right, don't do it for ulterior motives etc. I don't (personally) think that necessarily means you have to be married, and the matter of long-term commitment is of course up to every individual, but I do think 'no bad sex' means being as clear as you can be with each other about what you are both expecting from it. Oh, and did I mention, it might even be fun?

Am I getting what I want from this relationship?

On the one hand, if you're asking this question, already there's (maybe) a problem. On the other hand, the problem may be with how you're approaching the relationship. Of course we are not always going to like the same things, there are going to be arguments and sometimes we're going to think, "How did I get myself into this?" That's just normal. And it's also true that sometimes a relationship can be stultifying for one or both partners. If that's the case for you, then you probably need to seek some marriage guidance counselling. But are you looking at your partner as though s/he were a washing machine: "Is this machine giving me what I want?" Well, guess what – they're not a machine!

The Zen teacher Charlotte Joko Beck, is, as always, illuminating on this subject and I make no apology for quoting her at length:

> For instance, we meet a nice girl and, "Hmm, she looks like Channel 4; I know what to expect on Channel 4: a certain range of this and that; a little news – I can be pretty comfortable with a Channel 4 person." So we get together and for a while everything goes very well. There is a lot of comfort and agreement. It seems like a great relationship.
>
> But lo and behold, what happens after a while? Somehow Channel 4 has switched over to Channel 63, a lot of irritation and anger; sometimes Channel 49, all dreams and fantasies. And what am I doing during all this? See, I was pretending to be just a Channel 4 person. But no, it seems I like to spend a lot of time at Channel 33 with childhood cartoons, mostly about my dream prince or princess. And then I have other channels like Channel 19 – gloom, depression and withdrawal. And sometimes, just when I'm into gloom, depression and withdrawal, she's into fantasy and light; that doesn't fit very well...
> (*Everyday Zen* p81–82)

So this is the problem: we're trying to manipulate the other, like we do with the rest of the world, to make them fit with our idea of what should be; how they should fit in with our personal project. And sometimes the other doesn't seem to want to go in the same direction as you do – consider the following story:

The Talking Frog

An elderly man was walking down a country road one day when he espied a beautifully coloured frog. He stooped down to have a closer look, and, to his surprise, the frog started to talk to him,

"Hallo," she said (for it was definitely a she), "I am in fact a beautiful princess, and if you kiss me, then I will be transformed and we will be rich and happy and have lots of great sex."

At this, the old man scooped her up and put her in his pocket.

"At my age" he said, "I'd rather have a talking frog".

So what's the solution? Despite all this, Joko encourages us to work with relationships:

> ...aside from our formal sitting, there is no way that is superior to relationships in helping us see where we're stuck and what we're holding on to. As long as our buttons are pushed, we have a great chance to learn and grow. So a relationship is a great gift, not because it makes us happy – it often doesn't – but because any intimate relationship, if we view it as practice, is the clearest mirror we can find.

> You might say that relationships are the open door to our true self, to no-self. In our fear we always keep knocking at a painted door, one made of our dreams, our hopes, our ambitions; and we avoid the pain of the gateless gate, the open door of being with what is, whatever it is, here and now.
> (ibid. p84)

This may seem a little idealistic to many of you. That's right, it is! But it's something good to aim for, rather than another demand to place on ourselves. On a more prosaic level, we could say that it's just about feeling what we feel and trying to be open with each other about that, noticing which triggers are set off by the other's behaviour and not running away from them.

In my opinion, the central problem for many people is just as Joko describes, and I have attempted to portray (in the series of drawings which I reproduce again on page 384) the ways in which we are trying to get our juice from the other. It'll never work. We need to find ways of (individually) plugging in to Life itself, and fortunately for those of us in modern times, more spiritual and artistic technologies are available for doing this than ever before.

Yet, probably because of attachment issues from childhood and consequent beliefs in our own unlovability, we persist in trying to get the juice from our relationships. Not that it isn't there, but the intimacy can only happen when we stop grasping!

Great Intimacy

In a Big Mind workshop, the facilitator asked to speak to 'Great Intimacy'. Someone, speaking in that voice, said she was 'the connective tissue of the universe'. Another participant offered, "I am what people are seeking in sex." "Do they find you?" asked the facilitator.
"Rarely," said the participant.
"Are you there?" he asked.
"Always," was the response...

If on reading this you feel you want to explore relationship issues more, then Martin Crowe's *Overcoming Relationship Problems* may be the next step, or finding a good marriage guidance counsellor.

FAMILY RELATIONSHIPS

After (or possibly including) intimate relationships, family relationships are probably the ones that can cause us the most difficulty. So much is bound up in them: the formation of our personalities comes in large part from how we are treated by those who are in charge of our upbringing. While others may sometimes push our buttons, our parents installed them.

Much has been written on the different kinds of attachment that children experience at the hands of their parents and how this affects our adult relationships. Briefly, Ainsworth, building on the work of John Bowlby, identified patterns in children's responses after a brief separation from their mothers. Those who were *securely* attached were glad to see them. Of the two kinds of *insecure* attachment, the *ambivalently-insecure* expressed some hostility to the mother, while the *avoidant-insecure* showed no preference between their mother and another adult. It was thought that while the ambivalently-insecure derived from a lack of maternal availability, the avoidant-insecure came from neglect or abuse.

These different patterns of attachment are considered to have far-reaching effects in our adult lives, and are likely to be influential (to say the least) in the formation of our core beliefs, particularly those that relate to our connection with others. But what is connection? From a Zen perspective, we are actually interconnected with every other life form on the planet – but when you're depressed, for example, it certainly doesn't feel like that.

To get a greater sense of this interconnection, we can draw on two broadly different areas of study, which end up taking us to very similar places. First, consider our place in our immediate ecology: connections with other humans, certainly (even if not always felt very deeply), but also other life forms, from domestic pets to the cows you get your milk from to (if you live where I live) the seagulls that do their best to get to your rubbish before the refuse collection arrives, and the spider that lives in the top corner of my conservatory, not to mention the undoubted numbers of rats that I never see but are rumoured to outnumber us by several to one in urban areas...perhaps not a picture you like, but undoubtedly we're all interconnected. There is even our connection with air and water: we breathe in, there is some exchange of chemicals (although quite a lot stays the same), and we breathe out. Without that simple action we can't survive. But where did that air come from, and where is it going next? Similarly with water: we drink it; we wash in it; we're partly made of it. Whose water is it, anyway? Actually, it might be more helpful to consider ourselves as just a part of the air/water/earth/fire complex with delusions of separateness...

Remember the batteries drawing from chapter 8? Here it is again:

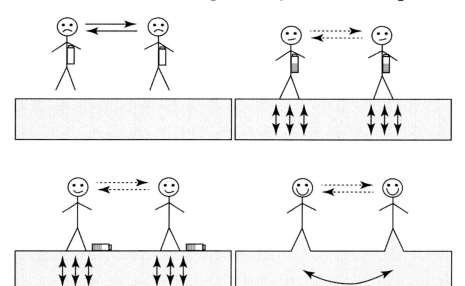

In Mahayana Buddhism, the structure of the universe is described in terms of the Net of Indra: a net in which all the intersections are multifaceted diamonds which reflect all the rest of it, and thus every part contains every other part. Universes pulsate in our cell structure. Tell me, which bit is 'you'?

So we are intimately interconnected with the rest of 'it', but because of the need to cultivate the sense of separateness to preserve safety (possibly compounded by attachment or other difficulties we experienced in our early lives), we have lost touch with our interbeing and feel unbearably lonely. This brings us back to emptiness in its 'bad' sense. And maybe it is just that shift from being frightened of emptiness to embracing it (as an experience of the deathless) that can transform all our relationships...

One of the greatest tensions that most of us experience in adult life is that between how we *actually* feel about other humans to whom we are related, and how we think we are *supposed to* feel. While for many that doesn't get worse than feeling that we have to put on a polite smile at Christmas, for some this is a real crisis, for example if they are being re-exposed to those who were abusive towards them when they were younger, yet they feel they have to be friendly or compliant. This, not surprisingly, is likely to bring up all kinds of conflicting emotions. While for those of us who are not in such a situation it might be easy to say, "Well, if you don't like them, then don't have anything to do with them", and while that may indeed be good advice, I think that underestimates the strength of the link that exists between children and parents.

Remembering the evolutionary psychology approach may be helpful here. For generations it has been vital for us to stay connected to our caregivers – that way we avoid being eaten, or attacked by members of other tribes. So 'loyal son or daughter' may be a program that goes back far beyond our personal history – which isn't to deny the attachment approach above. But those whose attachment has not been good may nonetheless have strong urges to retain links with, say, their former abusers, which then need to be explored in therapy. This is a huge issue, and well beyond the scope of a book such as this[23].

I should also mention another challenging area, which is that of the mother who for whatever reason has become emotionally disconnected from her child. Usually this is because of postnatal depression, an all-too-common occurrence. If this is your situation, there are two things that really need to happen:

---

23 But a start can be made by reading Jeff Young and Janet Klosko's *Reinventing Your Life*, an introductory self-help book on Schema Therapy.

1. ***Get some help***. Start with your GP or your midwife or health visitor. Don't be ashamed! Like depression (of which this is a variation) this is an illness, and doesn't say *anything* about what kind of a parent you'll be when you're better again.

2. Start making some time for you. Having got the help, make sure you have some time to do the things that remind you of your independent existence and the things you used to do before you had the baby. Think activity schedule/window.

It would be ridiculous in a book of this kind to cover the topic of family relationships thoroughly. But we can draw out a few strands: our connections with others have been influenced by a whole host of factors, most of which have never been in our control – evolution, simian scheming, cultural traditions, individual genetic variation, attachment with the mother, the behaviour of those who looked after us (sadly, sometimes a euphemism) when we were young, and on the back of all that, our (sometimes blundering) attempts to cope with whatever was going on. I think we need to give ourselves some compassion, don't you?

FRIENDSHIPS

Naturally, some of the same principles that apply to intimate and family relationships will also apply to our friendships. Are we just trying to get what we need from the other; using them to fulfil our needs? If we are, is this an open contract – like when people get together to form a sports team or a band – or are we pretending something? Or are we yet again trying to work out our unsatisfactory family relationships from childhood?

Yet *community* is one of the things that people bemoan the passing of. Basic friendliness may be one of the most important virtues, as in Louis Armstrong's *Wonderful World*: "I see friends passing by, saying 'How do you do?' They're really saying 'I love you...'"

So the same guidelines we talked about in intimate relationships apply here. Can we be open with each other? And, being clear about what we want and aware of how we feel (and what prejudices/schemas are lurking), just riding on a raft of basic friendliness so that our interactions are generous. It's OK to ask for help, and a privilege to be able to give it. And of course, in an ideal world it shouldn't be all one way, unless that is clearly agreed[24]. Even then, as in a friendship that arises from a caring situation, the 'carer' also gets to feel wanted and useful and may also get some companionship from the arrangement. Good friendships take the pressure off the couple relationship, too!

'Belonging' comes third on Maslow's Hierarchy of Needs[25], and whether or not you agree that this is the right place for it, it is certain that connection with other humans is vital for our wellbeing. Attachment is, after all, hardwired into our structure. And as the saying goes:
"God gave you your family; thank God you can choose your friends."

WORKING RELATIONSHIPS

These are only different from the above in that we *don't* choose who we work with, or at least not usually. So again, our buttons may be pushed more often, and we have to subjugate our preferences, at least between 9am and 5pm. Again this can be a great testing ground for how well our practice is going. Power relations, while present in all relationships, are more explicit here, which can sometimes be helpful, and sometimes a hindrance. If you're having a rough Monday morning and your boss asks you how you are, most of us wouldn't volunteer, "F***ing awful!"

So questions arise around staying with convention sufficiently to keep your job or prevent too much discord in the team, versus being true to yourself in your interactions. Finding common purpose helps, perhaps starting with the recognition that we're all human and desire to be happy! And for many people, it is the connection with others in the workplace that makes an otherwise tedious job bearable.

THE THERAPEUTIC RELATIONSHIP

If you've read this far in this book, there's a chance that you may be working with a therapist, or thinking about hiring one to help you through some difficulties. Much has been written about this, as you might expect, but most of it is for therapists. I will try to say something useful about what you should look for both in choosing a therapist and as the relationship progresses.

---

24 That said, also consider Kahlil Gibran (*The Prophet: Good and Evil*): *For when you strive for gain you are but a root that clings to the earth and sucks at her breast. Surely the fruit cannot say to the root, "Be like me, ripe and full and ever giving of your abundance." For to the fruit giving is a need, as receiving is a need to the root.*
25 The others are (working from the bottom): survival; security (belonging); self-esteem and self-actualisation.

The Rogerian triad

Carl Rogers, who is thought of as the father of counselling, named three factors which define a good therapeutic relationship or alliance: warmth, empathy and genuineness.

Warmth, or unconditional positive regard, is not about 'liking' because it's unconditional, but it does more or less equate to basic friendliness or lovingkindness. So you should get a sense that your therapist is warm towards you.

Empathy is not the same – it means really being able to connect with the inner reality of the person. It has nothing to do with being 'nice' – an empathic torturer would be much worse than an unempathic torturer, as Paul Gilbert seems to enjoy pointing out! So as the therapist gets to know you, hopefully you'll feel that they can get inside your head, and know something of what it is like to stand in your shoes. There is a Native American saying: "Never give anyone advice until you've walked a hundred miles in their moccasins."

Genuineness, or being 'congruent', means not pretending. So the therapist is prepared to grasp the nettle – deal with difficulties in the interactions – rather than just paper over the cracks.

BUDDHIST EQUIVALENTS

David Brazier, who has written on Buddhist psychotherapy, makes parallels between some of these Rogerian categories and the Buddhist cardinal virtues of lovingkindness, compassion, equanimity and sympathetic joy.

Equanimity, which can be defined as freedom from attachment to results, parallels genuineness – the therapist doesn't hold back because of what you might think of him/her. They can do this (in theory) because they can maintain a suitable level of detachment.

Lovingkindness and sympathetic joy are connected to warmth or unconditional positive regard. Sometimes we fall into the habit of feeling envious of others' achievements or wellbeing when we seem to lack it ourselves. Sympathetic joy is the counter to that – even if we ourselves are not having a great time, we are still able to enjoy and appreciate others' good fortune.

Lovingkindness or basic friendliness is that fundamental open-heartedness that is the basis of all connection with other people, or creatures for that matter. Both of these qualities are essential for therapy to happen, which doesn't mean that therapists are always going to manifest them consistently or perfectly – they're human too!

Compassion, which in this context means acting in the client's best interests, requires empathy – you have to be able to stand in the other's place to know what is helpful for them. But it may not be helpful to tell them (and not just because you might have got it wrong)! It may be useful to think, as we did when talking about compassion in the Big Mind process, of female and male compassion: nurturing *and* tough love. Both are about acting in the other's best interest.

RELATION TO METAPERSPECTIVE

For those of you who are interested in the theoretical side of this, we can see how these categories relate to the ideas of vertical and horizontal metaperspective alluded to earlier:

Warmth/friendliness is the basis for everything, but where we go from there depends on the task in hand. At first the therapist needs to stand back to see what is going on. This is detachment or *genuineness*, the world of horizontal metaperspective, and involves impartially noticing the interaction of components (thoughts, feelings, body sensations, behavioural tendencies etc.) in response to a situation or more generally, and encouraging you to do the same, *without getting caught up in the content*. Nonetheless there is still a sense of warmth; of holding and allowing – 'thoughts and feelings as my children', if you like.

But it may be that, once s/he has gained some kind of overview or formulation, then the two of you will together need to enter a particular schema, voice or mind-in-place. This is especially the place of *empathy*, where the therapist needs to be prepared to step right into your moccasins and visit the spirit or voice of whatever-it-is, and in so doing, show you that there are no no-go areas in your mind, and that if the time is right, you can visit anywhere. This is vertical metaperspective; the world of Big I Little I, where, secure in the knowledge that it is not the whole story, you can allow any part freedom of speech.

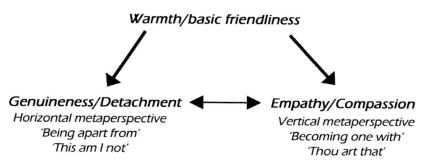

Elements of the therapeutic relationship
(Rogerian/Buddhist)

Warmth/basic friendliness

Genuineness/Detachment ⟷ Empathy/Compassion
Horizontal metaperspective   *Vertical metaperspective*
'Being apart from'   *'Becoming one with'*
'This am I not'   *'Thou art that'*

Edward Bordin

Another way of looking at the therapeutic relationship or alliance comes from Edward Bordin, who usefully broke it down into tasks, goals and bond.

The *goals* of therapy are the objectives that are agreed on after negotiation between the therapist and the client. They may need to be redefined as therapy progresses, and certainly should be reviewed. While clients often "just want to feel better", a good therapist will work with the client to try to define more specifically what that might look like, not just in terms of mood states, but also in terms of what you can now do differently, and in CBT, looking at strength of belief in particular thoughts/beliefs.

The *tasks* of therapy are the processes that need to be gone through in order to get to the goals. The first half of this book is all about those. In other kinds of therapy the tasks will be different; in fact what mostly differentiates one kind of therapy from another concerns the different kinds of task that client and therapist engage in.

The *bond* is the connection between client and therapist. As with intimate relationships above, it can be very hard for client and therapist to really see each other because of *projection* – a technical word from psychoanalysis. This is where we superimpose our feelings onto the personality of another because, consciously or unconsciously, they remind us of somebody who has affected us strongly. We then react to (e.g.) the therapist as though they were (e.g.) our mother or teacher, because they somehow resemble them in our minds. If the therapist asks you if they remind you of someone, then that is probably what they are trying to get at.

TRANSFERENCE AND COUNTER-TRANSFERENCE

Some therapists may talk about *transference* and *counter-transference*. These concepts also come originally from Freudian psychoanalysis, and refer to the bond; the personal dimension of the relationship, based on the idea that the client had to fall in love with the analyst. The working through of this relationship (which, of course, the analyst was not supposed to act on) was the medium through which change happened. Any feelings the analyst had towards the client were called counter-transference.

Most therapies now would not require the client to fall in love with the therapist (whew!) but we would not be human if, especially in long-term therapy, strong feelings were not sometimes evoked in both client and therapist; in fact if they aren't, you may not be working very deeply!

In CBT these are not considered to form the sole basis of change, but increasingly – and particularly through the work of Jeremy Safran – they are recognised as being more important than they used to be. So someone working in a Safranian way will look to point up *as it happens* how the problems you may be experiencing are actually showing up in the way you interact with the therapist. This can be helpful particularly around uncovering interpersonal strategies – 'security operations' – or safety behaviours you habitually use to avoid feeling difficult emotions; which have prevented you from processing 'stuff' and perhaps interfered with the quality of your non-therapy relationships.

In this way the therapy process becomes a (safe) laboratory in which you can experiment with new and different ways of relating. Sometimes this will go very deep, as you may be undergoing some kind of 're-parenting' process if your own experiences of early life were very unhelpful. This is sometimes referred to as 'family re-enactment' or even 'the corrective recapitulation of the primary family experience'. In many cases this will be about discovering that it is OK to feel what you feel and to be yourself without fear of reprisal, abuse, insult or humiliation.

PROBLEMS IN THE THERAPEUTIC RELATIONSHIP

As with any relationship, two humans are getting to know one another and from time to time, they will press each other's buttons. As trust develops, hopefully they can be more open with each other about what is going on. Sometimes this will just be normal (perhaps cultural issues of difference); sometimes it will relate to the client's problems, and that will be very fruitful to talk about. In fact, therapies where client and therapist have a problem, but confront and deal with it, have better outcomes than therapies where there is no problem! They have succeeded in working together through a difficult task, and that strengthens the bond.

On the other hand, sometimes you just won't get on with your therapist – you may be in a situation where you just get allotted a therapist. But if the chemistry is bad, and you've given it a shot, see if you can find a way to get another therapist. You don't want to spend your time as a client helping the therapist work through his or her counter-transference! On the *other* other hand, if this is the sixth therapist this has happened with, then maybe you need to ask some questions about how *you* relate to people.

There are, of course, some professional boundaries that the therapist shouldn't cross: different schools of therapy enforce these to different degrees. So while all schools would forbid sexual contact between therapist and client, some might see hugging as OK, while others wouldn't. What you're comfortable with is what's important.

Group dynamics

Sometimes and for a variety of good reasons, it can be more helpful to have therapy in a group. But in a group the relationships become more complex: there is the relationship between you and each of the other group members, as well as the dynamic that operates with the whole group and the relationship between each of you and the group leaders/facilitators. In group analysis and other primarily interactive unstructured groups, it is what happens in these relationships that forms the basis of change, just as it is the individual relationship in one-to-one psychodynamic therapy that is seen as the primary agent of change.

Group CBT does not usually operate in this way, although any therapist who ignores the relationships – what is usually referred to as the *group dynamics* – is likely to get in a right pickle! Some forms of group CBT work more in the relationship dimension than others. With those that do (and these will tend to be the less structured groups), there is more opportunity for the corrective recapitulation of the primary family experience.

Security operations

Many years ago, I attended a wonderful talk by the Tibetan Buddhist teacher Mike Hookham on the Bodhisattva Way. This is a Mahayana Buddhist ideal of someone who, despite having 'achieved' peace and happiness within him- or herself, doesn't disappear into some ethereal state, but stays around to help others deal with their unhappiness. Of course, in the early stages of training, it is much more about one's own interaction with the world.

Mike said – and I think he's right – that mostly we go around holding the world at arm's length. We daren't let it touch us, because we're scared of what might happen if we do. The bodhisattva path, said Mike, is learning to let your arms come down, which you can't do all at once, and for which you need a teacher to help you (see below). In groups particularly we get to explore this, and the different ways we keep the world – in this case the other group members – at arm's length. The interpersonal psychiatrist Harry Stack Sullivan called these strategies 'security operations'. In CBT we might call them *interpersonal* safety behaviours, in that they prevent us from finding out what genuine spontaneous interaction might be like.

Big I, Little I

```
| | | | | | |
  | | | |
  | | | |
  | | | |
  | | | |
| | | | | | |
```

The recognition that we are multifaceted, ever-changing individuals adds another dimension to relationship work, particularly in groups – which bit (sub-personality) of Person A is relating to which bit of Person B? One therapist I attended groups with often used to ask, "Who's your mother in the group?"

And which bit of you gets evoked by another's particular (challenging, annoying, submissive, flirtatious) behaviour? A Big Mind awareness can add a very powerful dimension to group therapy.

Spiritual teacher-student relationships
For the spiritually inclined, this can be the most important of all relationships. There is also a lot of hocus about it.

All the pitfalls that attend the therapeutic relationship can and will pop up here: projection; transference; counter-transference. As Jack Kornfield points out in his wonderful *After the Ecstasy, the Laundry*, spiritual teachers may have learned much about accessing the transcendent without ever having had any training in, or even being particularly good at, human relationships. The same is true of martial arts teachers:

they may be great at showing you how to use your body in effective and satisfying ways, and (hopefully) they will also be nice people. Does that mean you should necessarily seek their advice on who to marry? Or how to vote? Of course not.

On the other hand, the Way that can be shown to you by a fully qualified, reputable spiritual teacher can transform your life. So it is even more important to be careful about whom you entrust your life to – although you can undoubtedly learn much even from a teacher who may be personally flawed, or who in other ways turns out not to be right for you.

Different spiritual and religious traditions place different amounts of emphasis on how close the teacher-student relationship should be. In some, the teacher is merely a guide, a spiritual friend who has travelled a good way further along the path than yourself; at the other extreme, the teacher is seen as the embodiment of God or Buddha incarnate. I would suggest that you take this into account if you are seeking in this way. On the other hand, maybe it is about being open to the possibilities of being worked on by whoever the teacher is. And of course, in the end, the teacher is yourself (but not your ego)!

In the chapter on many selves in Part 1 we looked at the process of life as being a return to the source; here we have seen that we were never separate to begin with, however lonely we may feel. Once we can begin to allow the universe to work on us, rather than trying always to get it to follow our agenda, then this process of relinquishing our painful sense of separateness can proceed more easily. On the other hand, a clear sense of who you are is essential for working effectively in the world! So a valuable trick is to be able to shift more-or-less effortlessly between at-one-ness and clear selfhood according to the needs of the place you're in.

Further reading

Mark Rowlands (2009) *The Philosopher and the Wolf*, Granta
Colby Pearce (2009) *A Short Introduction to Attachment and Attachment Disorder*, Jessica Kingsley
Jeff Young and Janet Klosko (1998) *Reinventing Your Life*, Penguin
Kahlil Gibran (1926/1991) *The Prophet*, William Heinemann Ltd/Pan
Martin Crowe (2005) *Overcoming Relationship Problems*, Constable Robinson

John Gray (1992) *Men Are from Mars, Women Are from Venus*, HarperCollins[26]
Charlotte Joko Beck (1997) *Everyday Zen*, HarperCollins
John Rowan (1983) *The Reality Game*, Routledge
Irvin D. Yalom (2005) *The Theory and Practice of Group Psychotherapy* (fifth edition), Basic Books
David Brazier (2001) *Zen Therapy*, Constable Robinson
Jack Kornfield (2000) *After the Ecstasy, the Laundry*, Rider Books

---

26 This is included for interest, and doesn't mean I believe what it says 100%!

CHAPTER 28: CONCLUSIONS

Reviewing the journey – Fourth wave CBT summarised – Spiritual or religious? – Wider applications

REVIEWING THE JOURNEY

In Part 1 we looked at the various techniques that comprise the 'armoury' of fourth wave CBT: formulation; understanding of the function of thought, emotion and attention; and the various ways we can work with those components. These include doing thought-records (the ABC), cost-benefiting rules, and deeper work with schemas, those longstanding psycho-physiological patterns that can act as triggers to set off robotic reactions. We looked at ways of working with our attention, including mindfulness, to help us access different perspectives on our problems.

In Part 2 we have examined some of the major types of problem that people experience: depression and low self-esteem, the anxiety disorders, the body-related problems and trauma – and seen how to apply both conventional CBT techniques and more mindfulness- and compassion-based strategies. Some of these you may find perfectly possible to do by yourself; with others you may need or want to find a therapist to help you.

What is fourth wave CBT after all?

So, to summarise, what is fourth wave CBT? If you are offered some, what should you expect?

1. In common with traditional CBT, the therapist should be striving for what is known in the trade as *collaborative empiricism*. They should be working together with you to focus on working with your problems with a view to you getting a better life. Fourth wave embraces this and much else from traditional second wave CBT. There has been far too

much effective conventional CBT for us to want to throw the baby out with the bathwater.

2. But the longer-term goal of the thought-challenging techniques is not simply to 'get the right answer'. What we need to learn to do is mistrust our *automatic thinking* minds and 'relocate' into mindful, in-the-body awareness. That said, we don't want to disown our thinking mind either. Actually, like every other part, it is usually when it is disowned that it causes trouble! So as well as validating *deliberate* thinking, it is also helpful to balance the detachment with that sense of 'thoughts and feelings as my children'. You can learn a lot from your children.

3. We accept, more or less wholesale, the views put forward by Paul Gilbert in his Compassionate Mind approach. His emphasis (drawn from evolutionary psychology) on how our outdated equipment (old brain) is often in conflict with our new brain provides the context within which most of our 21st century struggles are worked out.

4. Fourth wave CBT is not just about thinking: as Jon Kabat-Zinn has said, "Mindfulness is not what you think." Metaperspective is about psychological *stance*: what you see is a product of where and how you're standing. The key question becomes: "Who or what am I identified with at this moment?"

5. You can expect some use of sub-personality work; whether this comes from techniques from Gestalt therapy, Leslie Greenberg's Emotion Focused Therapy, parts work in Neuro-Linguistic Programming, Shamanic-oriented techniques or the Big Mind process, a fourth wave practitioner should be able to work directly with different minds-in-place *as well as* helping you to work with the interaction of thoughts, body sensations, feelings and behaviour.

6. The focus of your fourth wave therapist should be as much on *where* your attention is focused – we could call it 'learning to operate the attention dial' – as on the *content* of your thoughts. With an awareness that you are the operator of your own attention dial, you can learn when it is a good idea to be absorbed in something and when it is better to be detached from it; or how to be absorbed in sensory awareness while detached from thoughts. When is it a good idea to have

observer perspective, and when do you just want to be part of whatever's going on? Moving freely and flexibly between different kinds of awareness, as well as noticing which part is dominant at any given time, helps us to be both sensitive and effective.

In short then, fourth wave CBT teaches us that we are not, initially, free agents, but as Gilbert has so eloquently pointed out, victims of our phylogenetic, family and personal histories: "we all just find ourselves here". We are trying to run Windows 8 on a modified Sinclair ZX; no wonder it doesn't work very well! Conventional CBT and mindfulness help us to uncover our programming (schemas; minds-in-place) and notice the conditions under which the programs get activated.

Discovering we are not our thoughts (we are the ones, living in bodies, who are aware of our thoughts) or feelings (ditto) enables us to (learn to) tolerate the emotions coming to the surface without getting (re-) traumatised by them. Using vertical metaperspective (empty chair; Big Mind) we can then listen to what they have to say and deal with any unfinished business (i.e. 'complete the Gestalt'). Accessing the transcendent sense of self without having to sign up to (or reject) any religious belief, we gain a sense of perspective against which difficulties become much less significant and more manageable. We have increased flexibility in terms of what modes we operate in, attentionally speaking.

Of course, a good therapeutic relationship (warmth, empathy, genuineness) is still necessary but not sufficient, and grasping the nettle in the session – working with what's 'hot' for you at the time – is more than ever a vital practice. If your therapist isn't doing this, bust them for it!

I think you can also expect that your therapist should be taking care of their own 'equipment': they should also have a personal meditation practice and some kind of body-discipline (whether yoga, chi gong, dance etc.), and to have had at least a period of personal psychotherapy. Fourth wave psychotherapists should not ask clients to do that which they would not do themselves.

SPIRITUAL OR RELIGIOUS?

There is obviously – in contrast to conventional CBT – an explicit spiritual dimension. Because mindfulness and the Big Mind have been such a strong influence, it would be easy to mistake it for a sort of Buddhism.

This *would* be a mistake. It may be that these techniques originated in Buddhism, but that doesn't mean they should be restricted to Buddhism[27]. One client of mine who particularly took to the Big Mind process found that it connected her back to her formal Jewish religious practice.

But I don't think that we have to be signed up to a religion in order to benefit from this way of looking at things. Our meditation group used to be called the 'Under Cover Dharma' group – no membership of any religion required. Stephen Batchelor talks eloquently about deliberate agnosticism. On the other hand, 'Buddha' is just a word for someone who has woken up, and that is the whole point: to wake up from the dream or nightmare of our programmed existence into moment-to-moment experienced reality, where we are a jewel in the net of Indra: the matrix of interbeing.

What characterises our programmed, schema-driven mind is duality: right/wrong, black/white and so on. Of course this is useful sometimes! But accessing the transcendent by whatever means does not mean denying everyday reality; the process is 'include and transcend': *the transcendent is the context which provides the ground for the dualistic figures and also includes them.*

WIDER APPLICATIONS

This both goes beyond therapy and has wider implications than therapy. As this approach gains ground, there are potential applications in education, environmental politics and the corporate world, which will need to change its priorities quite rapidly if we are to survive as a life-bearing planet at all. In this way there are links with *ecopsychology.*

A number of people, having gone through a course of this kind of CBT, have said something like, "If only we'd learned this stuff at school, it would have saved us so much suffering!" Hopefully the work on adapting mindfulness for children will continue to gain ground.

Yet this isn't something we can just learn and then it's 'job done'. This never-ending process is one of continual unsticking from or *unlearning* whatever we've become attached to; so don't ask *if* you're stuck, look and see *where* you're stuck!

---

27   One Zen Roshi, trained in Japan, is actually a Catholic nun and missionary. Apparently her (Buddhist) teacher said, "Although Zen grew within Buddhism, it can enhance any religion, so it can help you to be a better Catholic."

Nonetheless, insofar as we have stopped viewing ourselves as totally separate entities – not just theoretically, but experientially – then we can no longer look at the world as just something to exploit, because that would be like trying to exploit your own left foot, or (like the urban myth about the penniless amphetamine addicts) making your own blood into black pudding for something to eat.

So, aware of ourselves as plugged in to the Whole, it no longer makes sense to be motivated by greed. Why try and get that which you already are? And in that way, maybe *everybody* (not just humans) is allowed their place on the planet. So how can you live like this, out on the street?

In the end I guess it comes down to *not trying to mould the world according to my picture of it*, rather to recognise that the world *is as it is*, and then do whatever needs doing. So although we may have come to therapy in order to change some of our personal situations, and (helpfully) formulated some goals which helped us to get more of what we wanted *from* the world, maybe now we are ready (to paraphrase JFK's famous speech) to say, "Ask not what this world can do for you, but rather ask what you can do for this world." And not just this world, perhaps...

May you enjoy and develop as you learn to play your mind more skilfully, for your own benefit and that of all sentient beings!

Further reading:

Paul Gilbert (2009) *The Compassionate Mind*, Constable Robinson
D. Genpo Merzel (2007) *Big Mind, Big Heart, Finding Your Way*, Big Mind Publishing
Stephen Batchelor (1990) *The Faith to Doubt: Glimpses of Buddhist Uncertainty*, Parallax Press
www.mindfulnessinschools.org
Theodore Roszak, Mary E. Gomes and Allen D. Kramer (eds.) (2002) *Ecopsychology: Restoring the Earth, Healing the Mind*, Sierra Club Books

APPENDIX 1 : HOW DO YOU GET THIS STUFF?

Accessing CBT – Individual or group therapy – Mindfulness – Big Mind

Hopefully reading this book will enable you to deal effectively with what ails you. For others it will be more like a pointer *to* therapy, and perhaps will be of some use as an aid *in* therapy. So here we will discuss how to get therapy, and the different ways of working available. As it is unlikely that you will (yet!) be able to find a fourth wave therapist, we will also look at how to incorporate the different elements.

COGNITIVE BEHAVIOURAL THERAPY

Many people claim to offer CBT, on the basis of having done a few weekend courses to top up whatever their regular professional training is: counselling, clinical psychology, nursing, psychiatry etc. You may want to be more choosy than that! In the UK, CBT practitioners will usually be accredited by the British Association of Behavioural and Cognitive Psychotherapies (BABCP) or in the case of Rational Emotive Behaviour Therapists, the AREBT (Association of Rational Emotive Behaviour Therapists). These have now combined on a register at ***www.cbtregisteruk.com*** – other countries will have their own parallel organisations.

That said, just because a therapist has a qualification in CBT and accreditation with the appropriate organisation, it still doesn't necessarily mean you are going to be able to work well with that person. It may be that you get on better with someone whose main affiliation is with a different kind of therapy. I suggest you check out that they are registered with whatever their professional body is. But although in CBT the relationship is not seen as a *sufficient* condition for successful therapy, it is a *necessary* one; I have known some non-CBT therapists I would far rather talk to than some CBT therapists! In terms of the point of view of this book, Gestalt therapy is probably closer than most other modalities.

It may also be more important that the therapist has experience in what is troubling you, rather than what their theoretical orientation is.

INDIVIDUAL OR GROUP THERAPY

Most people like the *idea* of individual therapy much better than group therapy. That doesn't mean it necessarily works better. Of course there are certain kinds of problem that group therapy just isn't suited to: the content of PTSD, for example, is not appropriate (although CBT Skills and mindfulness groups can be very beneficial alongside one-to-one therapy). And one-to-one sessions can usually be slotted into a normal working life (an hour a week, most commonly), and comprise most of what is usually available.

Sometimes, however, a one-to-one session once a week is not enough. It can be more helpful, if resources allow, to have a more intensive course of treatment, especially if there is a lot of learning to be done. And although most people intuitively go for one-to-one because group therapy seems too exposing, those who *have* taken up group CBT, perhaps because that was what was available, have often been positively surprised by their experiences and the results. I referred in the relationship section to corrective recapitulation of the primary family experience, and this is one of the beneficial criteria which Irvin Yalom found to be present in group therapy. More immediately obvious for most participants are some of the others, of which the most important is, in my view, 'universality' – you are not alone in feeling like this or having these kinds of problems. If you are just having one-to-one therapy and your therapist seems relatively 'balanced' then you don't get a sense of this.

Another curative factor is 'instillation of hope'. This is particularly helpful in open groups, where new participants come into a situation where they can see for themselves that others have already gone a good way towards recovery. Closed groups (where the membership is set at the beginning of the agreed duration and nobody can come in once it's started) also have advantages in terms of greater intimacy and trust, or at least the potential for that.

These curative factors (of which there are many more[28]) came from Yalom's famous *Theory and Practice of Group Psychotherapy*, a classic in its field. But they were derived from an interactive unstructured form

---

28 The full list in the 1975 edition is: 1. Interpersonal input; 2. Catharsis; 3. Cohesiveness; 4. Insight; 5. Interpersonal output; 6. Existential awareness; 7. Universality; 8. Instillation of Hope; 9. Altruism; 10. Family re-enactment; 11. Guidance; 12. Identification.

of group therapy. Group CBT is not usually like this. Different therapists and different organisations run different kinds of CBT groups, with varying amounts of structure.

Aaron T. Beck, in a masterclass at Oxford which I was fortunate enough to be able to attend, described cognitive therapy as having three aspects: the therapeutic relationship, the cognitive and behavioural techniques and the psycho-educational element. The therapeutic relationship is necessary, as we have seen in all kinds of therapy. The cognitive and behavioural techniques are sometimes mistakenly thought of as the whole of CBT. But because of the poor start most of us have had in terms of our emotional education, a vital function of CBT groups is the psycho-educational aspect, and of course it is much more efficient to deliver this in a group format. So one kind of CBT group is just that, and consists mostly of the imparting of the sort of information to be found in this book, as well as tuition in how to practise it. ('How to' sessions on doing thought records, behavioural experiments, sitting mindfully etc.)

Other kinds of groups are disorder-specific. Because there is a specific protocol for working with a particular condition, the membership is limited to people who have that condition, and that is the sole area that is worked on. They will have titles like 'Coping with Depression' or 'Working with OCD'.

A third kind of group is the 'agenda', sometimes known as a 'core' group. This is basically individual therapy in a group format, where the therapist gets an agenda item from each person and goes around, working with each in turn. The idea is that there is enough commonality between the different problems that people will be suffering from for members to benefit from listening to the interaction between the therapist and the client who is working; yet because of the person-based agenda, it should give *each* participant a sense that their particular concerns on that day are being dealt with.

A fourth kind is where the group is less structured, probably closed, and more resembles a process group such as you might find in other kinds of group psychotherapy, but where the facilitator(s) will pull CBT techniques out of the hat as and when necessary, probably alongside other techniques.

Finally, there are of course the Mindfulness-Based Cognitive Therapy/ Stress Reduction group programmes, which are closed and last for eight, nine or sometimes ten weeks, and are primarily a skills training in mindfulness meditation. There are also various combinations including elements of all the above.

WHAT'S AVAILABLE

In the UK, the most widely available therapy on the National Health Service is the short-term CBT available under the Improving Access to Psychological Therapy (IAPT) initiative. This can either be 'low intensity' – either delivered in groups or on the telephone by Psychological Wellbeing Practitioners (PWPs) – or 'high intensity' usually short-term, protocol-based 1:1 CBT delivered by suitably qualified CBT therapists. At the time of writing, this will be unlikely to include much if any schema work or compassionate mind training. Mindfulness courses are, however, becoming more common on the NHS, and it is worth pestering your GP or local health professionals to see what is available.

Not surprisingly, more is available privately. Some private hospitals or other organisations offer particular combinations of individual and group therapy, with or without mindfulness, or occasionally Big Mind. Sometimes you can get your CBT from one place and take a mindfulness course somewhere else – mindfulness courses run by Breathworks or the Triratna sangha (formerly the Friends of the Western Buddhist Order) are reliable – a range of courses can be found on the **www.bemindful. co.uk** website. Again, although there are some great training courses in learning to deliver MBCT or MBSR, if I were looking to join a course I would be perhaps as interested in the instructor's own commitment to their personal practice as I would be in their formal training.

'If you have been intrigued by the many references to Big Mind in this book, check out **www.bigmind.org** for more discoveries.'

If you are in a situation where you do have some say over choosing your therapist (and usually you can have *some* influence), I would emphasise that you should not just put up with working with a therapist whom you are not happy with. I am not talking about professional misconduct, which of course is not acceptable and should be reported, but simply if you are not getting anything from the therapy process. Sometimes it happens, through nobody's fault. Change your therapist!

APPENDIX 2: BLANK FORMS AND CHARTS

ABC form
activity schedule
anger chaining form
anger diary
anger record
behavioural experiment record form
cost-benefit analysis
department store
formulation chart
hierarchy form
hot cross bun
OCD formulation
old model - new model
panic diary
perfect nurturer
positive log
problem and goal table
safety behaviours
schema awareness form
social anxiety thought record
task concentration training
vicious daisy
working backwards from safety behaviours
worry formulation

You can photocopy these forms for use as often as you need - enlarging any as appropriate.

The ABC Form

Activating event or trigger situation	Beliefs/negative automatic thoughts (NATs)	Co-productions	Dispute your beliefs & NATs and devise better alternatives	Effects of alternative thought...
Anything can be an 'A' – external or internal events	What went through your mind? What did 'A' mean to you?	What came with the thought?	Remember compassionate mind	...on your body, emotions and actions.
		Emotions: list and rate 0-100 intensity		Re-rate emotions 0-100 – any new emotions?
		Body sensations: list intensity 0-100		Body sensations: list intensity 0-100
		Behaviour: what did you do? Did it confirm beliefs in B?		New behaviour? Plan behavioural experiment(s)
	Remember: thinking errors?		What might I tell someone else in this situation?	

405

ACTIVITY SCHEDULE

Week beginning: / /

Rate each activity (0-10) for M (mastery = effort) and P (pleasure), according to how *challenging* or *pleasurable* the activity was for you.

Days→ Time	Monday	Tuesday	Wednesday	Thursday	Friday	Saturday	Sunday
6am – 8							
8 – 10							
10 – 12							
12 – 2pm							
2 – 4							
4 – 6							
6 – 8							
8 – 10							
10 – 12							
12 – 2am							
Overall mood rating (0-10)							

Anger Chaining Form

Type									Chain									Solutions								

Anger Diary

Day & Date	Intensity of Anger 0-10	Alcohol Units	Unwanted Behaviour	Went to work? Y/N	Minutes of Relaxation	% effort on new response
Mon						
Tue						
Wed						
Thur						
Fri						
Sat						
Sun						

Anger Record

Situation: What was I doing and with whom?	First signs: (body sensations, negative (hot) thoughts)	Meaning: Threat, rule of mine that was broken or sore spot touched	Emotion Anger (0-100) and other emotions?	What I did
Where did this meaning come from?	Is it still useful to believe this?	Different meaning?	Re-rate emotions	New behaviour

Behavioural Experiment Record Sheet

Theory you want to test	Planned experiment	Safety Behaviours you might use	What happens when you carry it out	Results	What can I do now?

Cost-benefit Analysis Form

In what ways does this rule make sense?	In what ways is this rule illogical?
How realistic is it to follow this rule?	How unrealistic is this rule?
What advantages are there for me or those I care about in following this rule?	What disadvantages are there for me and those I care about in following this rule?
Why would I recommend this rule as a guideline to those I care about?	Why wouldn't I recommend this rule as a guideline to those I care about?

Department Store

Family (immediate)	Relationship	Work	Health & appearance	Outdoor pursuits (walking, gardening)
Sexuality	Family (extended)	Days out	Financial	Housework & maintenance
Arts (doing): painting, dance, music etc.	Making or fixing things	Spiritual or religious	Academic	Holidays
Social/friends	Arts (visiting galleries, theatre, concerts)	Political involvement	Social action/ volunteering	Sports/ physical exercise

Formulation Chart

Early experiences

....
....
....
....

Core beliefs (what as a child I made of those early experiences)

I am...
....
....
Other people are.............................
....
The world is.....................................
....

Assumptions, Rules & Strategies (what we do because of the core beliefs – whatever we do to keep them (and painful early experiences) out of consciousness)

If.......................................then...
& therefore I should always...

If.......................................then...
& therefore I should always...

Critical incident(s) (whatever happened to stop you carrying out your rules or compensatory strategies):
....
....

Hot cross bun(s)

Hierarchy Form

Hierarchy

Situation	How scary? 0-100	Working on it? (Tick)	No longer gives anxiety (Tick)

Hot cross Bun

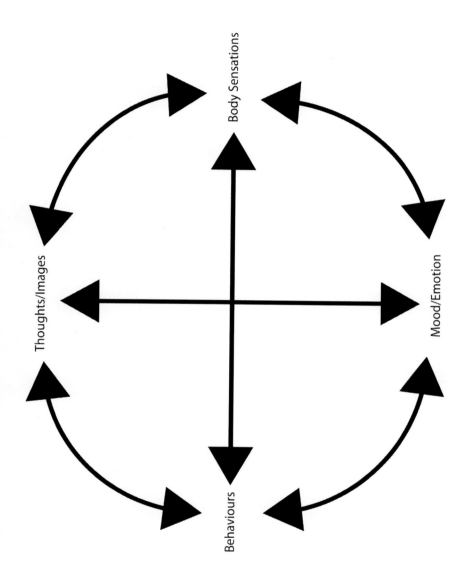

OCD Formulation

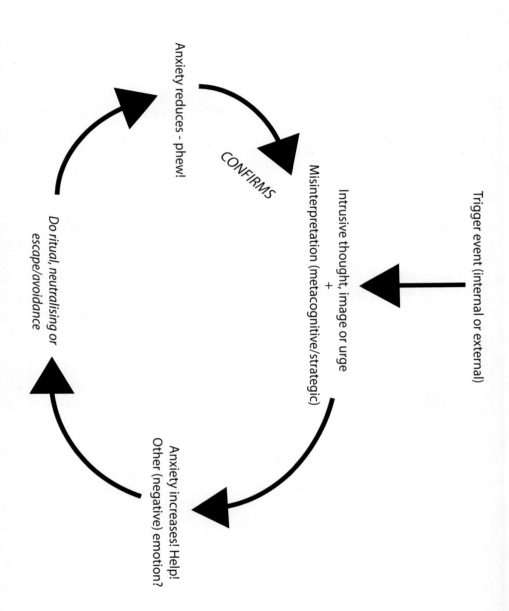

Trigger event (internal or external)

Intrusive thought, image or urge
+
Misinterpretation (metacognitive/strategic)

CONFIRMS

Anxiety increases! Help!
Other (negative) emotion?

Do ritual, neutralising or
escape/avoidance

Anxiety reduces - phew!

Old model - New model

Early experiences:

Old core beliefs	**New core beliefs**
Self:	Self:
World:	World:
Others:	Others:

Rules/Assumptions/Strategies:	**New rules/guidelines:**

Critical incident(s):

Thoughts:	Thoughts:
Feelings:	Feelings:
Body sensations:	Body sensations:
Behaviours:	Behaviours:

Panic Diary

Situation or trigger (Where, when, what was going through your mind, what were you focusing on?)	Anxiety Rate % intensity Time duration	Safety behaviours and avoidances What are you doing that prevents you finding out how it really is?	Is there a different (rational or 'mind-mind') interpretation (Theory B)?	New behaviour? Design experiment
Physical symptoms (What is 'body-mind' saying?) Heart racing Sweating Nausea Feeling faint/dizzy Shaking Choking Hot/cold Pain (where?) Feeling unreal Other: state what	Interpretation What does body-mind think these sensations mean (Theory A)?	Effect of safety behaviours/ avoidances Do they confirm Theory A?	What is body sensation *really* about – what is the actual threat in my life (if anything)?	Re-rate anxiety % intensity Time duration

Perfect Nurturer

Who is it?	
Appearance, clothing, complexion	
Tone of voice and other sounds	
Touch?	
Perfume?	
What are their particular qualities?	
What do they say?	

Positive Log

Examples of things I did or ways I behaved today or at any time in the past that show evidence that support my new belief that … … … … … …
… … … … … …… … … … …… … … … … …… … … … … …… … … … … …… … … … …

| Monday: |
| Tuesday: |
| Wednesday: |
| Thursday: |
| Friday: |
| Saturday: |
| Sunday: |

Problem & Goal Table

Problem	Goal

Safety Behaviour

Safety behaviour	Time spent on it/frequency

Schema Awareness Form

<u>Situation:</u>
What was I doing or thinking about before I became over-emotional and/or acted in a way that I later felt unhappy about?

<u>Thoughts and Images:</u>
What went through my mind at this time or shortly before it that led to such an upsurge of feeling? How much did I believe it at the time? (0-100)

<u>Emotion:</u>
What was the emotion I felt? How strong was it?

<u>Action:</u>
What did I do?

<u>Answer:</u>
I recognise that this was an activation of my .... Schema, which led to..
....
....

A more objective understanding of the situation might be...
....

And a more helpful way of acting might have been...
....
....

Standing back from the situation, how much do I now believe the original thoughts? Or the 'truth' of the core belief?[1]

Good luck!

---

[1] Remember the first law of Core Beliefs: **'They're not true'**

423

Social Anxiety Thought Record

Situation	Emotion	Negative Automatic Thoughts (NATs)	Meaning
What was I doing or thinking about? Who was I with?	*What emotion? How intense (0-100%)*	*How much did you believe them (0-100%)?*	*What did the NATs mean to you? What's the worst thing about that?* *What would that say about you if it were true? How did you see yourself in that situation? How old did you feel?*

Thinking errors?	Safety Behaviours & Effects	Alternative Thoughts	Results: What can I do now?
*Check the NATs **and** the meaning against the list*	*What did you do to prevent others seeing your anxiety or more helpful? How much do you who you 'really' are?*	*Is there another way of thinking about this that isn't distorted and is more helpful? How much do you believe the new version?*	*How could you test out which version is more useful? If you drop the safety behaviours, what happens?*

Task Concentration Training

Situation	Attention	Mood/Feeling	Exercise	Outcome
Who were you with? What was the task?	*What were you mainly focusing on?*	*How did you feel? (describe emotions and rate how intense 0 - 100%)*	*How did you try to redirect your attention to the task and environment?*	*How did the situation turn out?*
				How did you feel? (describe emotions and rate how intense 0 – 100%)
	How much attention (%) was directed at: 1. Self % 2. Task % 3. Environment % *(total should equal 100%)*		*How effective was it?*	*What did you do?*
				What did the other people do?

Vicious Daisy

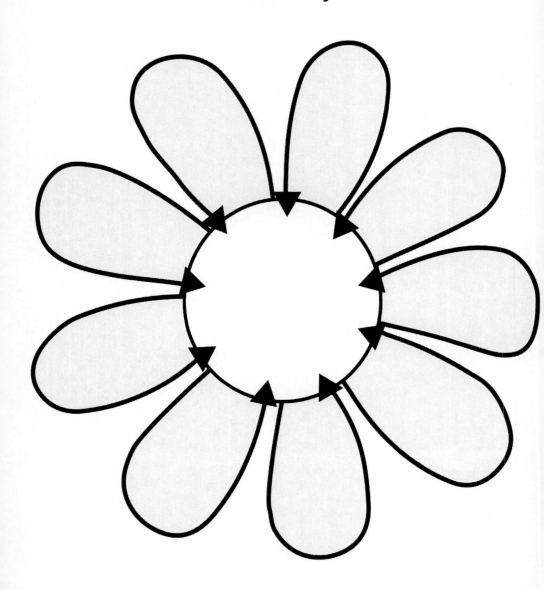

Working Backwards From Safety Behaviours

5. Early Experience	4. Core beliefs	3. Rules and Assumptions	2. Thoughts & Feelings if I didn't do it	1. Safety Behaviours
6. Compassionate View	7. Alternative Beliefs	8. Helpful Guidelines	9. Thoughts and Feelings	10. New Behaviours

Worry Formulation

Early frightening experience(s)	
Made you think you were (core belief):	*Weak? Vulnerable? Unlovable? Bad? Worthless?*
Rules about worrying	*If I worry, then. . .*
Other positive beliefs about worrying	*I can head off crises before they happen*
Negative beliefs about worrying	*It's out of control* *It's making me ill*
Critical Incident: what brought all this to a head? Any similarities to early experiences?	*Laid off work due to stress*
Symptoms:	*Thoughts:* *Body sensations:* *Behaviours:* *Emotions:*

BIBLIOGRAPHY

INTRODUCTION

Grant, A., Mills, J., Mulhern, R. & Short, N. (2004) *Cognitive Behavioural Therapy in Mental Health Care*, Sage, London.
Mao Shih An (1996) Statement made during a chi gong class at Acorn Day Centre, Oxford.
John Bowlby & Donald Winnicott. See e.g. Donald Winnicott & John Bowlby (2004) *Fifty Years of Attachment Theory*, Karnac, London.

CHAPTER 1

Greenberger, D. & Padesky, C. A. (1995) *Mind Over Mood*, Guilford New York.
Burns, D. (1980) *Feeling Good*, Harper Collins, New York.
Goleman, D. (1995) *Emotional Intelligence*, Bloomsbury, London.
For more Mulla Nasrudin stories, see (e.g.) Idries Shah (2004) *The Subtleties and the Exploits of Mulla Nasrudin*, Octagon, London.
Rachman, S., Radomsky, A.S. & Shafran, R. (2008) *Safety Behaviour: A Reconsideration Behaviour Research & Therapy* 46 163-173
Goscinny, R. & Uderzo, A. (various - the Asterix series). Orion

CHAPTER 2

REBT see e.g. Dryden, W. (1999) *How to Accept Yourself*, Sheldon, London.

CHAPTER 4

Fennell, M.J.V. & Teasdale, J.D. (1984) 'Effects of Distraction on Thinking and Affect in Depressed Patients', *British Journal of Clinical Psychology* 23, 65-66

Chapter 5

See Bennett-Levy, J., Butler, G., Fennell, M.J.V., Hackmann, A., Mueller, M. & Westbrook, D. (2004) *Oxford Guide to Behavioural Experiments in Cognitive Therapy*, Oxford University Press, Oxford.

Chapter 6

Wells, A. (2000) *Emotional Disorders & Metacognition: Innovative Cognitive Therapy*, Wiley, Chichester:
Task Concentration Training: see (e.g.) Mulkens, S., Bogels, S.M., deJong, P.J. & Louwers, J. (2001) 'Fear of Blushing: Effects of Task Concentration Training versus Exposure in Vivo on Fear and Physiology', *Journal of Anxiety Disorders* 15, 413-432
Wells, A. & Papageorgiou, C. (1998) 'Social Phobia: Effects of External Attention on Anxiety, Negative Beliefs, and Perspective Taking Behaviour Therapy' 29, 357-370

Chapter 7

Lake, F. (1966) *Clinical Theology*, Darton, Longman & Todd, London.
Burns, D. (1980) opus cit.
'Rules that protect'; 'possibility goals' I am indebted to Christine Padesky for these ideas; see padesky.com
Chuang Tzu: for an introduction to his writings, try: Watson, B. (translator) (1964) *Chuang Tzu*, Columbia University Press, New York.
Young, J. & Klosko, J. (1993) *Reinventing Your Life*, Penguin, Harmondsworth:

Chapter 8

See (e.g.) Teasdale, J.D. (1996) Clinically Relevant Theory: Integrating Clinical Insight with Cognitive Science in Salkovskis, P.M. (ed.) (1996) *Frontiers of Cognitive Therapy*, Guilford, New York.
Reich, Wilhelm (1949) *Character Analysis (3rd edition)*, Farrar, Straus & Giroux, New York.
Kabat-Zinn, Jon (2005) *Coming To Our Senses: Healing Ourselves and The World through Mindfulness*, Hyperion, New York.
Frantzis, B. (1998) *The Power of Internal Martial Arts and Chi*, Blue Snake Books, Berkeley.

Chapter 9

Jon Kabat-Zinn (1990) *Full Catastrophe Living*, Piatkus, London.

Segal, Z.V., Williams, J.M.G. & Teasdale, J.D. (2002) *Mindfulness-Based Cognitive Therapy for Depression*, Guilford, New York.

Linehan, M. M. (1993) *Cognitive-Behavioral Treatment of Borderline Personality Disorder*, Guilford, New York.

Hayes, S.C. with Smith, S. (2005) *Get Out of Your Mind and Into Your Life: The New Acceptance and Commitment Therapy*, New Harbinger, Oakland

Williams J. M. G., Teasdale, J.D., Segal, Z.V. & Kabat-Zinn, J. (2007) *The Mindful Way Through Depression: Freeing Yourself from Chronic Unhappiness*, Guilford, New York.

Beck, C. J. (1997) *Everyday Zen: Love and Work*, Harper, New York.

Zentatsu Baker-Roshi (1997) *Seeing and Observing Karma. Tree Planters*, Zeitschrift des Dharma Sangha Europe

Merzel, D.G. (2007) *Big Mind, Big Heart, Finding Your Way*, Big Mind Publications, Salt Lake City.

Ornstein, R. (1992) *The Evolution of Consciousness*. Simon & Schuster, New York: , in Teasdale, J.D. (1997) *The Mind-in-Place in Mood Disorders*, in Clark, D.M. & Fairburn, C.G. (1997) *Science and Practice of Cognitive Behaviour Therapy*, Oxford University Press, Oxford.

Gilbert, P. (2009) *The Compassionate Mind*, Constable, London: .

CHAPTER 10

For an introduction to Freud's work, try Freud, S. (1991) *Introductory Lectures on Psychoanalysis*. Penguin Freud Library; also Freud, S. (1995) *New Introductory Lectures on Psychoanalysis*, Norton, New York.

'Empty Chair' see e.g. Perls, F.S. (1992) *Gestalt Therapy Verbatim*, Gestalt Journal Press, Gouldsboro, ME.

Greenberg, L.S. & Paivio, S.C. (1997) *Working with Emotions in Psychotherapy*, Guilford, New York.

Stone, H. & Winkleman, S. (1985) *Embracing Our Selves: Voice Dialogue Manual*, Devorss & Company, Marina del Rey, CA.

Beck, A.T., Rush, A.J., Shaw, B.F. & Emery, G. (1979) *Cognitive Therapy of Depression*, Guilford, New York.

Dryden, W. (1998) *Developing Self-Acceptance*, Wiley, Chichester.

Lee, D.A (2005) *The Perfect Nurturer: A Model to Develop a Compassionate Mind within the Context of Cognitive Therapy*, in Gilbert, P. (ed.) (2005) *Compassion: Conceptualisations, Research and Use in Psychotherapy*, Routledge, London.

CHAPTER 11

Merzel, D.G. *op. cit.*

Wilber, K. (2000) *Integral Psychology*, Shambhala, Boston.

Chapter 12

Hanh, T.N. (1998) *The Heart of the Buddha's Teaching*, Rider Books London.

Part 2: Some Applications

References are in addition to those listed under Further Reading at the end of each chapter

Chapter 13 (Depression)

Goleman, D, *op. cit.*
Gilbert, P. (2009) *The Compassionate Mind*, Constable, London.
Teasdale, J.D. (1996) *Clinically Relevant Theory, op. cit.*

Chapter 18 (Worry)

de Ropp, R. S (2002) *The Master Game*, Gateways, Nevada City.
Wells, A (1997) *Cognitive Therapy of Anxiety Disorders: A Practice Manual and Conceptual Guide*, Wiley, Chichester.

Chapter 19 (OCD)

Salkovskis, P.M. & Kirk, J. (1997) Obsessive-compulsive disorder in Clark, D. M. & Fairburn, C. G. (1997) Science and Practice of Cognitive Behaviour Therapy, Oxford University Press, Oxford.

Chapter 20 (health anxiety)

Batchelor, S. (1997) *Buddhism Without Beliefs*, Bloomsbury, London.
Mary Oliver (1992) *House of Light*, Beacon Press, Boston.

Chapter 21 (social anxiety)

Clark, D.M. & Wells, A. (1995) *A Cognitive Model of Social Phobia.* in Heimberg R., Liebowitz,M., Hope, D.A. & Schneier, F.R. (eds) (1995) *Social Phobia, Diagnosis, Assessment and Treatment*, Guilford, New York.
Wells, A. (2000) *op. cit.*
Greenberg, L. S. & Paivio, S.C. (1997) *op.cit.*

CHAPTER 24 STRESS & PTSD

Ehlers, A. & Clark, D.M. (2000) *A Cognitive Model of PTSD*. Behaviour Research & Therapy 38, 1-27

CHAPTER 25 (BODY REGULATION DISORDERS...)

Williams et al. (2007) *op. cit.*
Mary Oliver (1986) *Wild Geese* in Dream Work. Grove Atlantic

CHAPTER 26 (PROBLEMS NOT ADDRESSED HERE)

Beck, A.T, Wright F.D., Newman, C.F. & Liese, B.S. (1993) *Cognitive Therapy of Substance Abuse*, Guilford, New York.
Beck, A.T., Freeman, A. & Associates (1990) *Cognitive Therapy of Personality Disorders*, Guilford, New York.

INDEX